Medical Care for Kidney and Liver Transplant Recipients

Editors

DAVID A. SASS
ALDEN M. DOYLE

MEDICAL CLINICS
OF NORTH AMERICA

www.medical.theclinics.com

Consulting Editors
DOUGLAS S. PAAUW
EDWARD R. BOLLARD

May 2016 • Volume 100 • Number 3

ELSEVIER

1600 John F. Kennedy Boulevard • Suite 1800 • Philadelphia, Pennsylvania, 19103-2899

http://www.theclinics.com

MEDICAL CLINICS OF NORTH AMERICA Volume 100, Number 3
May 2016 ISSN 0025-7125, ISBN-13: 978-0-323-44471-2

Editor: Jessica McCool
Developmental Editor: Alison Swety

Medical Clinics of North America (ISSN 0025-7125) is published bimonthly by Elsevier Inc., 360 Park Avenue South, New York, NY 10010-1710. Months of publication are January, March, May, July, September, and November. Business and editorial offices: 1600 John F. Kennedy Boulevard, Suite 1800, Philadelphia, PA 19103-2899. Periodicals postage paid at New York, NY, and additional mailing offices. Subscription prices are USD $260.00 per year (US individuals), $531.00 per year (US institutions), $100.00 per year (US Students), $320.00 per year (Canadian individuals), $690.00 per year (Canadian institutions), $200.00 per year (Canadian and foreign students), $390.00 per year (foreign individuals), and $690.00 per year (foreign institutions). To receive student/resident rate, orders must be accompanied by name of affiliated institution, date of term, and the signature of program/residency coordinator on institution letterhead. Orders will be billed at individual rate until proof of status is received. Foreign air speed delivery is included in all Clinics' subscription prices. All prices are subject to change without notice. **POSTMASTER:** Send address changes to *Medical Clinics of North America*, Elsevier Health Sciences Division, Subscription Customer Service, 3251 Riverport Lane, Maryland Heights, MO 63043. **Customer Service: Telephone: 1-800-654-2452** (U.S. and Canada); **1-314-447-8871** (outside U.S. and Canada). **Fax: 314-447-8029. E-mail: journalscustomerserviceusa@elsevier.com** (for print support); **journalsonlinesupport-usa@elsevier.com** (for online support).

Reprints. For copies of 100 or more of articles in this publication, please contact the Commercial Reprints Department, Elsevier Inc., 360 Park Avenue South, New York, NY 10010-1710. Tel.: 212-633-3874; Fax: 212-633-3820; E-mail: reprints@elsevier.com.

Medical Clinics of North America is also published in Spanish by McGraw-Hill Interamericana Editores S. A., P.O. Box 5-237, 06500 Mexico, D.F., Mexico.

Medical Clinics of North America is covered in *MEDLINE/PubMed (Index Medicus), Current Contents, ASCA, Excerpta Medica, Science Citation Index,* and *ISI/BIOMED.*

PROGRAM OBJECTIVE
The goal of the *Medical Clinics of North America* is to keep practicing physicians up to date with current clinical practice by providing timely articles reviewing the state of the art in patient care.

TARGET AUDIENCE
All practicing physicians and other healthcare professionals.

LEARNING OBJECTIVES
Upon completion of this activity, participants will be able to:
1. Review considerations for deciding who receives liver and kidney transplants.
2. Discuss the care and clinical management of transplant recipients.
3. Recognize preventative and therapeutic techniques for transplant complications.

ACCREDITATION
The Elsevier Office of Continuing Medical Education (EOCME) is accredited by the Accreditation Council for Continuing Medical Education (ACCME) to provide continuing medical education for physicians.

The EOCME designates this enduring material for a maximum of 15 *AMA PRA Category 1 Credit*(s)™. Physicians should claim only the credit commensurate with the extent of their participation in the activity.

All other health care professionals requesting continuing education credit for this enduring material will be issued a certificate of participation.

DISCLOSURE OF CONFLICTS OF INTEREST
The EOCME assesses conflict of interest with its instructors, faculty, planners, and other individuals who are in a position to control the content of CME activities. All relevant conflicts of interest that are identified are thoroughly vetted by EOCME for fair balance, scientific objectivity, and patient care recommendations. EOCME is committed to providing its learners with CME activities that promote improvements or quality in healthcare and not a specific proprietary business or a commercial interest.

The planning committee, staff, authors and editors listed below have identified no financial relationships or relationships to products or devices they or their spouse/life partner have with commercial interest related to the content of this CME activity:
Syed Amer, MBBS; Edward R. Bollard, MD, DDS, FACP; Jesse M. Civan, MD; Serban Constantinescu, MD, PhD; Christine Culkin, DNP, FNP-BC; Iliana Doycheva, MD; Alden M. Doyle, MD, MS, MPH; Sol Epstein, MD, FRCP, FACP; Jonathan M. Fenkel, MD; Anjali Fortna; Mythili Ghanta, MD; Ryan J. Goldberg, MD; William G. Greendyke, MD; Dina L. Halegoua-DeMarzio, MD; Vidhya Illuri, MD; Belinda Jim, MD, FNKF; Praveen Kandula, MD, MPH; Dianne LaPointe Rudow, DNP; Gregory Malat, PharmD, BCPS; Jessica McCool; Mrudula R. Munagala, MD, FACC; Premkumar Nandhakumar; Johan Daniël Nel, MBChB, MMed (Int Med), Cert Neph (CMSA); Marcus R. Pereira, MD, MPH; Anita Phancao, MD, FACC; Swati Rao, MD; Sheela S. Reddy, MD; David A. Sass, MD, FACP, FACG, AGAF, FAASLD; Megan Suermann; Karen M. Warburton, MD, FASN; Kymberly D. Watt, MD; Francis L. Weng, MD, MSCE.

The planning committee, staff, authors and editors listed below have identified financial relationships or relationships to products or devices they or their spouse/life partner have with commercial interest related to the content of this CME activity:
Mark E. Molitch, MD is a consultant/advisor for Novartis AG; Novo Nordisk A/S; Merck & Co., Inc.; Janssen Global Services, LLC; and Pfizer Inc., has research support from Bayer AG; Novartis AG; and Novo Nordisk A/S, and his spouse/partner has stock ownership in Amgen Inc.
Michael J. Moritz, MD has research support from Pfizer Inc. and Bristol-Myers Squibb Company.
Amisha Wallia, MD, MS has research support from Merck & Co., Inc.

UNAPPROVED/OFF-LABEL USE DISCLOSURE
The EOCME requires CME faculty to disclose to the participants:
1. When products or procedures being discussed are off-label, unlabelled, experimental, and/or investigational (not US Food and Drug Administration [FDA] approved); and
2. Any limitations on the information presented, such as data that are preliminary or that represent ongoing research, interim analyses, and/or unsupported opinions. Faculty may discuss information about pharmaceutical agents that is outside of FDA-approved labelling. This information is intended solely for CME and is not intended to promote off-label use of these medications. If you have any questions, contact the medical affairs department of the manufacturer for the most recent prescribing information.

TO ENROLL

To enroll in the *Medical Clinics of North America* Continuing Medical Education program, call customer service at 1-800-654-2452 or sign up online at http://www.theclinics.com/home/cme. The CME program is available to subscribers for an additional annual fee of USD $295.

METHOD OF PARTICIPATION

In order to claim credit, participants must complete the following:
1. Complete enrolment as indicated above.
2. Read the activity.
3. Complete the CME Test and Evaluation. Participants must achieve a score of 70% on the test. All CME Tests and Evaluations must be completed online.

CME INQUIRIES/SPECIAL NEEDS

For all CME inquiries or special needs, please contact elsevierCME@elsevier.com.

MEDICAL CLINICS OF NORTH AMERICA

FORTHCOMING ISSUES

July 2016
Pharmacologic Therapy
Douglas S. Paauw and Kim O'Connor,
Editors

September 2016
**Quality Patient Care: Making
Evidence-Based, High Value Choices**
Marc Shalaby and Edward R. Bollard,
Editors

November 2016
Practice-Based Nutrition Care
Scott Kahan and Robert F. Kushner, *Editors*

RECENT ISSUES

March 2016
Travel and Adventure Medicine
Paul S. Pottinger and
Christopher A. Sanford, *Editors*

January 2016
Managing Chronic Pain
Charles E. Argoff, *Editor*

November 2015
Dermatology
Roy M. Colven, *Editor*

RELATED INTEREST

Physician Assistant Clinics, January 2016 (Vol. 1, Issue 1)
Kidney Disease
Kim Zuber and Jane S. Davis, *Editors*
http://www.physicianassistant.theclinics.com/

THE CLINICS ARE AVAILABLE ONLINE!
Access your subscription at:
www.theclinics.com

Contributors

CONSULTING EDITORS

DOUGLAS S. PAAUW, MD, MACP
Professor of Medicine, Division of General Internal Medicine, Rathmann Family Foundation Endowed Chair for Patient-Centered Clinical Education; Medicine Student Programs, Professor of Medicine, University of Washington School of Medicine, Seattle, Washington

EDWARD R. BOLLARD, MD, DDS, FACP
Professor of Medicine, Associate Dean of Graduate Medical Education, Designated Institutional Official, Department of Medicine, Penn State-Hershey Medical Center, Penn State University College of Medicine, Hershey, Pennsylvania

EDITORS

DAVID A. SASS, MD, FACP, FACG, AGAF, FAASLD
Associate Professor of Medicine, Division of Gastroenterology and Hepatology, Thomas Jefferson University Hospitals, Medical Director, Liver Transplantation, Sidney Kimmel Medical College at Thomas Jefferson University, Philadelphia, Pennsylvania

ALDEN M. DOYLE, MD, MS, MPH
Associate Professor of Medicine, Division of Nephrology, Medical Director, Kidney and Pancreas Transplantation, Hahnemann University Hospital, Drexel University College of Medicine, Philadelphia, Pennsylvania

AUTHORS

SYED AMER, MBBS
Internal Medicine Resident, Division of Internal Medicine, Mayo Clinic, Phoenix, Arizona

JESSE M. CIVAN, MD
Assistant Professor, Department of Medicine, Thomas Jefferson University; Division of Gastroenterology and Hepatology, Medical Director, Jefferson Liver Tumor Center, Philadelphia, Pennsylvania

SERBAN CONSTANTINESCU, MD, PhD
Co-investigator, National Transplantation Pregnancy Registry, Gift of Life Institute; Associate Professor of Medicine, Medical Director, Kidney Transplant Program, Section of Nephrology, Hypertension and Kidney Transplantation, Temple University School of Medicine, Philadelphia, Pennsylvania

CHRISTINE CULKIN, DNP, FNP-BC
Nurse Practitioner, Solid Organ Transplantation, Hahnemann University Hospital, Philadelphia, Pennsylvania

ILIANA DOYCHEVA, MD
Gastroenterology Fellow, Division of Gastroenterology and Hepatology, Medical University-Sofia, Sofia, Bulgaria

ALDEN M. DOYLE, MD, MS, MPH
Associate Professor of Medicine, Division of Nephrology, Medical Director, Kidney and Pancreas Transplantation, Hahnemann University Hospital, Drexel University College of Medicine, Philadelphia, Pennsylvania

SOL EPSTEIN, MD, FRCP, FACP
Professor of Medicine and Geriatrics, Mount Sinai School of Medicine, New York, New York; Adjunct Professor, University of Pennsylvania School of Medicine, Philadelphia, Pennsylvania

JONATHAN M. FENKEL, MD
Division of Gastroenterology and Hepatology, Assistant Professor, Department of Medicine, Sidney Kimmel Medical College at Thomas Jefferson University, Philadelphia, Pennsylvania

MYTHILI GHANTA, MD
Medical Director, Pancreas Transplant Program, Section of Nephrology, Hypertension and Kidney Transplantation, Assistant Professor, Department of Medicine, Lewis Katz School of Medicine at Temple University, Philadelphia, Pennsylvania

RYAN J. GOLDBERG, MD
Renal and Pancreas Transplant Division, Saint Barnabas Medical Center, Livingston, New Jersey

WILLIAM G. GREENDYKE, MD
Instructor of Medicine, Division of Infectious Diseases, Columbia University College of Physicians and Surgeons, New York, New York

DINA L. HALEGOUA-DEMARZIO, MD
Division of Gastroenterology and Hepatology, Assistant Professor, Department of Medicine, Sidney Kimmel Medical College at Thomas Jefferson University, Philadelphia, Pennsylvania

VIDHYA ILLURI, MD
Fellow, Division of Endocrinology, Metabolism and Molecular Medicine, Northwestern University Feinberg School of Medicine, Chicago, Illinois

BELINDA JIM, MD, FNKF
Associate Professor of Clinical Medicine, Division of Nephrology, Department of Medicine, Jacobi Medical Center, Albert Einstein College of Medicine, Bronx, New York

PRAVEEN KANDULA, MD, MPH
Renal and Pancreas Transplant Division, Saint Barnabas Medical Center, Livingston, New Jersey

DIANNE LAPOINTE RUDOW, DNP
Associate Professor, Department of Population Health Science and Policy Director of the Zweig Family Center for Living Donation, Recanati Miller Transplantation Institute, Mount Sinai Hospital, New York, New York

GREGORY MALAT, PharmD, BCPS
Clinical Pharmacy Specialist, Solid Organ Transplantation, Hahnemann University Hospital, Drexel University College of Medicine, Philadelphia, Pennsylvania

MARK E. MOLITCH, MD
Martha Leland Sherwin Professor of Endocrinology, Division of Endocrinology, Metabolism and Molecular Medicine, Northwestern University Feinberg School of Medicine, Chicago, Illinois

MICHAEL J. MORITZ, MD
Chief, Transplant Services, Lehigh Valley Health Network, Allentown, Pennsylvania; Professor of Surgery, Morsani College of Medicine, University of South Florida, Tampa, Florida; Principal Investigator, National Transplantation Pregnancy Registry, Gift of Life Institute, Philadelphia, Pennsylvania

MRUDULA R. MUNAGALA, MD, FACC
Heart Failure and Transplant Cardiologist, Newark Beth Israel Medical Center, Newark, New Jersey

JOHAN DANIËL NEL, MBChB, MMed (Int Med), Cert Neph (CMSA)
Senior Specialist, Division of Nephrology, Department of Medicine, Tygerberg Hospital and University of Stellenbosch, Cape Town, Western Cape, South Africa

MARCUS R. PEREIRA, MD, MPH
Assistant Professor of Medicine, Division of Infectious Diseases, Columbia University College of Physicians and Surgeons, New York, New York

ANITA PHANCAO, MD, FACC
Heart Failure and Transplant Cardiologist, Integris Baptist Medical Center, Oklahoma City, Oklahoma

SWATI RAO, MD
Assistant Professor of Medicine, Section of Nephrology, Hypertension and Kidney Transplantation, Temple University School of Medicine, Philadelphia, Pennsylvania

SHEELA S. REDDY, MD
Division of Gastroenterology and Hepatology, Department of Medicine, Thomas Jefferson University, Philadelphia, Pennsylvania

DAVID A. SASS, MD, FACP, FACG, AGAF, FAASLD
Associate Professor of Medicine, Division of Gastroenterology and Hepatology, Thomas Jefferson University Hospitals, Medical Director, Liver Transplantation, Sidney Kimmel Medical College at Thomas Jefferson University, Philadelphia, Pennsylvania

AMISHA WALLIA, MD, MS
Assistant Professor of Medicine, Division of Endocrinology, Metabolism and Molecular Medicine, Northwestern University Feinberg School of Medicine, Chicago, Illinois

KAREN M. WARBURTON, MD, FASN
Associate Professor of Clinical Medicine, Division of Renal, Electrolyte and Hypertension, Penn Transplant Institute, Perelman School of Medicine, University of Pennsylvania, Philadelphia, Pennsylvania

KYMBERLY D. WATT, MD
Associate Professor, Division of Gastroenterology and Hepatology, Mayo Clinic and Foundation, Rochester, Minnesota

FRANCIS L. WENG, MD, MSCE
Renal and Pancreas Transplant Division, Saint Barnabas Medical Center, Livingston, New Jersey

Contents

Foreword: Medical Care for Kidney and Liver Transplant Recipients   xv

Edward R. Bollard

Preface: Long-Term Care of the Abdominal Organ Transplant Recipient: Pearls for the Primary Care Provider   xvii

David A. Sass and Alden M. Doyle

Liver and Kidney Transplantation: A Half-Century Historical Perspective   435

David A. Sass and Alden M. Doyle

> This article describes the evolution of solid organ kidney and liver transplantation and expounds on the challenges and successes that the early transplant researchers and clinicians encountered. The article highlights the surgical pioneers, delves into the milestones of enhanced immunosuppression protocols, discusses key federal legislative and policy changes, and expounds on the ongoing disparities of organ supply and demand and the need for extended criteria and live donor organs to combat these shortages. Finally, recent changes in organ allocation and distribution policies are discussed. The authors also spotlight novel interventions that will further revolutionize abdominal transplantation in the next 50 years.

From Child-Pugh to Model for End-Stage Liver Disease: Deciding Who Needs a Liver Transplant   449

Sheela S. Reddy and Jesse M. Civan

> This article reviews the historical evolution of the liver transplant organ allocation policy and the indications/contraindications for liver transplant, and provides an overview of the liver transplant evaluation process. The article is intended to help internists determine whether and when referral to a liver transplant center is indicated, and to help internists to counsel patients whose initial evaluation at a transplant center is pending.

Renal Transplantation in Advanced Chronic Kidney Disease Patients   465

Mythili Ghanta and Belinda Jim

> Kidney transplantation is the best option for patients with end-stage kidney disease. It is associated with better quality of life, lower medical costs, less hospitalization, and improved survival compared with wait-listed patients who remain on dialysis. Timely referral for transplantation is essential to reap the maximal benefit and should begin in the advanced chronic kidney disease stage prior to starting dialysis. Shortage of donor organs remains the biggest challenge to transplantation. With the improved success of kidney transplantation, candidate acceptance criteria continue to broaden. This article provides an overview of the pretransplantation multidisciplinary evaluation process detailing the factors that determine transplant candidacy.

Management of the Liver Transplant Recipient: Approach to Allograft Dysfunction   477

Jonathan M. Fenkel and Dina L. Halegoua-DeMarzio

Liver transplant (LT) recipients are living longer than ever today and many will experience some form of allograft dysfunction. The common causes of allograft dysfunction vary significantly depending on the timing since LT. Most allograft abnormalities are manageable with minimally invasive procedures, medications, and lifestyle modification. The most common differential diagnoses by time period after LT, and diagnostic and management considerations, are highlighted. Collaboration and comanagement of LT recipients between primary care and the transplant hepatologist is essential for optimizing recipient and allograft outcomes.

Acute and Chronic Allograft Dysfunction in Kidney Transplant Recipients   487

Ryan J. Goldberg, Francis L. Weng, and Praveen Kandula

Allograft dysfunction after a kidney transplant is often clinically asymptomatic and is usually detected as an increase in serum creatinine level with corresponding decrease in glomerular filtration rate. The diagnostic evaluation may include blood tests, urinalysis, transplant ultrasonography, radionuclide imaging, and allograft biopsy. Whether it occurs early or later after transplant, allograft dysfunction requires prompt evaluation to determine its cause and subsequent management. Acute rejection, medication toxicity from calcineurin inhibitors, and BK virus nephropathy can occur early or later. Other later causes include transplant glomerulopathy, recurrent glomerulonephritis, and renal artery stenosis.

The ABCs of Immunosuppression: A Primer for Primary Care Physicians   505

Gregory Malat and Christine Culkin

Immunosuppression use for prevention of allograft recognition/rejection has evolved to reflect an expanded understanding of the immune system, as well as a fine tuning of the goals of therapy. Immunosuppression in organ transplantation represents a balance between the desire to improve the health status of an individual affected by chronic conditions versus not imposing an unintended immunodeficiency leading to iatrogenic morbidity/mortality. This article discusses the selection and general dosing of immunosuppression in organ allograft recipients to allow providers to be comfortable in monitoring immunosuppressive therapy long term and the associated, expected posttransplant complications in allograft recipients.

Managing Cardiovascular Risk in the Post Solid Organ Transplant Recipient   519

Mrudula R. Munagala and Anita Phancao

Solid organ transplantation is an effective treatment for patients with end-stage organ disease. The prevalence of cardiovascular diseases (CVD) has increased in recipients. CVD remains a leading cause of mortality among recipients with functioning grafts. The pathophysiology of CVD recipients is a complex interplay between preexisting risk factors, metabolic sequelae of immunosuppressive agents, infection, and rejection. Risk modification must be weighed against the risk of mortality owing to rejection or infection. Aggressive risk stratification and modification before and after transplantation and tailoring immunosuppressive regimens are essential to prevent complications and improve short-term and long-term mortality and graft survival.

Diabetes Care After Transplant: Definitions, Risk Factors, and Clinical Management   535

Amisha Wallia, Vidhya Illuri, and Mark E. Molitch

Patients who undergo solid organ transplantation may have preexisting diabetes mellitus (DM), develop new-onset DM after transplantation (NO-DAT), or have postoperative hyperglycemia that resolves shortly after surgery. Although insulin is usually used to control hyperglycemia in the hospital, following discharge most of the usual diabetes oral and parenteral medications can be used in treatment. However, when there are comorbidities such as impaired kidney or hepatic function, or heart disease, special precautions may be necessary. In addition, drug-drug interactions, such as drugs interacting with CYP3A4 enzyme pathway, require additional consideration because of possible interaction with immunosuppressive drug metabolism.

De Novo Malignancies After Transplantation: Risk and Surveillance Strategies   551

Iliana Doycheva, Syed Amer, and Kymberly D. Watt

De novo malignancies are one of the leading causes of late mortality after liver and kidney transplantation. Nonmelanoma skin cancer is the most common malignancy, followed by posttransplant lymphoproliferative disorder and solid organ tumors. Immunosuppression is a key factor for cancer development, although many other transplant-related and traditional risk factors also play a role. In this review, the authors summarize risk factors and outcomes of frequently encountered de novo malignancies after liver and kidney transplantation to stratify recipients at highest risk. Future efforts in prospectively validated, cost-effective surveillance strategies that improve survival of these complex patients are greatly needed.

Metabolic Bone Disease in the Post-transplant Population: Preventative and Therapeutic Measures   569

Johan Daniël Nel and Sol Epstein

Post-transplant bone disease contributes significantly to patients' morbidity and mortality after transplantation and has an impact on their quality of life. This article discusses the major contributors to mechanisms causing bone loss, highlighting the role of preexisting disease in both kidney and liver failure and contributions from glucocorticoids and calcineurin inhibitors. Suggested monitoring and investigations are reviewed as well as treatment as far as the current literature supports, emphasizing the difference between kidney and liver recipients.

Infectious Complications and Vaccinations in the Posttransplant Population   587

William G. Greendyke and Marcus R. Pereira

Infections remain a major cause of mortality and morbidity after both kidney and liver transplantation, and internists increasingly play a major role in diagnosing and treating these infections. Because of immunosuppression, solid organ transplant recipients do not often demonstrate classic signs and symptoms of infection and have a broader variety of common and opportunistic infections, many of which are generally more difficult to diagnose and treat. Although these patients have many risk factors for infection, a major determinant is the time after transplant as it relates to levels of immunosuppression, healing, and hospital or environmental exposures.

Selection and Postoperative Care of the Living Donor   599

Dianne LaPointe Rudow and Karen M. Warburton

Live organ donors typically consult their primary care providers when considering live donation and then return for follow-up after surgery and for ongoing primary care. Live liver and kidney transplants are performed routinely as a method to shorten the waiting time for a recipient, provide a healthy organ for transplant, and increase recipient survival. Careful medical and psychosocial evaluation of the potential donor is imperative to minimize harm. This evaluation must be performed by an experienced live donor medical team. Routine health care with careful attention to weight maintenance, cardiovascular health, and prevention of diabetes and hypertension is paramount.

Long-Term Functional Recovery, Quality of Life, and Pregnancy After Solid Organ Transplantation   613

Swati Rao, Mythili Ghanta, Michael J. Moritz, and Serban Constantinescu

This article reviews the salient features of functional recovery, health-related quality of life (HR-QOL), and reproductive health, with special emphasis on pregnancy outcomes in kidney and liver recipients. Transplantation results in improved functional status and HR-QOL. Addressing factors that limit the optimal rehabilitation of transplant recipients can improve transplant outcomes. After successful transplantation, there is a rapid return of fertility, warranting counseling regarding contraception. Practitioners should be aware of the teratogenic potential of mycophenolic acid products. Posttransplant pregnancies are high risk, with increased incidences of hypertension, preeclampsia, and prematurity. Most pregnancies in kidney and liver recipients have successful maternal and newborn outcomes.

Index   631

Foreword

Medical Care for Kidney and Liver Transplant Recipients

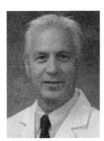

Edward R. Bollard, MD, DDS, FACP
Consulting Editor

As transplant medicine has evolved, so has the role of the generalist in the ongoing care of the patients receiving these vital organs. Liver and kidney transplantation, once considered a highly specialized area of surgery, has become quite common. The patient care it demands has resulted from not only the care related to the organ itself but also the types and degree of immunosuppression, as well as the inherent potential for complications that surround it. As the number of patients receiving cadaveric and living donor–related liver and kidney transplants has increased—and their life expectancy has lengthened—the need to involve the primary care physician in their care has become essential.

In this issue of the *Medical Clinics of North America*, Drs Sass and Doyle have assembled an exceptional panel of experts to address the common, yet complex, questions that present to the internal medicine physician whose patients undergo transplantation of these organs. The editors begin by providing the historical perspective to liver and kidney transplantation. The articles to follow address almost every aspect of the subsequent care of these patients (and donors), from determination of the time to transplant, discussion of immunosuppression and the potential short- and long-term complications, to the impact on quality of life and the potential for pregnancy in the transplanted patient.

If not now, then in the very near future, all of our practices will be providing longitudinal care to patients who have undergone liver and/or kidney transplantation. The articles in this issue present a breadth and depth of knowledge that will allow

Med Clin N Am 100 (2016) xv–xvi
http://dx.doi.org/10.1016/j.mcna.2016.03.004
0025-7125/16/$ – see front matter © 2016 Published by Elsevier Inc.
medical.theclinics.com

the internist or family practitioner to participate in the comprehensive, team-based care that is required in this unique and growing field of medicine.

Edward R. Bollard, MD, DDS, FACP
Department of Medicine
Penn State–Hershey Medical Center
Penn State University College of Medicine
500 University Drive
PO Box 850 (Mail Code H039)
Hershey, PA 17033-0850, USA

E-mail address:
ebollard@hmc.psu.edu

Preface

Long-Term Care of the Abdominal Organ Transplant Recipient: Pearls for the Primary Care Provider

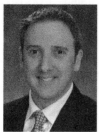   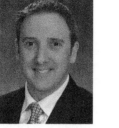

David A. Sass, MD, FACP, FACG, AGAF, FAASLD   Alden M. Doyle, MD, MS, MPH
Editors

Without the organ donor, there is no story, no hope, no transplant. But when there is an organ donor, life springs from death, sorrow turns to hope and a terrible loss becomes a gift.

—UNOS

It is our distinct privilege to be the guest editors of the May 2016 issue of *Medical Clinics of North America* entitled, "Medical Care for Kidney and Liver Transplant Recipients." This is the first time that a *Medical Clinics of North America* issue has been dedicated to the field of transplantation, and the timing is appropriate as we have just passed the half-century mark since the first successful kidney transplant. Our issue is aimed at the health care providers in primary care and internal medicine who care for patients who have undergone liver or kidney transplantation. Caring for such patients may present formidable challenges; thus, it is hoped that our collection of review articles will provide a useful framework for the treating physician to provide the comprehensive care that is needed to address the medical needs of this patient population.

In the first article, we expound on the tremendous advancements in the field of transplantation as well as the key federal legislative changes that have shaped transplant since the 1950s. Drs Civan and Reddy next discuss the indications for liver transplant evaluation and the evolution from Child-Pugh to MELD (model for end-stage liver disease) for organ allocation. Drs Jim and Ghanta similarly address the topic of timing of the kidney transplant evaluation in patients with advanced chronic kidney disease. Drs Fenkel and Halegoua-DeMarzio discuss an algorithmic approach to allograft

Med Clin N Am 100 (2016) xvii–xviii
http://dx.doi.org/10.1016/j.mcna.2016.03.003
0025-7125/16/$ – see front matter © 2016 Published by Elsevier Inc.

dysfunction in the liver transplant recipient, while Drs Goldberg and colleagues provide an overview of acute and chronic allograft dysfunction in kidney transplant patients.

Dr Malat and Christine Culkin, DNP summarize the basics of immunosuppression and provide a primer for the primary care provider. The next five review articles each deal with specific long-term complications of solid organ transplantation. An understanding on how to manage these is imperative in order to afford our patients the best chance at long-term survival. Drs Munagala and Phancao's review explores the realm of managing cardiovascular risk in the solid organ transplant recipient. Drs Molitch and colleagues discuss diabetes care, and Drs Watt and colleagues address risk for de novo malignancies and surveillance strategies. Drs Nel and Epstein review metabolic bone disease, while Drs Pereira and Greendyke address infectious complications and vaccinations.

The final two articles deal with other important aspects in the transplantation field. Dr Warburton and Dianne LaPointe Rudow, ANP discuss selection and postoperative care of the living kidney and liver donor, while Dr Constantinescu and colleagues delve into long-term functional recovery, quality of life, and fertility issues following solid organ transplantation.

In summary, readers of this issue of *Medical Clinics of North America* will find an informative and topical array of articles that should provide a solid foundation for primary care providers by which to care for the posttransplant recipient. We are deeply indebted to each of the authors and their respective coauthors for their truly invaluable contributions, and it has been our collective intent to provide a practical, stimulating resource that will be of value in your daily practice. We wish to extend our sincere gratitude to Jessica McCool and her editorial staff at Elsevier, particularly Alison Swety, for their assistance in compiling this issue. Finally, our love and heartfelt appreciation to our families, Allison, Lauren, and Aaron Sass, and Karen, Beckett, and Harper Doyle, for their support and encouragement in allowing us the time to devote many hours so that our labor of love could reach fruition.

David A. Sass, MD, FACP, FACG, AGAF, FAASLD
Division of Gastroenterology and Hepatology
Liver Transplantation
Sidney Kimmel Medical College
at Thomas Jefferson University
132 South 10th Street
Thompson Building, Suite 450
Philadelphia, PA 19107, USA

Alden M. Doyle, MD, MS, MPH
Division of Nephrology
Drexel University College of Medicine
Kidney and Pancreas Transplantation
Hahnemann University Hospital
245 North Broad Street
Suite 12318, New College Building
Philadelphia, PA 19102, USA

E-mail addresses:
david.sass@jefferson.edu (D.A. Sass)
alden.doyle@drexelmed.edu (A.M. Doyle)

Liver and Kidney Transplantation

A Half-Century Historical Perspective

David A. Sass, MD[a],*, Alden M. Doyle, MD, MS, MPH[b],*

KEYWORDS

- Kidney transplantation • Liver transplantation • Historical perspective
- Organ allocation • UNOS • Organ Procurement and Transplantation Network
- Evolution of immunosuppression

KEY POINTS

- Kidney and liver transplantation have enjoyed tremendous advancements over the past half-century.
- Over the past three decades there have been significant improvements in immunosuppressive regimens that are now being specifically tailored to the patient to better strike a balance between risk of rejection and infection.
- Use of ECD, DCD, and living donors has become common practice by many transplant centers to counter the disparity between organ supply and demand.
- Frequent communication between the primary care physician and transplant professionals is critical to successfully comanage kidney and liver transplant recipients.

INTRODUCTION

The dream of transplantation is an ancient one, captured vividly in the fantastic creatures of ancient mythology that combined components of different beasts for dramatic effect. The earliest attempts in humans were described around 1000 years ago in India and then later in Renaissance-era Italy, but these only involved autotransplantation of flaps, which skirted the formidable challenges that would later define the pioneering advances in solid organ transplantation: the development of

Disclosure Statement: The authors disclose no conflicts of interest.
[a] Liver Transplantation, Division of Gastroenterology and Hepatology, Thomas Jefferson University Hospitals, Sidney Kimmel Medical College at Thomas Jefferson University, 132 South 10th Street, Suite 480, Main Building, Philadelphia, PA 19107, USA; [b] Kidney and Pancreas Transplantation, Division of Nephrology, Hahnemann University Hospital, Drexel University College of Medicine, 245 North Broad Street, Suite 12318, New College Building, Philadelphia, PA 19102-1101, USA
* Corresponding author.
E-mail addresses: David.Sass@jefferson.edu; Alden.Doyle@drexelmed.edu

Med Clin N Am 100 (2016) 435–448
http://dx.doi.org/10.1016/j.mcna.2015.12.001
medical.theclinics.com

successful vascular anastomoses and the ability to cross between nonidentical immune systems.[1]

Today, a wide array of organs is successfully transplanted and kidney transplantation and liver transplantation (LT) are broadly considered the standard of care for suitable patients with end-stage kidney and/or liver disease. This article outlines some of the major milestones in the related fields of kidney transplantation and LT with a basic assumption that until such time as organs are able to be grown from a diseased patient's own stem cells, transplantation will continue to play a major role in health care. There is, furthermore, a real value for a wide spectrum of health care professionals to have a fundamental working knowledge of the historical evolution and current practice of solid organ transplantation. We focus on the major historical events that have transformed kidney transplantation and LT from a fantastical dream shared by the ancients to an everyday occurrence of modern medical practice. We have provided a comprehensive list (**Table 1**) of these historical transplant milestones chronologically as a quick and easy reference to the reader.

EARLY ATTEMPTS AT KIDNEY TRANSPLANTATION

In the early nineteenth century, Alexis Carrel published his work on vascular anastomoses, which involved the development of new sewing techniques and new suture material. Carrel[2] later reported using these techniques of anastomosis to successfully transplant kidneys of a dog into a different location (heterotopic) in the same animal's body. These kidneys would often function well, allowing the animals to maintain health and survive normally. His work also garnered national attention through publication in the lay press and could be argued to have been one of the primary drivers that planted the idea of organ transplantation in the imagination of the lay public.[3]

Numerous attempts by a variety of investigators at placing one animal's organs into another nonidentical (allogeneic) animal were met with early graft failure. Dr Emerich Ullman attached a dog's kidney into a goat and reported a brief period of urine output before the organ failed.[4] Dr Carrel himself described the idea of biologic incompatibility, bringing forward the next and perhaps greatest challenge of allogenic transplantation, crossing the immune barrier of self versus nonself.

The first known human-to-human kidney transplant was performed by Dr Yu Yu Yuronoy in 1936, which used a deceased donor organ. The kidney initially made urine and then quickly turned black and failed in what was assumed to be early rejection. Other attempts were made by different surgeons in Europe and the United States, helping to improve the technical aspects of the operation and to begin to establish the retroperitoneal position in the pelvis as the preferred location for a transplanted kidney. In Boston at the Peter Bent Brigham Hospital, a team led by Dr Joseph Murray transplanted 11 individual patients with kidneys, using a mixture of living and deceased donors, and had one patient survive for 5 months with a functioning allograft.[5]

SUCCESSFUL KIDNEY TRANSPLANTATION BEGINS

The era of successful human solid organ transplantation began with Dr Murray and his team in 1954 with the transplantation of a kidney between the identical twin Herrick brothers.[1] In this widely heralded success, both the donor and recipient did well and were able to lead healthy productive lives. This case spurred increased interest in transplantation as an answer to end-organ disease and led to a series of transplants

Table 1
Timeline of milestones in transplantation: a half century of progress

1936	First human-to-human kidney transplant attempted
1954	First successful kidney transplant performed between identical twins
1962	First successful deceased donor kidney transplant performed
1966	First successful kidney/pancreas transplant performed
1967	First successful liver transplant performed
1967–1968	Acceptance of brain death concept
1968	First successful isolated pancreas transplant performed First successful heart transplant performed SEOPF is formed as a membership and scientific organization for transplant professionals
1977	SEOPF implements the first computer-based organ matching system, dubbed UNOS
1981	First successful heart-lung transplant performed
1983	First successful single-lung transplant performed Cyclosporine, the first of several successful antirejection drugs, approved by the FDA
1984	National Organ Transplant Act passed UNOS separates from SEOPF and is incorporated as an independent, nonprofit organization committed to saving lives through uniting and supporting efforts of donation and transplantation professionals First successful combined liver/kidney transplant performed
1986	First successful double-lung transplant performed UNOS receives the initial federal contract to operate the OPTN and Scientific Registry of Transplant Recipients
1987	First successful intestinal transplant University of Wisconsin solution improves liver and other organ preservation
1987–1989	First successful transplantation of liver-containing multivisceral grafts
1988	First split-liver transplant performed
1989	First successful living-donor liver transplant performed Clinical introduction of FK506 (tacrolimus)-based immunosuppression
1990	First successful living-donor lung transplant performed
1992	UNOS helps found Donate Life America to build public support for organ donation
1994	Tacrolimus approved for use for liver transplantation by FDA
1995	UNOS launches its first Web site for all users with an interest in transplantation Mycophenolate mofetil approved for use by FDA
1998	First successful adult-to-adult living-donor liver transplant performed
1999	UNOS launches UNet, a secure, Internet-based transplant information database system for all organ matching and management of transplant data Mammalian target of rapamycin inhibitors (sirolimus) approved for use by FDA
2000	US Department of Health and Human Services publishes the Final Rule (federal regulation) for the operation of the OPTN
2001	For the first time, the total number of living organ donors for the year (6528) exceeds the number of deceased organ donors (6081)
2002	Introduction of the MELD/PELD system for liver organ allocation

(continued on next page)

Table 1 (continued)	
2006	UNOS launches DonorNet, a secure, Internet-based system in which organ procurement coordinators send out offers of newly donated organs to transplant hospitals with compatible candidates
2013	New rules for liver allocation including Share 15 and Share 35 go into effect
2014	New rules for kidney allocation go into effect

Abbreviations: FDA, Food and Drug Administration; MELD, Model for End-Stage Liver Disease; OPTN, Organ Procurement and Transplantation Network; PELD, Pediatric End-Stage Liver Disease; SEOPF, Southeast Organ Procurement Foundation; UNOS, United Network for Organ Sharing.

at different centers between identical twins and a renewed effort at solving the challenge of establishing tolerance for such a transplanted organ in an allogeneic host.

From the late 1940s into the 1950s immunology advanced rapidly, with the early characterization of immunologic memory and the discovery that nonidentical twin cattle that shared a placenta would be tolerant of each other's antigens and would not reject each other's skin grafts. Dr Peter Medawar, who later earned a Nobel Prize for his work, was able to promote tolerance in mice that were exposed to foreign antigens in utero.[6] He and others went on to characterize some of the principal components of immunologic memory, tolerance, and rejection that laid the foundations for the clinical studies of immunosuppression.[7]

After several failed attempts in the 1950s, the first successful allogeneic transplant was performed with the use of whole-body radiation plus corticosteroids to dampen immune response in two fraternal twin brothers in 1959 followed by nontwin siblings in 1960. In Boston in 1962, after the introduction of azathioprine, came the first successful use of a deceased donor kidney. Each of these efforts was aided by the major changes that were going on in nephrology, including advancement of the technology of hemodialysis, the development of the first dialysis catheters that allowed for continued safe access to the patient's bloodstream by nephrologist Dr Belding Scribner (Scribner Shunt), and the later development of the dialysis fistula by Dr Michael Brescia and James Cimino.[5]

TRANSPLANTATION DEBATE DRIVES CHANGES IN LAW AND POLICY

The use of deceased donor organs prompted a national debate and eventually led to a series of laws that allowed for the legal use of deceased donor organs.[8] This began with the Uniform Anatomic Gift Act in 1968; the President's Commission for the Study of Ethical Problems in Medicine and Biomedical Research Guidelines for Determination of Death, which established the initial definition of brain death; the National Transplantation Act in 1984, which prohibited the sale of organs; Required Request Rules to improve rates of donation after death; and the Final Rule issued by US Department of Health and Human Services (DHHS) to lay out the federal guidelines for organ sharing and the allocation of power among the organizations that are involved in solid organ transplantation including DHHS, the United Network for Organ Sharing (UNOS), and the Organ Procurement and Transplantation Network.[9]

NEXT MILESTONES MARKED BY ADVANCES IN IMMUNOSUPPRESSION

Other major milestones in transplantation stemmed from the discovery and introduction of new immunosuppressive agents. This began with total lymphoid irradiation, but alternatives were quickly sought because of the high burden of toxicity. Animal studies suggested that 6-mercaptopurine had promise, so this drug was used by researchers in bone marrow transplantation with some success and was later applied to canine models of kidney transplantation by the Boston team that included Dr Roy Calne and Dr Joseph Murray.[5] These researchers later found that the close relative of 6-mercaptopurine, azathioprine, had a better efficacy/toxicity profile and was found to be effective in humans.[5] Around the same time, in the early 1960s, corticosteroids became established initially as a way to treat rejection and then later, by Dr Thomas Starzl, as part of the maintenance immunosuppression regimen for patients who had received kidney allotransplants.[5] Dr Starzl was also the first to check laboratory parameters, such as the white blood cell count, and adjust the doses of his combination immunosuppression regimens, adopting what is commonplace today: individualization of dosing to the transplant patient to better strike a balance between risk of rejection and infection.[5] The discovery of the immunomodulatory properties of cyclosporine by Swiss physician Jean Borel in 1977, its clinical investigational introduction in 1978, and its Food and Drug Administration (FDA) approval as Sandimmune in 1983 were the most important immunosuppressive developments in organ transplantation.[10,11] Other major developments include the introduction of another calcineurin inhibitor, tacrolimus, in the early 1990s; then mycophenolic acid mofetil in 1995; and then the mammalian target of rapamycin inhibitors in 1999. In addition, there were several therapeutic antibodies that have played a major role in kidney transplantation and LT. The first of these was the polyclonal antithymocyte preparations, following which monoclonal anti-T-cell preparations (eg, OKT3) became available, and subsequently monoclonal and less immunogenic "humanized" preparations that targeted the interleukin-2 receptor were introduced. Even later, the anti-B-cell monoclonal antibody against CD-20 entered clinical practice; then the crossover of alemtuzumab (anti-CD52) from the world of bone marrow transplant for use with solid organ recipients; and then, most recently in 2011, the FDA approval of costimulatory blockers, such as belatecept, was introduced. The timeline for introduction and the mechanisms of action of all of the key immunosuppressive agents commonly used in the field of solid organ transplantation are covered in detail elsewhere in this issue (See Malat G, Culkin C: The ABC's of immunosuppression: a primer for the primary care physician, in this issue).

Today, LT and kidney transplantation is a largely successful enterprise and is widely considered the treatment of choice for suitable candidates with either end-stage kidney or end-stage liver disease (or both). Other solid organ transplants can be performed, including heart, lung, pancreas, and small bowel, but their use is more nuanced and beyond the scope of this review.

THE FASCINATING SAGA OF LIVER TRANSPLANTATION: MEMOIRS OF TWO SURGICAL PIONEERS

LT celebrated its fiftieth anniversary in 2013. Many of the personal histories and remembrances of the early struggles and later triumphs of LT are beautifully captured by two of the surgical founders in their respective published autobiographies. Starzl relates his life in *The Puzzle People*[12] and Calne[13] has produced a beautifully illustrated, nontechnical history in *Art, Surgery and Transplantation*. Over the last half-century, many transplant strategies have evolved worldwide regarding surgical techniques, immunosuppressive agents, organ allocation, donor selection, indications and contraindications, prophylaxis of infection, and prevention of recurrent diseases. This has led to LT becoming an accepted, mainstream, and well-established procedure that has saved innumerable lives. Today there are hundreds of LT centers in more than 80 countries worldwide.

GENESIS OF LIVER TRANSPLANTATION

The first report of LT did not appear until 1955 in a journal called *Transplantation Bulletin* where, in a one-page article, C. Stuart Welch of Albany Medical College in New York, reported on his efforts to transplant an auxiliary liver into the right paravertebral gutter of nonimmunosuppressed dogs without disturbing the native liver.[14] The livers withered quickly, a result Welch ascribed to rejection. The livers may well have atrophied in part because of the lack of portal blood. The concept of liver replacement (orthotopic transplantation) was first mentioned by Jack Cannon in a one-page account of the transplant activities in the surgery department of UCLA School of Medicine.[15] In 1958 Francis Moore described the standard technique of canine liver orthotopic transplantation.[16] It should be noted that Thomas Starzl had been working on a similar model and performed more than 200 canine transplants before his first attempt in humans. The two prerequisites for perioperative survival of the canine recipients were prevention of ischemic injury to the allograft by immersing the liver in a "preservation solution" and avoidance of damage to the recipient splanchnic and systemic venous beds, the drainage of which was obstructed during host hepatectomy and graft implantation. These early nonhuman experimental experiences expanded the available knowledge on many issues, such as venovenous bypass, organ preservation, tissue matching, and immunosuppression.

HUMAN LIVER TRIALS OF 1963

The first human to undergo an LT was a 3-year-old boy who suffered from biliary atresia. He died before the operation was completed on March 1, 1963. Dr Thomas Starzl who performed this first LT in Denver, Colorado, provides the details of the surgery in his memoir, *The Puzzle People*: "*Nothing* we had done in advance could have prepared us for the enormity of the task. Several hours were required just to make the incision and enter the abdomen. Every piece of tissue that was cut contained the small veins under high pressure that had resulted from obstruction of the portal vein by the diseased liver... his intestines and stomach were stuck to the liver in this mass of bloody scar. To make things worse, the patient's blood would not clot."[12]

The next two recipients transplanted by Starzl, both adults, died 22 and 7.5 days post-LT, respectively. They were transplanted for primary liver malignancies and were found at autopsy to have extrahepatic micrometastases.[17]

LIVER TRANSPLANTATION MORATORIUM AND LATER RESUMPTION

During the last half of 1963, two more LTs were performed in Denver and one each in Boston, Massachusetts[18] and Paris, France.[19] All patients received immunosuppression proposed for kidney transplantation (ie, azathioprine and corticosteroids). The longest surviving recipient of these first seven human LTs lived 23 days. Hence, the results were discouraging because ischemia-reperfusion injury and rejection inevitably progressed to liver failure or sepsis. After the deaths of these patients, there was a worldwide voluntary moratorium as clinical activity ceased for 3.5 years (January 1964 through the summer of 1967). As Starzl relates: "This self-imposed decision to stop did little to quiet polite but unmistakably disapproving discussions of an operation that had come to be perceived as too difficult to ever be tried again."[20] During the moratorium, problems contributing to the 1963 failures were addressed, such as achieving control of blood coagulation, improved organ preservation, infection containment, and avoidance where possible of venovenous bypasses.

July 1967 heralded the resumption of the human LT program by Starzl. There were multiple examples of prolonged human liver recipient survival under the "triple-drug" immunosuppression protocol with prednisone, azathioprine, and antilymphocyte globulin. The first case was a 19-month-old girl with hepatocellular carcinoma who survived more than 1 year with preserved liver function and died of disease recurrence.[21] In 1968, Calne in Cambridge, United Kingdom reported five cases of LT, detailing the technical difficulties encountered.[22] Starzl and Calne were later honored with the Lasker-DeBakey Clinical Medical Research Award in 2012 for these pioneering procedures. Success did not necessarily come quickly or easily. Over the next 10 years perhaps 200 LTs were performed worldwide, about half of these by Starzl. The technical problems that began to be solved over this period included bile duct reconstruction; coagulation support; and refinement of the donor procedure, including acceptance of the concept of "brain death" in the United States in 1968. This landmark for LT development allowed donor organ preservation in ideal, physiologic conditions and resulted in better graft quality and survival.[23]

The discovery and introduction of cyclosporine had a profound effect on the entire field of transplantation and for LT, there was no exception. In 1979 Calne used cyclosporine for the first time in two patients post-LT,[24] paving the way for LT to be transformed from a curiosity into a therapy.

NATIONAL INSTITUTES OF HEALTH APPROVAL OF LIVER TRANSPLANTATION AS A "VALID THERAPY"

In June 1983, the National Institutes of Health held a consensus development conference on LT in Bethesda, Maryland. Four groups from four countries (United States, England, Germany, and The Netherlands) presented outcome data on 531 cases. It had been 20 years since the first LT, and in the eyes of most physicians (and all insurance companies), the procedure was seen as dangerous and experimental. The cumulative message from these 531 cases was that end-stage liver disease was no longer a death sentence. The panel of experts agreed that LT had become a "clinical service" rather than an experimental procedure and approved it as a valid therapy for treating patients with cirrhosis and liver failure.

Five years after the National Institutes of Health conference, there were 616 patients awaiting LT in the United States. Ten years later the number had ballooned to more than 12,000. In 1989, Starzl and colleagues[25] reported survival of 1179 patients who had undergone LT with a 1- and 5-year survival of 73% and 64%, respectively.

CONVERSION TO TACROLIMUS

In the late 1980s Dr Starzl set in motion in his laboratory in Pittsburgh, preclinical studies of FK-506 (tacrolimus) that eventually led to its substitution for cyclosporine and fast-track approval by the FDA in November 1993.[26] In the early 1990s, tacrolimus was clinically investigated in human LT recipients with cyclosporine-refractory rejection.[27] Approximately 75% of such allografts were rescued with the conversion to tacrolimus.[28] The sequential increment in graft and patient survival in LT with the introduction of the calcineurin-inhibitors compared with the precalcineurin immunosuppressive era was impressive. The greater potency and equivalent safety of tacrolimus compared with cyclosporine resulted in significant conversion to tacrolimus-based immunosuppression for liver, kidney, pancreas, and thoracic organ transplantation.[29] Tacrolimus also provided a major boost to overcome the immunologic hurdle of intestinal and multivisceral transplantation in patients with short-gut syndrome.[30] The first successful transplantation of liver-containing multivisceral grafts was in 1988.

Novel immunosuppressive agents that also became available during this time, such as antilymphocyte drugs (OKT3, antithymocyte globulin), a new antiproliferative agent (mycophenolate mofetil), and sirolimus, have allowed clinicians the freedom to tailor a combination immunosuppressive regimen based on the recipient's toxicity risks and degree of allograft tolerance.

ORGAN PROCUREMENT AND PRESERVATION

Removal of an organ from the body creates an obligatory ischemic insult whose sequelae may be subclinical organ dysfunction including delayed or permanent non-function. Organ immersion or the "slush" technique became the dominant standard of postprocurement storage from the 1980s to the present day. The development of the University of Wisconsin solution in 1987 by James Southard and Folkert Belzer of the University of Wisconsin, Madison, was the major historical landmark advance in graft flush solutions and has emerged as the preferred solution.[31]

DISPARITY BETWEEN ORGAN SUPPLY AND DEMAND

One of the unintended consequences of the widespread success and acceptance of kidney transplantation and LT is a growing disparity between the numbers of patients who need organs and the availability of suitable organs. The recent Scientific Registry for Transplant Recipient report of June 2014 cataloged more than the previous 12 months that there were 11,600 kidney transplants performed, 106,007 patients wait-listed for transplant, and 37,644 new patient registrations.[32] This disparity has driven up wait times for kidneys and has resulted in an increasing death rate while on the wait list. The major shortage of suitable organs has prompted a large effort among the lay and professional communities to address this growing problem. These efforts have included public awareness campaigns, lobbying for changes in donor registration and donor acceptance laws, and increased use of "marginal donors." The severity of the shortage and its impact on waiting times and wait list mortality has led UNOS and the rest of the transplant community to carefully consider more equitable systems for organ sharing and have led to recent major policy adjustments for kidney and liver transplants.

For kidney transplantation the organ shortage has led to a drive to use a much wider array of organ donors then were initially considered and an ongoing discussion regarding which organs are suited for which type of wait-listed patients. Examples include the use of "expanded criteria" donors who may be older or have comorbidities that are associated with less organ longevity; "Public health service elevated risk" donors who have increased risk of blood-borne infections, such as human immunodeficiency virus and hepatitis viruses; and donors who have died from cardiac death (donation after cardiac death [DCD]) where cessation of circulatory function must be documented and which leads to ischemic injury to the organs in the perimortem period. Some centers have put two expanded criteria kidneys into a single recipient or have used en bloc infant kidneys that remain attached by their native renal arteries to the aorta, which is oversewn and then anastomosed en bloc to the recipient.

In addition, there has been a broad push to expand the use of living donors, which are generally associated with some of the best patient and graft survival rates. The use of living donors is now widely accepted and performed at almost all kidney transplant centers. Although generally safe for the donor, recent studies have noted some risks that have to be weighed carefully. There is currently an active debate how to remove financial disincentives for potential living donors through potential legislation or changes in insurance carriers' policy. For donor issues and others, (See Rudow DL, Warburton KM: Selection and postoperative care of the living donor, in this issue).

For those patients with end-stage liver disease, the story of organ shortage and efforts to combat this shortage is similar. The number of patients awaiting primary or repeat LT in the United States has tripled to 18,000 in the last two decades.[33–35] Over the same period, organ availability increased from 1700 to 6200 grafts annually. The discrepancy between supply and demand and the increasing organ scarcity has motivated select transplant centers to relax customary restrictions to donation, creating the term "extended-criteria" donors (ECD) or "marginal" donors. As early as 1986, Makowka and colleagues[36] identified the impending organ shortage and reported the feasibility of systematically using livers from older donors and donors with biochemical or histopathologic evidence of liver injury. Older donor age, donor hepatic steatosis, donor hypernatremia, prolonged cold ischemia times, donors with positive hepatitis B and C serologies, known donor malignancy, and those with "high-risk" lifestyles are all examples of such ECDs. DCD donor, formerly known as "non-heart-beating donor," is another type of ECD. The number of LTs performed using DCD donors in the United States grew from 0.5% (in 1999) to 4.5% (in 2008), making it the most rapidly expanding component of the donor pool.[37]

DCD has a fundamentally different recovery technique based on cardiopulmonary criteria rather than neurologic criteria for brain death. Organs may be retrieved in "controlled" or "uncontrolled" fashion, with "controlled" DCD livers having a better chance of organ recovery.[38] To standardize procurement protocols and refine reporting of data, updated practice guidelines for organ procurement have been published by UNOS, the Institute of Medicine, and the Society of Critical Care Medicine,[39] and in 2009 the American Society of Transplant Surgeons issued recommendations on controlled DCD based on evidence and expert opinion.[40]

Another way the liver transplant community has tried to address the shortage of suitable organs is through advancements in surgical technique including the increased use of living donors. Live donor LT (LDLT) was developed in the same context as the split liver. In 1989, in Sao Paulo, Brazil, Raia and coworkers[41] described the first attempt at a living donor graft in a child. One year later, Strong and colleagues[42] performed the first successful LDLT using a left lateral segment graft. In 1993, Hashikura and colleagues[43] reported the first successful left lobe LDLT in an adult, followed 3 years later by the first successful adult-to-adult right lobe LDLT, reported by Lo and coworkers.[44] Beyond its technical complexity, a major concern about LDLT is the morbidity and risk of death for the donors. It has been shown that right donor hepatectomy may carry a higher morbidity than for the left lateral segment.[45] The mortality risk to the donor has been quoted at 0.4% to 0.5%. Beyond the risks to the donors, there are some challenges related to the recipient's surgery, including small for size syndrome, biliary complications, hepatic artery reconstruction, and optimization of venous drainage. Domino liver transplant (DLT) involves transplantation using grafts from patients with metabolic liver diseases, such as familial amyloidotic polyneuropathy. The familial amyloidotic polyneuropathy World Transplant Register includes experience of more than 1000 domino transplants performed in 21 countries until the end of 2011.[46] DLT seem to have similar outcomes to traditional deceased donor LTs[47] with a low risk of transmitting the metabolic disease through the transplanted liver.[48]

THE EVOLUTION OF LIVER ORGAN ALLOCATION AND DISTRIBUTION POLICIES

In the early decades of transplantation (1960s through 1980s), organs were allocated based on local transplant institutions and in the early 1990s, wait list time became a major criterion. In the latter 1990s in the United States, the listing criteria were substituted by government-regulated policies, which later established priority for candidate recipients based on disease severity, according to a medical status system (status 1, emergent transplant; status 2, patient in intensive care unit; status 3, inpatient, non–intensive care unit patient; status 4, outpatient). In the late 1990s through the early 2000s, the Child-Turcotte-Pugh score was also incorporated but this score was problematic in that it emphasized subjective measures of urgency leading to large disparities in waiting times across geographic regions.

As a result, in 1998 DHHS issued a regulation known as "the OPTN final rule" to ensure the allocation of scarce organs be based on common medical criteria, not accidents of geography, and provided a framework within which the transplant system would operate.[49] During the subsequent 4 years the Model for End-Stage Liver Disease (MELD)/Pediatric End-Stage Liver Disease (PELD) system was developed, studied, and finally implemented in February 2002.[50] This system prioritizes candidates based on risk of death while awaiting LT and has proven to be a highly objective and reliable predictor of most liver candidates' short-term (3-month) risk of dying without receiving an LT. Since the incorporation of MELD/PELD for transplant organ allocation, various "MELD exception categories" have been introduced and in 2006 MELD exception guidelines were published providing recommendations from the MELD Exception Study Group and Conference (MESSAGE).[51]

In addition to changes in organ allocation, there have also been several geographic distribution policies that changed the liver wait list priority algorithm. The most recent change was implemented on June 18, 2013. Under "Share 35" deceased donor livers are offered first to all candidates in the region with MELD of 35 or higher, regardless of donation service area, before being offered to other local candidates and then regional candidates. The Share 35 policy was implemented to decrease wait list mortality for the most urgent MELD/PELD, non–status 1 candidates. The policy was not intended to decrease the variance in the median MELD at transplant. Based on preliminary analysis, the policy is working as intended, without impacting the overall post-LT survival in the postimplementation era.[52]

THE EVOLVING ROLE OF TRANSPLANT CENTER

As kidney transplantation and LT have become more widely used and enjoy improved graft and patient survival, there are a growing number of patients who are alive with a functioning liver and/or kidney graft. This has broad implications for society and the health system that cares for them. These patients are in all segments of society, are often able to work and have children, and encounter a new host of issues that are associated with long-term use of immunosuppression. Many of these patient issues, (See Rao S, Ghanta M, Moritz MJ, et al: Long-term functional recovery, quality of life and pregnancy after solid organ transplantation, in this issue).

One of the consequences of an increased prevalence of kidney and liver recipients among the US population is that primary and specialty providers are much more likely to encounter and provide medical care for them in their regular practice. We therefore believe that a working knowledge of the major issues of transplant care are relevant for nontransplant specialized physicians and other caregivers. This increased prevalence has also led transplant centers to evolve the way they care for their patients, moving away from operating in isolation toward a model that explicitly expects patients to have primary care physicians and that this relationship is maintained through improved lines of communication and referral. Challenges remain because often varied providers are in different health systems, or have differential access to electronic medical records, so calls, letters, and the sharing or key medical data is of paramount importance.

THE FUTURE OF TRANSPLANTATION

There is a plethora of exciting scientific work that may fundamentally alter how transplantation is conceived of and practiced. One area of active research is the continued development of new immunosuppressive agents. The recent addition of several agents that allow more effective suppression of humoral immunity (eg, rituximab that targets B cells, bortezimib that targets plasma cells) has served as a potent reminder about how intertwined effective T- and B-cell responses can be and have raised the hope of tackling some of the more pernicious and hard to treat consequences of the long-term activation of humoral allogeneic responses. There is also hope to be able to combine different agents in more specific ways that increase efficacy while minimizing toxicity. Of particular concern is the marked, if not universal long-term kidney toxicity associated with the use of calcineurin inhibitors (cyclosporine and tacrolimus) that are believed to play a large part in limiting longer kidney allograft survival and is the most important single factor leading to the development of kidney disease in recipients of nonrenal solid organs including liver allografts.

There is also continued hope toward achieving the long-term goal of tolerance that would obviate ongoing immunosuppression with all of its inevitable direct and indirect toxicities. At least in some animal models this has been possible and the mechanisms of different kinds of tolerance, much of which is active and mediated by specific specialized types of immune cells, is becoming better understood.

Another area is the ongoing trials of xenotransplantation where the more formidable barriers of putting tissue from one species into another has been attempted. There has been some success using germ-free (gnobiotic) colonies of pigs that have been genetically modified to reduce some of the most difficult to manage antigens (eg, some carbohydrate moieties). Despite some progress, there is a lingering fear that viruses (eg, retroviruses) that lay dormant within the porcine or monkey donors may be unwittingly introduced into the human population, which are especially alarming given the experience with the zoonotic sourced infections of human immunodeficiency virus and more recently Ebola.

Finally, there has been real progress toward the goal of growing replacement organs in tissue culture. This was highlighted at some of the recent national transplant meetings where examples of beating, functional human hearts have been grown using a noncellular scaffolding of proteins as a sort of tissue matrix that helps guide the repopulation by differentiated human stem cells. Although not ready for clinical deployment, the sight of such a beating and potentially functional human heart gave even an expert transplant professional audience some pause.

REFERENCES

1. Tilney NL. Transplant: from myth to reality. New Haven (CT): Yale University Press; 2003.
2. Carrel A. LaTechnique operatoire des Anasomoses Vasculaires et la Transplantation des Visceres. Lyon Med 1902;98:859–64.
3. Carrel A. Landmark article, Nov 14, 1908: results of the transplantation of blood vessels, organs and limbs. By Alexis Carrel. JAMA 1983;250:944–53.
4. Nagy J. A note on the early history of renal transplantation: Emerich (Imre) Ullmann. Am J Nephrol 1999;19:346–9.

5. Papalois VE, Hakim NS, Najarian JS. The history of kidney transplantation. In: Hakim NS, Papalois VE, editors. History or organ and cell transplantation. London: Imperial College Press; 2003. p. 76–99.

6. Billingham RE, Brent L, Medawar PB, et al. Quantitative studies on tissue transplantation immunity. Proc R Soc Lond B Biol Sci 1954;143:43–58.

7. Billingham RE, Brent L, Medawar PB. Actively acquired tolerance of foreign cells. Nature 1953;172:603–6.

8. Papalois VE, Matas AJ. The history of the concept of brain death and organ preservation. In: Hakim NS, Papalois VE, editors. History of organ and cell transplantation. London: Imperial College Press; 2003. p. 64–73.

9. Available at: http://optn.transplant.hrsa.gov/governance/about-the-optn/history-nota/. Accessed September 2, 2015.

10. Kahan B. Cyclosporine. N Engl J Med 1989;321(25):725–38.

11. Starzl TE, Iwatsuki S, Shaw BW Jr, et al. Immunosuppression and other nonsurgical factors in the improved results of liver transplantation. Semin Liver Dis 1985;5(4):334–43.

12. Starzl TE. The puzzle people: memoirs of a transplant surgeon. Pittsburgh (PA): University of Pittsburgh Press; 1992.

13. Calne R. Art, surgery and transplantation. London: Williams and Wilkins Europe; 1996.

14. Welch CS. A note on transplantation of the whole liver in dogs. Transplant Bull 1955;2:54.

15. Cannon JA. Brief report. Transplant Bull 1956;3:7.

16. Moore FD, Wheeler HB, Demissianos HV, et al. Experimental whole organ transplantation of the liver and spleen. Ann Surg 1960;152:374–87.

17. Starzl TE, Marchioro TL, von Kaulla KN, et al. Homotransplantation of the liver in humans. Surg Gynecol Obstet 1963;117:659–76.

18. Moore FD, Birtch AG, Dagher F, et al. Immunosuppression and vascular insufficiency in liver transplantation. Ann N Y Acad Sci 1964;120:729–38.

19. Demirleau J, Noureddine M, Vignes, et al. Tentative d'homogreffe hepatique. [Attempted hepatic homograft]. Mem Acad Chir (Paris) 1964;90:177 [in French].

20. Starzl TE, Fung JJ. Themes of liver transplantation. Hepatology 2010;51(6):1869–84.

21. Starzl TE, Groth CG, Brettschneider L, et al. Orthotopic homotransplantations of the human liver. Ann Surg 1968;168:392–415.

22. Calne RY, Williams R. Liver transplantation in man. I. Observations on technique and organization in five cases. Br Med J 1968;4:535–40.

23. Landmark article Aug 5, 1968: a definition of irreversible coma. Report of the Ad Hoc Committee of the Harvard Medical School to examine the definition of brain death. JAMA 1984;252:677–9.

24. Calne RY, Rolles K, White DJ, et al. Cyclosporin A initially as the only immunosuppressant in 34 recipients of cadaveric organs: 32 kidneys, 2 pancreases and 2 livers. Lancet 1979;2(8151):1033–6.

25. Starzl TE, Todo S, Tzakis AG, et al. Liver transplantation: an unfinished product. Transplant Proc 1989;21:2197–200.

26. Starzl TE, Todo S, Fung J, et al. FK506 for human liver, kidney and pancreas transplantation. Lancet 1989;334:1000–4.

27. Fung JJ, Todo S, Jain A, et al. Conversion of liver allograft recipients with cyclosporine related complications from cyclosporine to FK506. Transplant Proc 1990;22(1):6–12.

28. Fung JJ, Todo S, Tzakis A, et al. Conversion of liver allograft recipients from cyclosporine to FK506-based immunosuppression: benefits and pitfalls. Transplant Proc 1991;23:14–21.
29. Fung JJ, Todo S, Jain A, et al. The Pittsburgh randomized trial of tacrolimus versus cyclosporine for liver transplantation. J Am Coll Surg 1996;183:117–25.
30. Todo S, Tzakis AG, Abu-Elmagd K, et al. Intestinal transplantation in composite visceral grafts or alone. Ann Surg 1992;216:223–33.
31. Todo S, Nery J, Yanaga K, et al. Extended preservation of human liver grafts with UW solution. JAMA 1989;261:711–4.
32. SRTR OPO-Specific reports archives. Available at: www.srtr.org. Accessed September 2, 2015.
33. OPTN and SRTR. Annual reports. Available at: www.optn.org. Accessed September 2, 2015.
34. Harper AM, Baker AS. The UNOS OPTN waiting list: 1988-1995. Clin Transplant 1995;69–84.
35. Sass DA, Reich DJ. Liver transplantation in the 21st century: expanding the donor options. Gastroenterol Clin North Am 2011;40:641–58.
36. Makowka L, Gordon RD, Todo S, et al. Analysis of donor criteria for the prediction of outcome in clinical liver transplantation. Transplant Proc 1987;19:2378–82.
37. Thuluvath PJ, Guidinger MK, Fung JJ, et al. Liver transplantation in the United States, 1999-2008. Am J Transplant 2010;10:1003–19.
38. Reich DJ, Munoz SJ, Rothstein KD, et al. Controlled non-heart beating donor liver transplantation: a successful single center experience, with topic update. Transplantation 2000;70:1159–66.
39. Reich DJ, Hong JC. Current status of donation after cardiac death liver transplantation. Curr Opin Organ Transplant 2010;15:316–21.
40. Reich DJ, Mulligan DC, Abt PL, et al. ASTS recommended practice guidelines for controlled donation after cardiac death organ procurement and transplantation. Am J Transplant 2009;9:2004–11.
41. Raia S, Nery JR, Miles S. Liver transplantation from live donors. Lancet 1989;2:497.
42. Strong RW, Lynch SV, Ong TH. Successful liver transplantation from a living donor to her son. N Engl J Med 1990;322:1505–7.
43. Hashikura Y, Makuuchi M, Kawasaki S, et al. Successful living-related partial liver transplantation to an adult patient. Lancet 1994;343:1233–4.
44. Lo CM, Fan ST, Liu CL, et al. Extending the limit on the size of adult recipient in living donor liver transplantation using extended right lobe graft. Transplantation 1997;63:1524–8.
45. Umeshita K, Fujiwara K, Kiyosawa K, et al. Operative morbidity of living liver donors in Japan. Lancet 2003;362:687–90.
46. The Familial Amyloidotic Polyneuropathy World Transplant Registry and the Domino Liver Transplant Registry. Available at: http://www.fapwtr.org/ram_domino.htm. Accessed September 2, 2015.
47. Sebagh M, Yilmaz F, Karam V, et al. Cadaveric full-size liver transplantation and the graft alternatives in adults: a comparative study from a single center. J Hepatol 2006;44:118–25.
48. Adams D, Lacroix C, Antonini T, et al. Symptomatic and proven de novo amyloid polyneuropathy in familial amyloid polyneuropathy domino liver recipients. Amyloid 2011;18(Suppl 1):174–7.
49. Available at: http://optn.transplant.hrsa.gov/policiesAndBylaws/final_rule.asp. Accessed September 2, 2015.

50. Freeman RB, Wiesner RH, Harper A, et al. The new liver allocation system: moving toward evidence-based transplantation policy. Liver Transpl 2002;8(9):851–8.

51. Freeman RB, Gish RG, Harper A, et al. MELD exception guidelines: results and recommendations from MELD Exception Study Group and Conference (MESSAGE) for the approval of patients who need liver transplantation with diseases not considered by the standard MELD formula. Liver Transpl 2006;12(Suppl 3): S128–36.

52. Edwards E, Harper A, Hirose R, et al. MELD/PELD 35+ candidates benefit from regional sharing [abstract]. Am J Transplant 2015;15(Suppl 3). Available at: http://www.atcmeetingabstracts.com/abstract/meldpeld-35-candidates-benefit-from-regional-sharing/. Accessed September 2, 2015.

From Child-Pugh to Model for End-Stage Liver Disease
Deciding Who Needs a Liver Transplant

Sheela S. Reddy, MD, Jesse M. Civan, MD*

KEYWORDS

- Liver transplantation • Organ allocation • MELD score • Cirrhosis
- Hepatocellular carcinoma

KEY POINTS

- Patients with acute liver injury with hepatic encephalopathy and coagulopathy require immediate transfer to a liver transplant center for urgent evaluation for liver transplant.
- Patients with cirrhosis and Model for End-stage Liver Disease score greater than 15, or with clinically decompensated cirrhosis, should be referred to a transplant center for transplant evaluation.
- Patients with hepatocellular carcinoma (HCC), including very early HCC and also HCC beyond the Milan Criteria, should be referred to a transplant center for evaluation.

INTRODUCTION

Liver transplant is a lifesaving intervention for patients with acute liver failure, decompensated cirrhosis, and hepatocellular carcinoma (HCC) within certain criteria. However, careful assessment of the indication for transplant, and suitability of the individual patient for transplant, are necessary to balance the anticipated benefit of liver transplant against anticipated risk, and to take into account societal considerations of allocation of a scarce resource.

According to the most recent data provided by the Scientific Registry of Transplant Recipients/Organ Procurement and Transplantation Network (OPTN), in 2013 there were 5921 liver transplants performed in adults across the United States, leaving

Disclosures: The authors have no relevant financial disclosures or other potential conflicts of interest to report.
Author Contributions: S.S. Reddy contributed to the concept of the article and to the writing of the article. J.M. Civan contributed to the concept of the article and the writing of the article, and takes responsibility for the overall content.
Division of Gastroenterology & Hepatology, Department of Medicine, Thomas Jefferson University, Suite 480 Main Building, 132 South 10th Street, Philadelphia, PA 19107, USA
* Corresponding author.
E-mail address: Jesse.Civan@jefferson.edu

Med Clin N Am 100 (2016) 449–464
http://dx.doi.org/10.1016/j.mcna.2015.12.002
0025-7125/16/$ – see front matter © 2016 Elsevier Inc. All rights reserved.

12,407 patients active on the liver transplant waiting list as of 12/31/13.[1] During the year 2013, in addition to the 5921 patients undergoing liver transplant, 589 patients were removed from the list because of clinical improvement and no longer needing transplant.[1] However, 1767 patients died while awaiting transplant, 1223 patients were removed from the liver transplant waiting list because they were deemed too sick to be able to undergo liver transplant, and a further 1072 patients were removed for other reasons from the waiting list.[1] It is reasonable to hypothesize that most patients removed from the transplant list for reasons of either being too sick to transplant or for other reasons died of complications relating to their liver disease not long thereafter. Thus, approximately 4000 people who were, at least for a period of time, suitable candidates for transplant died for want of an available donor organ. These deaths highlight the solemn responsibility of internists in consultation with transplant hepatologists to ensure that patients appropriate for liver transplant are evaluated expeditiously, and that contraindications to transplant candidacy are identified if present.

HISTORICAL PERSPECTIVE: EVOLUTION OF ORGAN ALLOCATION POLICY

The first successful liver transplant was performed in 1963 by the pioneering surgeon Thomas Starzl. However, it was not until the advent of cyclosporine in the late 1970s and adoption of this through the 1980s that adequate immunosuppression could be attained resulting in good outcomes in terms of 1-year survival,[2] and a national policy regarding organ allocation became necessary.

Through this time period, and up until 1998, organ allocation was based on each patient's blood type, time on waiting list, and the physical location of the patient (out of hospital, in hospital, in an intensive care unit [ICU]). Thus, in this era, organ allocation was decided almost entirely by physician behavior and was not directly tied to severity of liver disease or anticipated mortality without transplant, and therefore it was extremely subjective. A consequence of this was overuse of ICUs across the country in order to facilitate access of patients to liver transplant, and this raised obvious concerns about fairness and equity in terms of access to transplants. In an attempt to establish a more uniform and fair allocation policy, the US government passed the Transplantation Act in 1987, which established the OPTN, and United Network for Organ Sharing (UNOS).[3]

In 1998, the Child-Turcotte-Pugh (CTP) score was adopted to guide organ allocation. The CTP score is based on 5 parameters: serum bilirubin level, serum albumin level, prothrombin time, degree of encephalopathy, and severity of ascites[4] (**Table 1**). Thus, organ allocation became dependent on objective measures that were directly related to the severity of liver disease. However, assessment of 2 of these 5 criteria, namely severity of hepatic encephalopathy and ascites, remained subjective to a degree. Furthermore, although these objective parameters were used to stratify patients' medical need for transplant, it did so into a small number of distinct categories, and time on the transplant list remained a critical determinant of access to organs for transplant within each of these categories. It was observed that deaths on the waiting list at that time did not correlate well with time on the transplant waiting list, indicating that further optimization of the organ allocation policy was needed.[5]

In 2002, the Model for End-stage Liver Disease (MELD) score was adopted to replace the CTP score in determining organ allocation. This scoring system, developed and validated at the Mayo Clinic, was originally devised as a prognosticator in cirrhotic patients undergoing a transjugular intrahepatic portosystemic shunt procedure.[6] The

Table 1		
The Child-Pugh classification		
Calculation of Child-Pugh Score		
Encephalopathy	None	1 point
	Grade 1/2	2 points
	Grade 3/4	3 points
Ascites	Absent	1 point
	Slight	2 points
	Moderate/large	3 points
Bilirubin level	<2 mg/dL	1 point
	2–3 mg/dL	2 points
	>3 mg/dL	3 points
Albumin level	>3.5 g/dL	1 point
	2.8–3.5 g/dL	2 points
	<2.8 g/dL	3 points
International Normalized Ratio	<1.7	1 point
	1.7–2.3	2 points
	>2.3	3 points
Assignment of Child-Pugh Classification From Child-Pugh Score		
5–6 points		Child class A
7–9 points		Child class B
10–15 points		Child class C

MELD score is based on 3 parameters that are entirely objective: serum total bilirubin level, serum creatinine level, and International Normalized Ratio (INR).[6] (**Fig. 1**). Although the formula for calculating the MELD score is complex, several on-line, freely accessible calculators are available, including one provided on the OPTN Web site (http://optn.transplant.hrsa.gov/converge/resources/MeldPeldCalculator.asp).

Adoption of the MELD score carried 3 main benefits compared with the CTP score. First, subjective measures were eliminated, increasing fair access to transplants. Second, the importance of renal function was recognized, because creatinine level is a component of the MELD score but not the CTP score. With the creatinine level being the most heavily weighted of the 3 MELD variables, a distinct advantage was granted to the patients presenting with type 1 hepatorenal syndrome (HRS) who have a rapidly increasing serum creatinine level. This advantage was a clear distinction from the CTP score, in which patients presenting with acute kidney injury were not given any additional transplant priority despite HRS type 1 conferring the worst prognosis for survival of all the complications seen in the cirrhotic patient population. Third, adoption of the MELD system introduced considerably more granularity in the characterization of the degree of liver disease and urgency for transplant because the components of the MELD score are continuous variables, whereas those of the CTP score are ordinal variables. For example, a patient with an INR of 3.4 receives no incremental priority compared with a patient with an INR of 2.4 in the CTP score, whereas the MELD score is higher for the patient with the higher INR. The same is true for patients with total bilirubin levels higher than 3 mg/dL, because the MELD score provides a clear advantage as a continuous variable.

$$MELD = 6.43 + 10 \times [\, 0.957 \times \ln(creatinine) + 0.378 \times \ln(bilirubin) + 1.12 \times \ln(INR)]$$

Fig. 1. The MELD score.

Adoption of the MELD score resulted in several demonstrable benefits. Median MELD scores at time of transplant increased, indicating that patients with the greatest medical urgency for transplant were being better prioritized.[3] Furthermore, this occurred while reducing median time on the waiting list, and without reduction in 1-year outcomes of either patient or graft survival.[3]

Although the introduction of the MELD score in organ allocation policy was a significant step forward, the MELD score does not adequately reflect the risk of death without liver transplant for specific subpopulations of patients. This shortcoming resulted in the creation of MELD exceptions. MELD exceptions refer to the allocation of a higher MELD score than that calculated from the patient's laboratory values, in recognition of a particular diagnosis that has been established as placing the patient at high risk of death without transplant. Most frequently used is the MELD exception for HCC, in recognition that even patients with well-compensated cirrhosis are at high risk of death without transplant, and they are therefore allocated additional priority. The MELD exception for HCC in particular has been controversial, and the policy has been revised twice since its advent in 2002 because it was thought that the exception policy that was initially implemented overly prioritized patients with HCC to the detriment of patients without HCC.[7] At the time of this writing, further refinements of the HCC MELD exception policy are under debate within the transplant community. Additional MELD exception categories are discussed later in this article.

One of the unanswered challenges to the current organ allocation policy is the significant regional variation in mismatch between organ supply and demand, resulting in variation in median MELD scores at time of transplant, and time on transplant waiting list. The consequence of this is significant regional inequities in the risk of death while awaiting transplant.[8,9]

The most recent change to the organ allocation scheme was the implementation of the Share-35 initiative. To put this initiative into context, first it must be noted that the United States is divided into 11 geographic regions that cross state lines. The nation's OPTN consists of 59 Donation Service Areas (DSAs). A DSA consists of an Organ Procurement Organization (OPO), at least 1 transplant center, and 2 or more hospitals (reference: http://www.srtr.org). In general, when organs become available from a donor, they are offered to the sickest patient within the OPO where the organ was obtained. After Share-35, organs can only be offered within an OPO to a patient with a MELD score of less than 35 if there is not a patient within that OPO's larger region with a MELD score exceeding 35 of the appropriate blood type and in need of that organ. However, the scale of the United States' geographic boundaries, and the limited time that a donor organ can remain out of the body for transport (cold ischemia time), make it impossible to completely eliminate such geographic disparities.

As long as organ demand exceeds available organ supply, which is the foreseeable future, there will be ongoing debate on how to further minimize inequities and maximize efficiency in organ allocation policy.

INDICATIONS FOR TRANSPLANT

The primary indications for liver transplant are acute liver failure, decompensated cirrhosis, and HCC defined within certain parameters.[10] In 2013, indications for adult transplant in the United States were acute hepatic failure in 3.9% of cases, HCC in 19.4%, and decompensated cirrhosis or other indications for the remaining 76.7%.[1] Patients with chronic liver disease secondary to viral hepatitis C represented 25% of all patients undergoing transplant in 2013, and those with chronic liver disease secondary to alcohol represented 18.4%.[1]

The presence of cirrhosis alone is not an indication for liver transplant, because well-compensated cirrhotic patients may have good prognosis without transplant, with median survival of 12 years.[11,12] Those patients who die of the complications of cirrhosis generally do so after transitioning from a period of compensated cirrhosis to a period of decompensated cirrhosis, heralded by clinically evident signs and symptoms, at which point there is a window of opportunity to evaluate the patient for liver transplant.

Nonetheless, it is advisable for internists to refer any patient with newly diagnosed cirrhosis to a specialist to ensure thorough work-up of the underlying cause, for consideration of whether liver transplant might be indicated, and for longitudinal management, including screening for HCC and gastroesophageal varices, in addition to medical management of any clinical manifestations of cirrhosis.

Indications: Acute Liver Failure

Acute liver failure is a clear indication for liver transplant evaluation, and is defined as an acute liver injury accompanied by hepatic encephalopathy, coagulopathy (INR>1.5), absence of underlying cirrhosis, and illness of less than 26 weeks' duration.[13] The term acute liver failure encompasses the subgroup of patients with fulminant liver failure, defined as illness of less than 8 weeks' duration. Although patients with both duration of illness less than 8 weeks and greater than or equal to 8 weeks may require a liver transplant to survive, this distinction is important because UNOS/OPTN policy allows for listing of patients only with fulminant liver failure (<8 weeks' duration) as status 1, whereas patients with duration of illness greater than 8 weeks could be listed for transplant from their MELD scores. Patients listed under status 1 are prioritized for transplant when an organ becomes available over all patients listed by MELD score.

In the United States, drug-induced liver injury accounts for most cases of acute liver failure, with acetaminophen toxicity accounting for 39% of all cases of adult transplant for acute liver failure, and other drugs accounting for an additional 13%.[14] The specific cause of acute liver failure remains unknown in 18% of cases.[14] The prognosis of acute liver failure in the absence of liver transplant is poor. Various prognostic models are available, most notably the King's College criteria.[15] However, it is critical for the internist to be aware that although models such as the King's College criteria have good sensitivity in identifying patients with poor transplant-free prognosis, they have not been proved to be able to identify patients with good transplant-free prognosis.[13] Therefore, it is critical that all patients with acute liver failure be transferred expeditiously to a transplant center, preferably to the ICU setting. Furthermore, because some particular causes of acute liver failure carry such poor prognosis, American Association for the Study of Liver Diseases (AASLD) guidelines call for expeditious listing for transplant, regardless of any reassuring clinical factors. Examples of this include acute liver failure secondary to *Amanita* mushroom poisoning, autoimmune hepatitis, and Wilson disease.[13] Because of the high mortality associated with acute liver failure, transfer to a transplant center should not necessarily be delayed in patients not yet meeting all criteria for acute liver failure. For example, patients with acute liver injury and increasing INR may be well served with transfer to a transplant center even if encephalopathy is not yet evident.

A full discussion of the medical management of patients with acute liver failure is beyond the scope of this article. The authors refer internists caring for patients with acute liver failure or suspected impending acute liver failure to the current AASLD practice guideline, which can be found on the AASLD Web site at www.aasld.org. This article highlights only that if a reversible cause of acute liver failure is identified, then treatment of the underlying cause should be given in parallel with evaluation for transplant (N-acetylcysteine for acetaminophen toxicity, corticosteroids for autoimmune hepatitis, antivirals for viral hepatitis B, acyclovir for herpes or varicella virus, penicillin G for *Amanita* mushroom poisoning).[13] N-acetylcysteine may be beneficial in acute liver failure even if not caused by acetaminophen toxicity, and should be considered especially in patients with early-stage encephalopathy, in whom potential benefit seems greatest.[16]

Indications: Cirrhosis

In contrast with acute liver failure, in which context transplant-free survival is low and transplant evaluation is indicated for all patients, not all patients with chronic liver disease resulting in cirrhosis necessarily require liver transplant. Although overall survival is lower in cirrhotic patients overall compared with the general population,[17] prognosis is good in patients with well-compensated cirrhosis, with median survival on the order of 12 years.[11,12] The benefits of liver transplant in well-compensated cirrhotic patients must be balanced against the anticipated risk, keeping in mind an overall 87% 1-year survival following liver transplant.[18]

Cirrhotic patients for whom liver transplant evaluation is indicated generally are in 3 broad categories: those with high MELD score, those with low MELD score but clinical manifestations of decompensated liver disease, and those with HCC. Patients with HCC are discussed later.

In a seminal article, Merion and colleagues[19] showed that a MELD score of 15 identified patients who were likely to benefit from transplant, such that patients with MELD score greater than or equal to 15 were more likely to survive with transplant than without, but those with MELD score less than 15 were more likely to die of complications of liver transplant than to die of complications of cirrhosis without transplant. Thus, MELD score greater than or equal to 15 is recognized as an indication for transplant evaluation, independent of clinical manifestations of decompensated cirrhosis.[10]

In contrast, development of clinically decompensating events, such as jaundice, ascites, hepatic encephalopathy, or variceal hemorrhage, should prompt an evaluation for liver transplant, independent of MELD score. Patients without any clinical manifestations of cirrhosis initially may develop new-onset ascites at a rate of approximately 7% per year and new varices at a rate of 4.4% per year.[11] The advent of the first clinically decompensating event heralds a significant increase in the risk of death over the following year, from around 1% in the very well compensated to 20% in patients with ascites and varices, and further to 57% in patients with ascites who have experienced variceal hemorrhage.[11] Therefore, the first clinically decompensating event requires consideration for referral of the patient to a transplant center. However, progression of the clinical course is not necessarily inexorable, and complications of cirrhosis may respond to medical management and treatment of the underlying cause. For example, patients with alcohol-induced cirrhosis may show substantial clinical stabilization with sustained abstinence from alcohol, and likewise patients with viral hepatitis after successful antiviral therapy.

Indications: Complications of Cirrhosis

Although patients with decompensated cirrhosis are generally listed for transplant from their calculated MELD score, there are 2 specific complications of cirrhosis that carry such significant increased risk of mortality that patients qualify for automatic MELD exceptions. These complications are hepatopulmonary syndrome[20] and portopulmonary hypertension.[21]

Hepatopulmonary syndrome is a hypoxic condition caused by abnormal intrapulmonary vasodilation and arteriovenous shunting arising in the context of cirrhosis and portal hypertension.[22] Under current UNOS/OPTN policy, patients with evidence of hepatopulmonary syndrome are eligible for automatic MELD exception if Pao_2 is less than 60 mm Hg on room air in the absence of another known cause of primary lung disease.[23]

Portopulmonary hypertension is a form of pulmonary arterial hypertension occurring in association with portal hypertension, characterized by mean pulmonary arterial pressure greater than 25 mm Hg with left ventricular end diastolic pressure less than 15 mm Hg.[22] Under current UNOS/OPTN policy, patients with evidence of portopulmonary hypertension are eligible for automatic MELD exception points if the mean pulmonary arterial pressure is less than 35 mm Hg.[23]

The AASLD recommends screening all patients undergoing liver transplant evaluation for both hepatopulmonary syndrome and portopulmonary hypertension.[10]

In 2006, a working group considered, but recommended against, automatic MELD exceptions for hepatic encephalopathy,[24] ascites,[25] or variceal bleeding[26] while acknowledging the role of case-by-case review by regional review boards (RRBs).

Indications: Hepatocellular Carcinoma

Cirrhosis is the single most important risk factor for developing HCC. HCC, in turn, occurs at an incidence of up to 5% annually in patients with cirrhosis and chronic hepatitis C virus, and up to 8% annually in patients with hepatitis B virus–related cirrhosis.[27] Depending on staging, HCC may be either an indication for, or contraindication to, liver transplant.

Historically, outcomes of liver transplant for patients with HCC were so poor that the role of liver transplant in this patient population was in jeopardy. However, in a seminal article, Mazzaferro and colleagues[28] showed that a subgroup of patients could be identified whose posttransplant outcomes were equivalent to those of patients undergoing transplant without HCC. This subgroup of patients was characterized by the absence of extrahepatic metastases, absence of macrovascular invasion, and tumor burden restricted either to a single tumor no more than 5 cm in maximal diameter, or alternatively either 2 or 3 tumors none of which exceed 3 cm in maximal diameter.[28] These criteria became known as the Milan Criteria. Although alternative, broader criteria have since been proposed, including most notably the University of California, San Francisco criteria,[29] the Milan Criteria continue to dictate candidacy for liver transplant at most US centers as dictated by UNOS.[27] Thus, patients with HCC within the Milan Criteria should be referred for liver transplant evaluation, regardless of MELD score or degree of clinical decompensation.[10]

Metastatic HCC is an absolute contraindication to liver transplant. However, tumor burden exceeding the Milan Criteria is not necessarily, with many centers using downstaging protocols. At present there is no uniform standard to dictate which patients are candidates for downstaging, what treatments are optimal to achieve downstaging, or how to define the success of downstaging.[30–32] Thus, patients with HCC beyond the Milan Criteria should also be referred to a transplant center to determine whether, with tumor-directed therapy, the patient may at a later date become a candidate for liver transplant. Because of the lack of uniform standards for downstaging, rates of success of downstaging protocols to convert patients into transplant candidates have variously been reported from 24% to 90%.[33]

Current UNOS/OPTN policy grants automatic MELD exception to patients with HCC who are within the Milan Criteria. However, only patients with definite evidence of HCC and clinical stage T2 (1 tumor between 2 cm and 5 cm in maximal diameter, or either 2 or 3 tumors each between 1 cm and 3 cm in maximal diameter) qualify for this automatic HCC MELD exception.[34] Therefore, internists are cautioned against referring patients with newly diagnosed HCC directly for antitumor therapy (eg, for transarterial embolization therapy by an interventional radiologist) until after the patient is first referred to a transplant center for evaluation, because treatment of very early HCC may jeopardize access of the patient to liver transplant, which in turn represents definitive curative intervention.

Indications: Cholangiocarcinoma

There is a limited role for transplant in patients with cholangiocarcinoma (CCA), restricted to those with early-stage CCA who are unresectable given underlying liver disease or because of anatomic location.[10,35] Liver transplant is indicated for patients meeting strict criteria, who undergo an appropriate protocol of neoadjuvant chemotherapy, associated with 5-year survival of up to 82%.[36] Patients meeting criteria are eligible for MELD exception, but transplant for this indication is available only at selected transplant centers.[10]

Indications: Other

Liver transplant may be considered for other indications not resulting in either acute liver failure or cirrhosis. Three rare genetic disorders are recognized indications for liver transplant with automatic MELD exception priority: primary hyperoxaluria, familial amyloidotic polyneuropathy, and cystic fibrosis.[10,37]

Familial amyloidotic polyneuropathy is a condition caused by a mutation in the transthyretin (TTR) gene, resulting in deposition of an abnormal protein throughout the body, leading to profound sensorimotor peripheral polyneuropathy, as well as autonomic dysfunction. After liver transplant, patients experience stabilization of the polyneuropathy because the newly grafted liver produces the normal form of the transthyretin protein.[38]

Primary hyperoxaluria is a genetic disorder resulting in deficiency of the enzyme peroxisomal alanine:glyoxylate aminotransferase, which in turn leads to overproduction of oxylate, which is deposited in the kidney, ultimately causing renal failure.[39] Patients with renal failure from primary hyperoxaluria benefit from combined liver/kidney transplant,[39] and liver transplant is indicated preemptively to prevent development of end-stage kidney disease.[10]

There are other potential indications for liver transplant, and individual transplant centers have discretion to list for transplant patients with other unusual indications. However, in the absence of automatic exception priority for such other indications, transplant centers and patients depend on case-by-case review of narrative appeals to RRBs for MELD exception, in order to secure access to an available organ. Examples of such indications that are not recognized for automatic MELD exception, but which could be considered on a case-by-case basis, include primary sclerosing cholangitis with recurrent life-threatening bouts of cholangitis, polycystic liver disease resulting in severe impairment of quality of life,[40,41] epithelioid hemangioendothelioma,[35,42] high-output cardiac failure secondary to hepatic involvement of hereditary hemorrhagic telangiectasia,[43] and metastatic neuroendocrine tumor.[35]

TRANSPLANT EVALUATION PROCESS

Evaluating a patient for liver transplant is a multidisciplinary process, involving at minimum a hepatologist, transplant surgeon, anesthesiologist, social worker, and financial specialist. Often, consultation is needed with 1 or more additional subspecialists.

Extensive medical testing, particularly cardiovascular testing, is conducted to ensure that the patient is likely to survive the transplant surgery. Additional testing, both medical and psychosocial, is geared toward assessing the probability of a reasonably good anticipated longer-term survival. Examples include screening for malignancies, and identification of psychiatric illness or psychosocial problems that may prevent adequate adherence to the necessary posttransplant medication regimen and follow-up. **Box 1** provides a summary of contraindications to liver transplant candidacy, and **Box 2** provides a summary of the evaluation process.

Cardiopulmonary Evaluation

Significant uncontrolled cardiovascular or pulmonary disease may preclude liver transplant. Such disease may either be a preexisting medical comorbidity or may represent new or evolving extrahepatic sequelae of liver disease. For example, cirrhosis is a high cardiac-output state that can lead to increased left ventricular wall thickness and diastolic dysfunction.[44] Hepatopulmonary syndrome and portopulmonary hypertension are examples of cardiopulmonary manifestations or complications of portal hypertension that, if sufficiently severe, could contraindicate liver transplant (discussed earlier).

All patients undergoing evaluation for liver transplant should be screened with transthoracic echocardiography and cardiac stress test, preferably stress echocardiogram.[10,45] If cardiac ischemia is detected on this evaluation, cardiac catheterization may be needed. The decision to proceed with cardiac catheterization takes into account the severity of coronary artery disease, the implication of a prolonged course of antiplatelet therapy delaying transplant surgery, the risk of induced contrainduced nephropathy, and increased risk of bleeding complications of cardiac catheterization in this population with coagulopathy and thrombocytopenia.[10,45,46]

Box 1
Contraindications to liver transplant

Absolute:

- Severe cardiopulmonary disease
- Active malignancy (other than HCC, or cholangiocarcinoma, meeting specific criteria)
- Active drug or alcohol use
- Uncontrolled severe psychiatric disease
- Uncontrolled acquired immunodeficiency syndrome
- Severe pulmonary hypertension
- Active bacterial or fungal infection (other than infection confined to the liver in certain circumstances)

Relative:

- Morbid obesity or severe cachexia
- History of recent extrahepatic malignancy (depending on treatment history and risk of recurrence)
- Lack of psychosocial support
- Severe psychiatric illness (eg, history of suicide attempts)

Box 2
Evaluation process

Financial

- Insurance coverage of liver transplant surgery
- Insurance coverage for lifelong immunosuppressive therapy

Psychosocial

- Adequacy of social support
- Screening for active drug/alcohol abuse
- Adequacy of treatment of any history of prior drug/alcohol abuse

Cancer screening

- Colonoscopy[a]
- PAP smear[a]
- Mammogram[a]
- Prostate-specific antigen

Cardiac

- Transthoracic echocardiogram with bubble study
- Stress test (preferably stress echocardiogram)

Vascular

- Carotid Doppler ultrasonography[b]

Pulmonary

- Arterial blood gas on 100% fraction of inspired oxygen
- Full pulmonary function tests
- Chest radiograph

Dental

- Exclude active dental infection

Radiographic

- Contrast-enhanced cross-sectional imaging of liver and hepatic vasculature

Multidisciplinary subspecialty consultations

- Hepatology
- Transplant surgery
- Anesthesiology
- Psychiatry[b]
- Addictions specialist[b]

[a] As per age-appropriate screening guidelines for the general population.
[b] Depending on risk factors.

If significant pulmonary hypertension is identified on echocardiogram, further evaluation with right heart catheterization is indicated. Mean pulmonary arterial pressures exceeding 35 mm Hg contraindicate proceeding with liver transplant, unless this can be treated with medical therapy (eg, diuresis, vasodilator therapy).[10,47–49]

Oncological Evaluation

All cirrhotic patients undergoing evaluation for liver transplant are at risk for HCC. HCC that is within the Milan Criteria may expedite liver transplant because such patients qualify for automatic HCC MELD exception, whereas HCC that is outside the Milan Criteria contraindicates transplant at most centers. All patients should be brought up to date on age-appropriate routine cancer screening such as colonoscopy for colorectal cancer, PAP smear for cervical cancer, and mammogram for breast cancer, based on the screening guidelines for the general population.[10] Patients with extrahepatic malignancy must undergo curative therapy, and generally undergo a subsequent period of recurrence-free observation, before undergoing liver transplant.[10] For many solid organ malignancies, a 5-year cancer-free period is required following curative therapy. However, for certain malignancies with an especially good prognosis and low risk of recurrence, a shorter period of observation may be sufficient, which is generally ascertained on a case-by-case basis in consultation with medical oncology. The Israel Penn International Transplant Tumor Registry provides a consultative service in which transplant centers may submit a detailed oncological history through this organization's Web site (http://ipittr.uc.edu), and in return receive a report with an estimated likelihood of recurrent cancer after transplant. In the absence of evidence-based guidelines on this issue, assessment of adequacy of prior cancer treatment remains center dependent.

Infectious Disease Evaluation

An extensive serologic evaluation is indicated to assess exposure and immunity to various viruses, to determine the indication for vaccinations, and for antiviral prophylaxis immediately following liver transplant. All patients naive to hepatitis A or B should be vaccinated. Live/attenuated viral vaccines are contraindicated after transplant in the context of potent immunosuppression, and therefore any such live vaccines due or overdue should be administered before transplant.[50] Other vaccinations that should be provided before transplant include pneumococcal, influenza, diphtheria/pertussis/tetanus, and human papilloma virus.[50]

All patients under evaluation for liver transplant should be screened for tuberculosis (TB) and for syphilis, and should preferably be treated before transplant.[10] Although active mycobacterial infection contraindicates transplant, some patients with latent TB may have liver disease that is too badly decompensated to safely allow antimycobacterial therapy with the preferred regimens of either isoniazid/pyridoxine or rifampin, and therefore in some cases treatment of latent TB may be deferred until after transplant.[10]

Although not universally indicated, patients in endemic areas should be screened for coccidiomycosis and strongyloides infection, and treated before transplant if there is evidence of active infection.[10]

All patients should be screened for human immunodeficiency virus (HIV). HIV in itself is not a contraindication to transplant, but adequate control of HIV is necessary. In the absence of a universally accepted definition of adequate control of HIV, policies of individual centers vary. Detectable HIV viremia and CD4 counts less than 100 cells/mm^3 are universally accepted as evidence of inadequate control,[10,51,52] although many centers use more stringent criteria with CD4 counts greater than 200 cells/mm^3.

Nutrition

Both very cachectic and morbidly obese patients are at risk for worse outcomes following liver transplant.[53–56] Some very cachectic patients may benefit from supplemental enteral nutrition to protect their candidacy for liver transplant, although there are no established criteria to identify patients who would clearly benefit from this.[57,58] Morbid obesity with body mass index (BMI) greater than 40 is considered a relative, although not absolute, contraindication to transplant and merits, at minimum, nutritional counseling.[10] However, caution is needed in using the BMI as a screening tool, because anasarca often complicates end-stage liver disease, and therefore the BMI may fail to detect even severe protein-calorie malnutrition at one extreme, or may grossly overestimate obesity at the other.

Drug/Alcohol Addiction

Active drug and/or alcohol abuse is a contraindication to liver transplant. The need for ongoing methadone maintenance therapy for patients under active treatment of opioid dependence is not considered a contraindication to transplant.[10] For patients with alcohol-induced liver disease, it remains highly controversial how best to assess whether the patient has been adequately treated for alcohol dependence. In many centers, a sustained period of 6 months of complete abstinence from all alcohol, in conjunction with a formal program of counseling, are required before a patient can be listed for transplant.[10,59] Evaluation for liver transplant before achieving this traditional 6-month period of sustained sobriety has been proposed, and, although controversial, is an option at some centers.[60]

One way that internists can help their patients with alcoholic liver disease in need of liver transplant evaluation is to prevail on the patients to engage in a formal program of alcohol abuse counseling/treatment as early in the process as possible. When patients are already actively engaged in such treatment, psychosocial clearance may be facilitated, improving the patients' chances of successfully navigating the process without delay during which the patients would remain at risk for further life-threatening medically decompensating events.

SUMMARY

In conclusion, evaluation of patients in need of a liver transplant is a complex, multidisciplinary process. Policy regarding optimal allocation of available organs to patients on the transplant list continues to evolve, sometimes with spirited debate. Internists play a critical role in first identifying an indication for liver transplant and making referral to a transplant center, or perhaps as a first step to a gastroenterologist/hepatologist. Internists also have an opportunity to help all patients in need of liver transplant by talking to their patients and community members about organ donation, participation in advocacy organizations, and through the political process that affects national policy.

REFERENCES

1. Kim WR, Lake JR, Smith JM, et al. OPTN/SRTR 2013 annual data report: liver. Am J Transplant 2015;15(Suppl 2):1–28.
2. Starzl TE, Klintmalm GB, Porter KA, et al. Liver transplantation with use of cyclosporin A and prednisone. N Engl J Med 1981;305(5):266–9.
3. Wiesner R, Lake JR, Freeman RB, et al. Model for End-stage Liver Disease (MELD) exception guidelines. Liver Transpl 2006;12(S3):S85–7.
4. Pugh RN, Murray-Lyon IM, Dawson JL, et al. Transection of the oesophagus for bleeding oesophageal varices. Br J Surg 1973;60(8):646–9.
5. Freeman RB Jr, Edwards EB. Liver transplant waiting time does not correlate with waiting list mortality: implications for liver allocation policy. Liver Transpl 2000; 6(5):543–52.

6. Malinchoc M, Kamath PS, Gordon FD, et al. A model to predict poor survival in patients undergoing transjugular intrahepatic portosystemic shunts. Hepatology 2000;31(4):864–71.

7. Wiesner RH. Evolving trends in liver transplantation: listing and liver donor allocation. Clin Liver Dis 2014;18(3):519–27.

8. Gentry SE, Massie AB, Cheek SW, et al. Addressing geographic disparities in liver transplantation through redistricting. Am J Transplant 2013;13(8):2052–8.

9. Yeh H, Smoot E, Schoenfeld DA, et al. Geographic inequity in access to livers for transplantation. Transplantation 2011;91(4):479–86.

10. Martin P, DiMartini A, Feng S, et al. Evaluation for liver transplantation in adults: 2013 practice guideline by the American Association for the Study of Liver Diseases and the American Society of Transplantation. Hepatology 2014;59(3): 1144–65.

11. D'Amico G, Garcia-Tsao G, Pagliaro L. Natural history and prognostic indicators of survival in cirrhosis: a systematic review of 118 studies. J Hepatol 2006;44(1): 217–31.

12. Zipprich A, Garcia-Tsao G, Rogowski S, et al. Prognostic indicators of survival in patients with compensated and decompensated cirrhosis. Liver Int 2012;32(9): 1407–14.

13. Lee WM, Stravitz RT, Larson AM. Introduction to the revised American Association for the Study of Liver Diseases position paper on acute liver failure 2011. Hepatology 2012;55(3):965–7.

14. Bernal W, Wendon J. Acute liver failure. N Engl J Med 2013;369(26):2525–34.

15. O'Grady JG, Alexander GJ, Hayllar KM, et al. Early indicators of prognosis in fulminant hepatic failure. Gastroenterology 1989;97(2):439–45.

16. Lee WM, Hynan LS, Rossaro L, et al. Intravenous N-acetylcysteine improves transplant-free survival in early stage non-acetaminophen acute liver failure. Gastroenterology 2009;137(3):856–64, 864.e1.

17. Fleming KM, Aithal GP, Card TR, et al. All-cause mortality in people with cirrhosis compared with the general population: a population-based cohort study. Liver Int 2012;32(1):79–84.

18. Berg CL, Steffick DE, Edwards EB, et al. Liver and intestine transplantation in the united states 1998-2007. Am J Transplant 2009;9(4 Pt 2):907–31.

19. Merion RM, Schaubel DE, Dykstra DM, et al. The survival benefit of liver transplantation. Am J Transplant 2005;5(2):307–13.

20. Fallon MB, Mulligan DC, Gish RG, et al. Model for End-stage Liver Disease (MELD) exception for hepatopulmonary syndrome. Liver Transpl 2006;12(S3): S105–7.

21. Krowka MJ, Fallon MB, Mulligan DC, et al. Model for End-stage Liver Disease (MELD) exception for portopulmonary hypertension. Liver Transpl 2006;12(S3): S114–6.

22. Hoeper MM, Krowka MJ, Strassburg CP. Portopulmonary hypertension and hepatopulmonary syndrome. Lancet 2004;363(9419):1461–8.

23. HRSA/OPTN; Policy 9: allocation of livers and liver-intestines. 2015. Available at: http://optn.transplant.hrsa.gov/ContentDocuments/OPTN_Policies.pdf. Accessed August 31, 2015.

24. Ham J, Gish RG, Mullen K. Model for End-stage Liver Disease (MELD) exception for hepatic encephalopathy. Liver Transpl 2006;12(S3):S102–4.

25. Biggins SW, Colquhoun S, Gish RG, et al. Model for End-stage Liver Disease (MELD) exception for ascites. Liver Transpl 2006;12(S3):S88–90.

26. Sheiner P, Gish RG, Sanyal A. Model for End-stage Liver Disease (MELD) exception for portal hypertensive gastrointestinal bleeding. Liver Transpl 2006;12(S3): S112-3.

27. Bruix J, Sherman M, American Association for the Study of Liver Diseases. Management of hepatocellular carcinoma: an update. Hepatology 2011;53(3): 1020-2.

28. Mazzaferro V, Regalia E, Doci R, et al. Liver transplantation for the treatment of small hepatocellular carcinomas in patients with cirrhosis. N Engl J Med 1996; 334(11):693-9.

29. Yao FY, Ferrell L, Bass NM, et al. Liver transplantation for hepatocellular carcinoma: expansion of the tumor size limits does not adversely impact survival. Hepatology 2001;33(6):1394-403.

30. Yao FY, Breitenstein S, Broelsch CE, et al. Does a patient qualify for liver transplantation after the down-staging of hepatocellular carcinoma? Liver Transpl 2011;17(Suppl 2):S109-16.

31. Sharr WW, Chan SC, Lo CM. Section 3. current status of downstaging of hepatocellular carcinoma before liver transplantation. Transplantation 2014;97(Suppl 8): S10-7.

32. Yu CY, Ou HY, Huang TL, et al. Hepatocellular carcinoma downstaging in liver transplantation. Transplant Proc 2012;44(2):412-4.

33. Toso C, Mentha G, Kneteman NM, et al. The place of downstaging for hepatocellular carcinoma. J Hepatol 2010;52(6):930-6.

34. Wald C, Russo MW, Heimbach JK, et al. New OPTN/UNOS policy for liver transplant allocation: standardization of liver imaging, diagnosis, classification, and reporting of hepatocellular carcinoma. Radiology 2013;266(2):376-82.

35. Grossman EJ, Millis JM. Liver transplantation for non-hepatocellular carcinoma malignancy: indications, limitations, and analysis of the current literature. Liver Transpl 2010;16(8):930-42.

36. Heimbach JK, Gores GJ, Haddock MG, et al. Liver transplantation for unresectable perihilar cholangiocarcinoma. Semin Liver Dis 2004;24(2):201-7.

37. Freeman RB Jr, Gish RG, Harper A, et al. Model for End-stage Liver Disease (MELD) exception guidelines: results and recommendations from the MELD Exception Study Group and conference (MESSAGE) for the approval of patients who need liver transplantation with diseases not considered by the standard MELD formula. Liver Transpl 2006;12(12 Suppl 3):S128-36.

38. Herlenius G, Wilczek HE, Larsson M, et al, Familial Amyloidotic Polyneuropathy World Transplant Registry. Ten years of international experience with liver transplantation for familial amyloidotic polyneuropathy: results from the Familial Amyloidotic Polyneuropathy World Transplant Registry. Transplantation 2004;77(1): 64-71.

39. Jamieson NV, European PHI Transplantation Study Group. A 20-year experience of combined liver/kidney transplantation for primary hyperoxaluria (PH1): the European PH1 Transplant Registry experience 1984-2004. Am J Nephrol 2005; 25(3):282-9.

40. Swenson K, Seu P, Kinkhabwala M, et al. Liver transplantation for adult polycystic liver disease. Hepatology 1998;28(2):412-5.

41. van Keimpema L, Nevens F, Adam R, et al. Excellent survival after liver transplantation for isolated polycystic liver disease: an European Liver Transplant Registry study. Transpl Int 2011;24(12):1239-45.

42. Cardinal J, de Vera ME, Marsh JW, et al. Treatment of hepatic epithelioid hemangioendothelioma: a single-institution experience with 25 cases. Arch Surg 2009; 144(11):1035–9.
43. Dupuis-Girod S, Chesnais AL, Ginon I, et al. Long-term outcome of patients with hereditary hemorrhagic telangiectasia and severe hepatic involvement after orthotopic liver transplantation: a single-center study. Liver Transpl 2010;16(3): 340–7.
44. Torregrosa M, Aguade S, Dos L, et al. Cardiac alterations in cirrhosis: reversibility after liver transplantation. J Hepatol 2005;42(1):68–74.
45. Lentine KL, Costa SP, Weir MR, et al. Cardiac disease evaluation and management among kidney and liver transplantation candidates: a scientific statement from the American Heart Association and the American College of Cardiology Foundation: endorsed by the American Society of Transplant Surgeons, American Society of Transplantation, and National Kidney Foundation. Circulation 2012; 126(5):617–63.
46. Azarbal B, Poommipanit P, Arbit B, et al. Feasibility and safety of percutaneous coronary intervention in patients with end-stage liver disease referred for liver transplantation. Liver Transpl 2011;17(7):809–13.
47. Krowka MJ, Plevak DJ, Findlay JY, et al. Pulmonary hemodynamics and perioperative cardiopulmonary-related mortality in patients with portopulmonary hypertension undergoing liver transplantation. Liver Transpl 2000;6(4):443–50.
48. Hollatz TJ, Musat A, Westphal S, et al. Treatment with sildenafil and treprostinil allows successful liver transplantation of patients with moderate to severe portopulmonary hypertension. Liver Transpl 2012;18(6):686–95.
49. Swanson KL, Wiesner RH, Nyberg SL, et al. Survival in portopulmonary hypertension: Mayo Clinic experience categorized by treatment subgroups. Am J Transplant 2008;8(11):2445–53.
50. Danzinger-Isakov L, Kumar D, AST Infectious Diseases Community of Practice. Guidelines for vaccination of solid organ transplant candidates and recipients. Am J Transplant 2009;9(Suppl 4):S258–62.
51. Fox AN, Vagefi PA, Stock PG. Liver transplantation in HIV patients. Semin Liver Dis 2012;32(2):177–85.
52. Di Benedetto F, Tarantino G, Ercolani G, et al. Multicenter Italian experience in liver transplantation for hepatocellular carcinoma in HIV-infected patients. Oncologist 2013;18(5):592–9.
53. Dick AA, Spitzer AL, Seifert CF, et al. Liver transplantation at the extremes of the body mass index. Liver Transpl 2009;15(8):968–77.
54. Leonard J, Heimbach JK, Malinchoc M, et al. The impact of obesity on long-term outcomes in liver transplant recipients–results of the NIDDK liver transplant database. Am J Transplant 2008;8(3):667–72.
55. Nair S, Verma S, Thuluvath PJ. Obesity and its effect on survival in patients undergoing orthotopic liver transplantation in the United States. Hepatology 2002; 35(1):105–9.
56. Reichman TW, Therapondos G, Serrano MS, et al. "Weighing the risk": obesity and outcomes following liver transplantation. World J Hepatol 2015;7(11): 1484–93.
57. Sanchez AJ, Aranda-Michel J. Nutrition for the liver transplant patient. Liver Transpl 2006;12(9):1310–6.
58. Langer G, Grossmann K, Fleischer S, et al. Nutritional interventions for liver-transplanted patients. Cochrane Database Syst Rev 2012;(8):CD007605.

59. O'Shea RS, Dasarathy S, McCullough AJ, Practice Guideline Committee of the American Association for the Study of Liver Diseases, Practice Parameters Committee of the American College of Gastroenterology. Alcoholic liver disease. Hepatology 2010;51(1):307–28.

60. Mathurin P, Moreno C, Samuel D, et al. Early liver transplantation for severe alcoholic hepatitis. N Engl J Med 2011;365(19):1790–800.

Renal Transplantation in Advanced Chronic Kidney Disease Patients

 CrossMark

Mythili Ghanta, MD[a],*, Belinda Jim, MD[b]

KEYWORDS

- Kidney transplant • New kidney allocation system
- Pretransplantation evaluation process • Factors affecting transplant candidacy
- Wait times • Wait-list mortality

KEY POINTS

- Kidney transplantation (KT) is the optimal modality of treatment for patients with end-stage kidney disease (ESKD).
- Timely referral for transplantation is essential to maximize benefit and should begin when patients' estimated glomerular filtration rate (eGFR) drops to less than 20 mL/min/m^2.
- Improved success of KT has broadened candidacy.
- Pretransplantation evaluation is a detailed, multidisciplinary process.

INTRODUCTION

KT is the optimal modality of treatment for patients with ESKD and, if successful, is associated with improved quality of life, lower medical costs, and improved survival. Better results are associated with shorter periods of time on dialysis, and the best results are achieved with preemptive transplantation.[1] Thus, timely preparation for KT is crucial to reap the maximal benefit, with preparations beginning during stage IIIb or stage IV chronic kidney disease and referral for transplant evaluation when the glomerular filtration rate (GFR) drops to less than 20 mL/min/1.73 m^2.

KIDNEY ALLOCATION SYSTEM

The new kidney allocation system (KAS) was implemented in United States in December 2014.[2] The objective of the new KAS is to improve outcomes of deceased donor (DD) KT with better matching of allograft and recipient survival. In the new KAS,

Disclosure Statement: The authors disclose no conflict of interest.
[a] Department of Medicine, Lewis Katz School of Medicine at Temple University, 3440 N Broad St, Kresge West Suite 100, Philadelphia, PA 19046, USA; [b] Division of Nephrology, Department of Medicine, Jacobi Medical Center, Albert Einstein College of Medicine, 1400 Pelham Parkway, Bronx, NY 10461, USA
* Corresponding author.
E-mail address: mythilighanta@gmail.com

Med Clin N Am 100 (2016) 465–476
http://dx.doi.org/10.1016/j.mcna.2015.12.003
0025-7125/16/$ – see front matter © 2016 Elsevier Inc. All rights reserved.

DDs are characterized by a percent scale (0%–100%) using the Kidney Donor Profile Index (KDPI), which takes into account the 10 donor variables that have an impact on the long-term survival of the allograft: the lower the KDPI the better the quality of the donor organ.[3] Recipients are characterized by an Estimated Post-Transplant Survival Score (EPTS). The top 20% of DD kidneys with the highest expected graft life are preferentially allocated to the top 20% EPTS recipients, before offering to the remaining candidates. Variables used to calculate KDPI and EPTS are shown in **Table 1**. The new KAS is projected to add approximately greater than 8000 life years annually, with improved transplant rates in sensitized and minority recipients. The new KAS awards wait time points for adults on dialysis from the time of initiation of dialysis rather than from the date of wait listing (WL) and for preemptive patients at the time of listing if the GFR remains less than 20 mL/min/1.73 m^2. Hence, patients do not lose wait time for late referrals.

KIDNEY TRANSPLANT WAIT LIST

Median wait times for KT have increased from 3 years in 2003 to 4.5 years in 2009 and continue to rise.[2] The current KT WL has more than 100,000 registrants. Donation rates and transplant rates have remained stagnant in the past 5 years. Although approximately 34,000 patients are added to the WL each year, only 17,000 KTs are performed annually. Additionally, approximately 5000 patients die while waiting for KT each year. These sobering statistics highlight the critical shortage of donor organs as the major challenge to KT today and underscore the critical priority of allocating this precious resource justly and equitably.

RECIPIENT EVALUATION

There is a wide variation in the perceptions of nephrologists in terms of referral patterns for KT. Furthermore, transplant centers have varying thresholds in accepting and declining patients with comorbidities. Contraindications for KT are listed in **Box 1**. Despite these contraindications, most patients should be deemed potential transplant candidates until proved otherwise and should be referred for KT evaluation. KT evaluation involves multidisciplinary teams, including transplant nephrologists, surgeons, nurse coordinators, social workers, dieticians, financial coordinators, and psychologists.

Table 1
Kidney Donor Profile Index and Estimated Post-Transplant Survival Score

Donor Factors for Kidney Donor Profile Index Calculation	Recipient Factors for Estimated Post-Transplant Survival Score Calculation
Age	Age
Height	Time on dialysis
Weight	Current diabetes mellitus
Ethnicity	Prior solid organ transplant
History of hypertension	—
History of diabetes	—
Cause of death	—
Serum creatinine mg/dL	—
Anti-HCV antibody positivity	—
Donation after cardiac death donor	—

Box 1
Contraindications for kidney transplant

Active or metastatic malignancy

Untreated active infection

Active illicit drug use

Severe psychiatric illness interfering with medication adherence

Irreversible extrarenal disease limiting life span, for example: severe chronic obstructive pulmonary disease

Advanced dementia

HIV with CD4 counts less than 200/μm or AIDS-defining illness

Morbid obesity (see text)

Severe CVD limiting life span (see text)

Severe PVD (see text)

Primary amyloidosis with extrarenal disease

Abbreviations: AIDS, acquired immune deficiency syndrome; CVD, cardiovascular disease; PVD, peripheral vascular disease.

PATIENT EDUCATION

Potential candidates are encouraged to attend a detailed education session prior to formal evaluation. Topics covered in this session involve description of surgical procedure, lifelong need for immunosuppressive therapy, benefits of living donation, and wait times for DD KT in the region as well as different types of DDs. **Boxes 2** and **3** summarize the basic kidney transplant evaluation.

EVALUATION OF FACTORS AFFECTING TRANSPLANT CANDIDACY
Cardiovascular Disease

Cardiovascular disease (CVD) is the leading cause of death with a functioning KT, accounting for approximately 30% of deaths.[4] Hence, CVD screening remains the

---

Box 2
History and physical examination

1. Focus on establishing the etiology of the native kidney disease.

2. Assess for cardiovascular disease.

3. Age-appropriate cancer screening and immunologic risk assessment

4. Assess the impact of comorbid conditions on KT outcomes.

5. Residual urine output should be documented because it assists with assessment of allograft function immediate post-KT.

6. Family history is important in assessment of living related donors and relates to patients primary disease.

7. Dental history is pertinent.

8. A thorough physical examination is performed, including documentation of femoral and pedal pulses. **Box 3** details the basic evaluation.

Box 3
Basic evaluation of kidney transplant recipient

Laboratory evaluation

HIV Ab, HBsAg, HBsAb, HCVAb, CMV, EBV, HSV, VZV, RPR

Complete blood cell count with differential, comprehensive metabolic panel, prothrombin time, partial thromboplastin time

Urinalysis and urine culture

PSA – men > age 50

Blood type, tissue typing, PRA

Serum and urine drug screen

PPD

Electrocardiogram, cardiac work-up (see text)

Chest radiograph, abdominal imaging (see text)

Papanicolaou smear, colonoscopy, mammogram (per guidelines for screening in general population)

Abbreviations: CMV, cytomegalovirus; EBV, Epstein-Barr virus; HBSAb, hepatitis B surface antibody; HBSAg, hepatitis B surface antigen; HSV, herpes simplex virus; PPD, purified protein derivative (tuberculin); PRA, panel reactive antibody titer; PSA, prostate-specific antigen; RPR, rapid plasma reagin (syphilis); VZV, varicella zoster virus.

---

essential focus of KT evaluation. Patients with severe unrevascularized critical coronary lesions are often denied for KT due to limited life expectancy and significant risk for perioperative fatal myocardial infarction. In general, candidates with advanced ischemic or nonischemic cardiomyopathy are considered ineligible for KT alone; combined heart KT needs to be considered in some of these situations.

ESKD patients frequently remain asymptomatic from their CVD and have several risk factors for CVD and, furthermore, DD transplant surgery is commonly performed several years after initial evaluation. Thus, CVD risk stratification guidelines applicable to general population may not be relevant to ESKD patients. The prevalence of angiographic significant coronary lesions in pre-KT patients could range between 40% and 90% based on the risk factor profile. The American Heart Association and the American College of Cardiology published an expert consensus statement on CVD work-up specifically pertinent to pre-KT and liver transplant patients in 2012.[5] Risk factors for CVD include advanced age, diabetes, longer duration of dialysis, prior history of coronary artery disease, peripheral vascular disease (PVD), cerebrovascular accidents (CVAs), decompensated congestive heart failure, or poor functional capacity.

Studies have highlighted the variable pre-KT CVD evaluation practices in the United States across centers. A majority of centers start with noninvasive stress testing whereas approximately 15% of centers advocate for cardiac catheterizations in high-risk patients. Noninvasive stress testing is an imperfect tool in patients with renal failure but positive findings on a stress test could be used as a prognostic marker. The method of stress testing is transplant center specific but generally involves some combination of exercise stress, radionuclide-nuclear stress, and dobutamine stress echocardiogram and cardiac catheterization. Further cardiac testing once a patient remains on a WL is also center specific and a matter of debate; in general, high-risk patients are subjected to an annual stress test. Revascularization along with aggressive medical management should be considered pretransplant when high anatomic risk critical coronary lesions are identified.

It is reasonable to perform an echocardiogram prior to transplant listing. Pulmonary hypertension (PHTN) is frequently encountered during KT evaluation and can be associated with volume overload states, especially for patients on dialysis.[6] PHTN secondary to volume overload is correctable with aggressive ultrafiltration and challenging estimated dry weight. Repeat echocardiogram or right heart catheterization could be performed to ensure improvement of pulmonary artery pressures after these strategies prior to wait listing in this subset of patients. These patients should be screened for sleep apnea or underlying cardiopulmonary etiologies leading to PHTN. Right heart catheterization is a useful tool for work-up of PHTN. KT might not be safe or beneficial in patients with severe primary PHTN; however, a subset of these patients, especially if they are young, might benefit from combined lung KT.[6]

Recurrent Glomerulonephritis

Recurrent glomerulonephritis is the third leading cause of KT loss.[7] At 10 years post-KT, recurrent glomerulonephritis contributes to 5% to 8% of graft loss. Risk of recurrence needs to be discussed and native renal biopsy should be reviewed pre-KT. **Table 2** summarizes the recurrence risk.

Peripheral Vascular Disease

The prevalence of PVD in ESKD patients is high, approximately 30% or higher.[8] Significant disease in the iliac vessels may make the anastomosis of the kidney allograft vessels difficult or impossible. Moreover, there is the concern of ischemia to the ipsilateral lower extremity as a result of steal phenomenon by the grafted kidney. The goal of PVD evaluation pre-KT should focus on estimation of the extent of aortoiliac occlusive disease to avoid critical limb ischemia post-KT. Additionally, PVD is a marker of increased mortality and poor quality of life; hence, patients with advanced PVD might not achieve the anticipated benefits post-KT.

Patients with claudication, nonhealing ulcers, a history of amputation, and feeble femoral pulses need further evaluation. Current practice guidelines recommend endovascular or surgical correction of symptomatic PVD prior to KT.[9] Vascular imaging with Doppler ultrasound, measurement of ankle brachial index, CT scan or MR angiogram of pelvic vasculature, and invasive angiography are used as needed.

Cerebrovascular Disease

Patients with a history of CVA/transient ischemic attack and/or audible carotid bruit should undergo carotid Doppler ultrasound to evaluate for carotid stenosis. Review of available prior brain imaging studies at the time of CVA with detailed neurologic examination provides valuable prognostic information. Patients with epilepsy on antiepileptics with potential drug interactions with post-KT immunosuppressive agents need to discuss alternative agents with fewer interactions prior to KT. In patients with autosomal dominant polycystic kidney disease (ADPKD), there may be an increased risk for cerebral aneurysm, so patients with a family history of intracranial aneurysms or a personal history of unexplained headaches should undergo testing with an MR angiogram of the brain.

Older Age

In general, there is no upper age limit for KT. The KTs performed in older patients have almost tripled in the past decade.[2] There is still a survival advantage over the age of 60 with KT compared with remaining on dialysis. Older patients have a higher risk of

Table 2
Recurrent glomerular disease

Disease	Recurrence Rate Post–Kidney Transplant	Important Facts
IgA nephropathy	With protocol biopsies 50%–60%	—
	Without protocol biopsies 15%–50%	Histological changes are not associated with graft dysfunction in >50% of recipients with recurrence.
Primary FSGS	20%–50%	Can recur with in first 24 hours post-KT; risk factors for recurrence are young age, white race, and rapid progression of native disease. Genetic forms with mutations of podocyte-specific proteins do not recur.
Type 1 MPGN	20%–50%	Risk factors for recurrence include living related transplant, low complement levels, monoclonal gammopathy.
Type 2 MPGN (dense deposit disease)	80%–100%	—
Membranous nephropathy	3%–30%	Differentiate from de novo disease.
ANCA vasculitis	7%–17%	Achieve clinical remission for 6 months prior to KT.
Lupus nephritis	Histologic recurrence 30% Clinically significant recurrence 10%	ANA, complements are checked pre-KT. SLE has to remain in clinical remission prior to KT. Check antiphospholipid antibodies in patients with history of thrombosis or miscarriages.
Atypical HUS	10%–40%	Check for mutations of complement regulatory proteins pre-KT. Consider eculizumab induction and preemptive plasmapheresis. Small subgroup might benefit from combined liver KT. Living related donors should be screened for the mutations as well.
Anti-GBM disease	Rare	Achieve clinical and serologic remission prior to KT.
Alport syndrome	Risk for de novo anti-GBM disease (<10%)	Aggressively screen living related donors.
Primary oxalosis	—	Consider liver KT.

Abbreviations: ANA, antinuclear antibody; ANCA, antineutrophil cytoplasmic antibody; FSGS, focal segmental glomerulosclerosis; GBM, glomerular basement membrane; HUS, hemolytic uremic syndrome; MPGN, membranoproliferative glomerulonephritis; SLE, systemic lupus erythematosus.

death related to CVD, death with functioning transplant and longer hospitalizations. The risks of infection and malignancy after immunosuppression exposure also increase in the older population. Although graft survival rates were similar between KT recipients age greater than 80 and those in the age 60 to 69 range, there was higher risk of death with functioning graft in the octogenarian group.[10]

Active Infection

Infections are the major cause of morbidity and mortality post-KT. Careful screening for latent or active infections is an essential part of the transplant evaluation. Active bacterial infections (such as diabetic foot infections) should be completely treated prior to KT. Latent tuberculosis and syphilis need appropriate treatment prior to KT. Patients living in or with history of recent travel to endemic areas should be screened for coccidioidomycosis; azole prophylaxis may be needed in cases with established infection. An immunization history should be obtained and patients encouraged to remain up to date with the age-appropriate vaccinations, including influenza and pertussis. Live attenuated vaccines (such as Varicella vaccine) cannot be administered after KT and should be given 4 to 6 weeks prior to KT.

HIV

KT of HIV-infected (HIV+) individuals in the pre–highly active antiretroviral therapy (HAART) era was disappointing with inferior patient and graft survival.[11] Less than 25% of US centers offer KT to HIV-infected patients. In the post-HAART era, KT in HIV+ individuals is well tolerated and is now associated with better outcomes than with hepatitis C–positive patients.[12] Prerequisites for KT are rigorous, including a CD4 count greater than 200 cells/μL, an undetectable viral load on a stable HAART regimen, and the absence of AIDS-defining illness. Formal infectious disease consultation is obtained pre-KT at most centers. The largest US experience with HIV+ KT comes out of a National Institutes of Health–sponsored trial where the 3-year patient and graft survival rates in HIV+ KT patients were reported at 88% and 73.7%, respectively, comparable to the uninfected, older KT recipients and better than the HIV+ patients on the WL.[13] A higher rate of acute rejection in the first year was reported compared with the noninfected patients. Fortunately, the HIV infection seemed well controlled post-KT. Those patients coinfected with HIV and hepatitis C (HCV), however, continue to have worse outcomes than HIV monoinfected patients.[12]

Hepatitis C

KT is considered the best treatment option for patients with HCV infection, because it is associated with greater survival advantage than for those remaining dialysis dependent. There seems, however, to be lower patient survival on dialysis and post-KT in HCV-infected patients compared with patients without HCV. A recent analysis of paired DD kidneys where 2 kidneys were derived from the same donor into either an HCV+ or HCV-negative (HIV−) recipient showed that HCV+ recipients conferred increased risks of death-censored graft loss* (adjusted hazard ratio 1.24; 95% CI, 1.04–1.47) and inferior patient survival (adjusted hazard ratio 1.24; 95% CI, 1.06–1.45).[14]

All potential KT candidates should be screened with anti-HCV antibody and/or active viremia with nucleic acid amplification technique (in areas of high prevalence) prior to KT. HCV-infected patients are commonly viremic pre-KT due to ineffectiveness of interferon based antiviral therapy, which contributes to inferior post-KT outcomes. Whether antiviral therapy needs to be offered pre-KT is not clear. With the advent of new interferon-free anti-HCV regimens, eradication of active HCV infection post-KT is possible, which might translate to improvement of post-KT outcomes. Viral load and genotype determination are performed on all HCV-infected patients. Liver biopsy remains the gold standard test for evaluation of patients with active HCV infection and should be performed on all patients because normal liver function tests do not imply normal histology. The risk of post-KT progression of liver disease exists but is small and largely dependent on pre-KT liver pathology. Annual evaluation is needed for WL patients to ensure that the liver disease has not progressed and may warrant a repeat biopsy if the wait times exceed 3 to 5 years. Patients with established decompensated cirrhosis should be evaluated for combined liver-KT. Wedge hepatic vein pressures should remain less than 10 mm Hg to proceed with kidney alone transplant. Stable patients with compensated cirrhosis can undergo KT alone. In patients with cirrhosis, the alpha fetoprotein level should be periodically measured with liver imaging to screen for hepatocellular carcinoma.

Transplanting kidneys from HCV+ donors to HCV+ recipients can shorten wait times. Despite its initial controversy, retrospective data show that 5-year and 10-year graft survival rates were 84.8% and 72.7% respectively, in HCV+ to HCV+ transplants versus 86.6% and 76.5% respectively, in the HCV− to HCV+ group ($P = .25$).[15] The 2 groups had comparable rates of decompensated liver disease. There is, an increased risk of post-transplant diabetes, CVD, glomerulonephritis, infections, and hematologic neoplasia in patients with active HCV infection post-KT.

Hepatitis B

Although hepatitis B virus (HBV) antigenemia is not a contraindication for KT, patients need to be evaluated with liver biopsy and assessment of viral replication prior to KT. Reactivation of the infection with worsening of liver disease in the setting of immunosuppression should be discussed with all potential recipients. Patients with mild liver disease based on the pathology can be transplanted with antiviral therapy pre-KT and post-KT. Imaging of the liver to screen for hepatocellular carcinoma is warranted. The outcomes of KT in patients infected with hepatitis B in the pre–antiviral therapy era were inferior primarily secondary to hepatic complications. With the advent of effective anti-HBV nucleotide analogs, outcomes have dramatically improved.[16]

Noncompliance and Substance Abuse

The risk for noncompliance should be sought because it is one of the major reasons for graft failure. This may not always be easy to decipher and thus requires a multidisciplinary approach of a psychiatrist or psychologist and social worker. Major psychiatric illness affecting compliance is a risk factor for graft loss. In patients with cognitive deficits, adequate social support needs to be established prior to proceeding with KT. Patients with active history of substance abuse are usually not considered good candidates for KT and need to obtain clearance from a drug rehabilitation program prior to initiating work-up. Smoking cessation is encouraged pre-KT. Pulmonary function tests are performed pre-KT when emphysema is suspected pre-KT. Consider low-dose CT scan chest to screen for lung malignancy in patients above age 55 who have greater than 30 pack years of smoking.

Obesity

Morbid obesity is a major barrier for KT and is the third leading cause of remaining inactive status on the transplant list.[19] Approximately 60% of patients have a body mass index (BMI) greater than 30 kg/m^2 at the time of KT. Obesity is a risk factor for delayed graft function, wound complications, prolonged hospitalization, acute rejection, increased costs, CVD, and graft loss.[20] Current evidence, however, does not provide a clear BMI cutoff that precludes KT, and exact guidelines remain a matter of some controversy, which is reflected in a wide range of varying thresholds for upper-limit BMI to offer KT ranging between 35 kg/m^2 and 42 kg/m^2. Bariatric surgery could be offered to patients who fail weight loss by conservative measures where morbid obesity is prohibitive of KT.[21]

Highly Sensitized Patients

Potential KT recipients may have preformed anti-HLA antibodies from childbirth, prior transfusions, or previous transplants that raise the risk of rejection, making matching of potential organs more difficult and associated with inferior graft and patient survival.[22] To evaluate for these antibodies, the panel reactive antibody titer (PRA) is performed on all pre-KT recipients. More than 30% patients on the WL are sensitized. Desensitization (removal or reduction of antibody titer), kidney paired exchange, or a combination of both techniques, positive cross-match KT have made KT an option for these patients. High-quality support from a histocompatibility laboratory with identification of antibody specificity and strength is the key to this approach. Despite potent induction protocols involving use of 1 or more of these agents—rituximab, plasmapheresis, eculizumab, bortezomib, and intravenous immunoglobulin—sensitized patients remain at high risk for antibody mediated rejection post-KT and need close monitoring.

Repeat Transplanted Candidates

Recent reports reveal that approximately 10% of KTs performed annually are repeat transplants (RTs) and 15% of current WL patients are waiting for a RT.[2] RT involves longer wait time due to high PRA and is a risk factor for acute rejection and inferior graft survival. Despite these risks, it still provides survival advantage compared with remaining on dialysis. The clinical course of the first transplant needs to be known, because it is the major determinant of RT survival; primary KT loss within the first 1 to 3 years is a major risk factor for graft loss with repeat KT. Prior transplant outcomes, such as acute rejection, delayed graft function, and hospitalization, seem to recur in retransplants.[23] Shorter time spent on dialysis prior to RT is associated with improved outcome. Patients evaluated for an RT must undergo an evaluation as stringent as the original assessment, especially now that patients are older, with a higher risk of CVD and/or malignancy.

Other Important Factors

Prior history of malignancy, urological issues and underlying hypercoagulable states are encountered and need careful work up prior to KT to optimize outcomes. **Boxes 4**, **5** and **6** summarize work up focusing on these issues.

Simultaneous Kidney Pancreas Transplantation

Pancreas transplantation offers the most physiologic glycemic control in both type 1 and type 2 diabetics. The most common modality of pancreas transplantation is

---

Box 4
Thrombophilias

1. Thrombophilias can lead to devastating complications, such as KT thrombosis, if unrecognized pre-KT.

2. Obtain hypercoagulable evaluation for patients with a history of recurrent deep vein thrombosis or dialysis access thrombosis or women with miscarriages.

3. Screen for prothrombin gene mutation, factor V Leiden mutation, antiphospholipid antibodies, and proteins C and S deficiencies.

4. Assess the presence of inferior vena caval filters or history of deep venous thrombosis, which extends to the proximal iliac veins, which may compromise KT venous anastomosis.

Box 5
Urologic problems

1. Urologic problems are common in KT candidates and could be masked in oligoanuric dialysis patients.

2. Patients with congenital urologic anomalies, voiding problems, incontinence, or recurrent urinary tract infections require formal urologic evaluation with voiding cystourethrography and/or urodynamic studies.

3. Microscopic hematuria and sterile pyuria may warrant a cystoscopy.

4. In some cases of severe bladder dysfunction, which cannot be remedied by self-catheterization, bladder diversion with ileal conduit could be performed 6 to 8 weeks prior to KT; KT ureter could then be anastomosed to the diversion.

5. Urinalysis and urine cultures should be checked in patients with considerable residual urine volume.

6. Benign prostatic hypertrophy is common in older male dialysis patients and could necessitate medical or surgical interventions pre-KT or post-KT.

7. Patients on dialysis are at increased risk for renal cell carcinoma; they should undergo imaging of the native kidneys with either an ultrasound, CT scan, or MRI pre-KT.

8. In patients with ADPKD, a unilateral or bilateral native nephrectomy may be needed if the kidneys are massively enlarged or if a patient has significant hematuria or infected cyst or stones.

---

simultaneous pancreas-kidney transplantation (SPK). SPK provides comparable long-term KT survival compared with living donor transplantation.[24] Type 1 or type 2 diabetics with eGFR less than 20 ml/min/m2 or ESKD qualify to be listed for SPK. Eligibility criteria for type 2 diabetics include BMI less than 30 kg/m2, C-peptide levels less than 10 ng/ml, and insulin requirements less than 70 units/d or 1 unit/kg/d who are presumed to have minimal insulin resistance benefit from SPK. A majority of transplant centers pursue left heart catheterization as part of SPK work-up. Pancreas

---

Box 6
Malignancy

1. Immunosuppression is a risk factor for both de novo and recurrent malignancy.

2. Most of the guidelines for KT in patients with prior malignancies come from the Israel Penn International Transplant Tumor Registry.

3. In general, a 2-year waiting period between treatment of cancer and KT is appropriate.

4. A longer wait time of 5 years is preferred for breast, colorectal, symptomatic or greater than 5-cm renal cell carcinomas and for lymphomas.

5. The shorter the interval between the treatment of malignancy and KT, the higher the risk of recurrence.[17]

6. No wait time is needed for incidental renal cell carcinomas and bladder and cervical in situ cancer.

7. Patients with prostate cancers treated with prostatectomy could be safely transplanted with less than 2 years of wait time.[18]

8. Patients with benign monoclonal gammopathy need serial surveillance to rule out evolution to myeloma prior to KT.

transplantation involves complex arterial anastomosis, often excluding patients with a heavy smoking history or severe PVD.

SUMMARY

All patients with ESKD should be considered for KT until proved otherwise. With more and more centers achieving success with KT, the eligibility criteria have broadened tremendously in the recent past. Once considered absolute contraindications for KT, HIV, for example, no longer is so. The main goal of transplant evaluation lies in identifying conditions that limit life expectancy where KT might not offer much benefit as well as identifying factors that need to be corrected to ensure the safety and success of the KT.

REFERENCES

1. Huang Y, Samaniego M. Preemptive kidney transplantation: has it come of age? Nephrol Ther 2012;8:428–32.
2. Matas AJ, Smith JM, Skeans MA, et al. OPTN/SRTR 2013 annual data report: kidney. Am J Transplant 2015;15(Suppl 2):1–34.
3. Rao PS, Schaubel DE, Guidinger MK, et al. A comprehensive risk quantification score for deceased donor kidneys: the kidney donor risk index. Transplantation 2009;88:231–6.
4. Ghanta M, Kozicky M, Jim B. Pathophysiologic and treatment strategies for cardiovascular disease in end-stage renal disease and kidney transplantations. Cardiol Rev 2015;23:109–18.
5. Lentine KL, Costa SP, Weir MR, et al. Cardiac disease evaluation and management among kidney and liver transplantation candidates: a scientific statement from the American Heart Association and the American College of Cardiology Foundation. J Am Coll Cardiol 2012;60:434–80.
6. Issa N, Krowka MJ, Griffin MD, et al. Pulmonary hypertension is associated with reduced patient survival after kidney transplantation. Transplantation 2008; 86(10):1384–8.
7. Ivanyi B. A primer on recurrent and de novo glomerulonephritis in renal allografts. Nat Clin Pract Nephrol 2008;4:446–57.
8. Gill R, Shapiro R, Kayler LK. Management of peripheral vascular disease compromising renal allograft placement and function: review of the literature with an illustrative case. Clin Transplant 2011;25(3):337–44.
9. Snyder JJ, Kasiske BL, Maclean R. Peripheral arterial disease and renal transplantation. J Am Soc Nephrol 2006;17:2056–68.
10. McAdams-DeMarco MA, James N, Salter ML, et al. Trends in kidney transplant outcomes in older adults. J Am Geriatr Soc 2014;62:2235–42.
11. Swanson SJ, Kirk AD, Ko CW, et al. Impact of HIV seropositivity on graft and patient survival after cadaveric renal transplantation in the United States in the pre highly active antiretroviral therapy (HAART) era: an historical cohort analysis of the United States Renal Data System. Transpl Infect Dis 2002;4:144–7.
12. Sawinski D, Forde KA, Eddinger K, et al. Superior outcomes in HIV-positive kidney transplant patients compared with HCV-infected or HIV/HCV-coinfected recipients. Kidney Int 2015;88(2):341–9.
13. Stock PG, Barin B, Murphy B, et al. Outcomes of kidney transplantation in HIV-infected recipients. N Engl J Med 2010;363:2004–14.
14. Xia Y, Friedmann P, Yaffe H, et al. Effect of HCV, HIV and coinfection in kidney transplant recipients: mate kidney analyses. Am J Transplant 2014;14:2037–47.

15. Morales JM, Campistol JM, Dominguez-Gil B, et al. Long-term experience with kidney transplantation from hepatitis C-positive donors into hepatitis C-positive recipients. Am J Transplant 2010;10:2453–62.
16. Yap DY, Chan TM. Evolution of hepatitis B management in kidney transplantation. World J Gastroenterol 2014;20:468–74.
17. Penn I. Evaluation of transplant candidates with pre-existing malignancies. Ann Transplant 1997;2:14–7.
18. Tillou X, Chahwan C, Le Gal S, et al. Prostatectomy for localized prostate cancer to prepare for renal transplantation in end-stage renal disease patients. Ann Transplant 2014;19:569–75.
19. Segev DL, Simpkins CE, Thompson RE, et al. Obesity impacts access to kidney transplantation. J Am Soc Nephrol 2008;19(2):349–55.
20. Hill CJ, Courtney AE, Cardwell CR, et al. Recipient obesity and outcomes after kidney transplantation: a systematic review and meta-analysis. Nephrol Dial Transplant 2015;30(8):1403–11.
21. Freeman CM, Woodle ES, Shi J, et al. Addressing morbid obesity as a barrier to renal transplantation with laparoscopic sleeve gastrectomy. Am J Transplant 2015;15:1360–8.
22. Iyer HS, Jackson AM, Zachary AA, et al. Transplanting the highly sensitized patient: trials and tribulations. Curr Opin Nephrol Hypertens 2013;22:681–8.
23. Heaphy EL, Poggio ED, Flechner SM, et al. Risk factors for retransplant kidney recipients: relisting and outcomes from patients' primary transplant. Am J Transplant 2014;14:1356–67.
24. Kandaswamy R, Skeans MA, Gustafson SK, et al. OPTN/SRTR 2013 annual data report: pancreas. Am J Transplant 2015;15(Suppl 2):1–20.

Management of the Liver Transplant Recipient
Approach to Allograft Dysfunction

Jonathan M. Fenkel, MD*, Dina L. Halegoua-DeMarzio, MD

KEYWORDS

- Liver transplantation • Allograft dysfunction • Acute cellular rejection • Hepatitis
- Immunosuppression

KEY POINTS

- Early recognition of liver allograft dysfunction is key to preventing graft failure.
- The differential diagnosis of allograft dysfunction depends on the timing after transplantation, with anatomic and infectious issues being most common in the first month.
- Acute cellular rejection occurs in approximately 15% of liver transplant recipients, with most episodes occurring between the third and twelfth month.
- Recurrent diseases, including hepatitis C and nonalcoholic fatty liver disease, are the most common causes of allograft dysfunction after the first year.

INTRODUCTION

Due to improved outcomes after liver transplant (LT) over the last 30 years, many patients with end-stage liver disease and acute liver failure have been granted a second chance at life. This improvement in survival post-LT is largely due to advances in surgical techniques, careful selection of donors and recipients, fine-tuned immunosuppression, and aggressive management of infections. With more than 6000 LTs performed annually in the Unites States, it can be estimated that with an increasing number of long-term survivors, primary care physicians will be seeing a larger number of LT recipients in their practice.[1,2] Primary care physicians must be able to recognize and optimally manage key complications, including detection of allograft dysfunction. This article provides an overview of issues pertinent to the diagnosis and management of allograft dysfunction in LT recipients.

Disclosure Statement: The authors have nothing to disclose.
Division of Gastroenterology and Hepatology, Department of Medicine, Sidney Kimmel Medical College at Thomas Jefferson University, 132 South 10th Street, Suite 480, Main Building, Philadelphia, PA 19107, USA
* Corresponding author.
E-mail address: jonathan.fenkel@jefferson.edu

Med Clin N Am 100 (2016) 477–486
http://dx.doi.org/10.1016/j.mcna.2016.01.001
0025-7125/16/$ – see front matter © 2016 Elsevier Inc. All rights reserved.

medical.theclinics.com

DEFINITION OF ALLOGRAFT DYSFUNCTION

Liver allograft dysfunction may be identified by either clinical or laboratory findings. In many instances, laboratory findings may be more specific (ie, abnormal liver function tests) and are detected earlier than clinical manifestations.[3] If liver enzymes (alanine aminotransferase, aspartate aminotransferase, alkaline phosphatase) or function tests (bilirubin, international normalized ratio [INR]) are elevated 1.5 or more times the upper limits of normal, further evaluation is warranted. Clinical manifestations include poor mental function, hypoglycemia, acidosis, jaundice, poor bile output when a T-tube is present, acholic stools, ascites, and bleeding. It is possible to have none of these clinical findings and yet for the LT recipient to have significant graft dysfunction. For this reason, diagnostic investigation should be pursued for any rise in or failure to normalize aminotransferase enzymes, alkaline phosphatase enzyme, serum bilirubin, and/or the coagulation profile (prothrombin time [PT] and INR).

DIFFERENTIAL DIAGNOSIS

Liver allograft dysfunction is a serious complication that can result in loss of the donor organ. Salvage of the organ depends on accurate diagnosis and prompt treatment. The approach to the patient with graft dysfunction is highly dependent on timing posttransplant (**Table 1**).

Less than 1-month Posttransplant

Early graft dysfunction

To offer grafts to as many LT candidates as possible, the transplant professional community has had to expand its organ pool. One of the main results of this is variability in early graft function.[4] Almost all LT recipients have significant laboratory elevations immediately posttransplant and some degree of early graft dysfunction is common. Laboratory trends in this period are especially important with regard to the aminotransferase enzymes. An early peak, usually in the first or second postoperative day, is expected and then a consistent decline to the normal range is the typical course.[5] Values in the aminotransferases greater than the 3000 range are worrisome that the injury causing the enzyme elevation may be too significant for the liver to reasonably recover. In instances in which this occurs within the first 2 days of transplantation, early diagnosis of primary nonfunction or hepatic artery thrombosis (HAT) must be considered. If either of these 2 conditions occurs within 1 week of transplant, the recipient may be relisted for a second transplant with the highest priority (United Network for Organ Sharing Status 1 listing).

Table 1		
Common cause of liver allograft dysfunction depending on posttransplant period		
<1 mo Post-LT	**1–12 mo Post-LT**	**>1 y Post-LT**
Early graft dysfunction	Rejection (acute or chronic)	Rejection (acute or chronic)
Vascular complications (ie, HAT, vascular impairment)	Recurrence of primary disease (ie, HCC, HCV)	Recurrence of primary disease (ie, HCC, HCV, alcoholism)
Biliary complications (ie, bile leak, strictures)	Vascular complications	Development of de novo liver disease (ie, NAFLD)
Infection (ie, sepsis)	Infection (ie, CMV)	—

Abbreviations: CMV, cytomegalovirus; HAT, hepatic artery thrombosis; HCC, hepatocellular carcinoma; HCV, hepatitis C virus; NALFD, nonalcoholic liver disease.

Vascular complications

Persistently abnormal liver tests can be reflective of a vascular complication, which occurs in up to 10% of LT recipients, usually within the first month after LT. One of the most severe complications, HAT, may cause ischemic destruction of the bile ducts leading to biliary strictures or bilomas. Secondary infection of a biloma may result in a hepatic abscess. Percutaneous or endoscopic stenting of the biliary strictures formed due to biliary ischemia, as well as percutaneous drainage of any existing bilomas, may lead to restoration of normal function but patients may require retransplantation. If HAT is identified within the first week, usually manifested by acute and dramatic increase in serum transaminase levels, the graft may be occasionally salvaged by thrombectomy, thrombolytic therapy, or surgical revascularization.[6] Portal and hepatic vein thrombosis can also occur and may manifest symptomatically as recurrent ascites or variceal hemorrhage. There is no universal approach to the treatment of these problems; however, vascular stenting or anastomotic revision may be considered and patients should be referred back to the transplant center for urgent evaluation and treatment.[7]

Biliary complications

Biliary complications represent some of the more frequent problems encountered by the post-LT patient with an incidence rate of 10% to 25%.[8,9] Recipients of livers from donors after cardiac death (DCD) have the highest rate of biliary complications (60%), which has limited this potential source of donor organs.[10] Live donor LT recipients may also experience a higher frequency of biliary complications than their deceased donor counterparts. Post-LT biliary complications can also be related to a T-tube used by some surgeons to stent the biliary anastomosis and allow access to the biliary system. The various types of biliary complications seen include bile leaks, bilomas, anastomotic strictures, diffuse biliary strictures, sludge, bile casts, and stones. All of these can occur in the early posttransplant period. It ought to be noted that a liver ultrasound is not as sensitive a test for diagnosing bile duct obstruction in the post-LT recipient as it is in a nontransplant patient because the transplanted bile duct does not dilate to the same degree as the native bile duct. Most biliary complications can be treated by endoscopic retrograde cholangiopancreatography (ERCP) or percutaneous transhepatic cholangiogram and may require serial procedures for a period of time.[11]

Infectious complications

Posttransplant infections, including sepsis, may develop in up to 20% of LT recipients during the first month after transplantation and can lead to graft dysfunction in the immunosuppressed patient.[12] Due to this risk, prophylaxis against infections is routinely given to patients in the early postoperative period. Pneumonia, catheter-related infections, and wound infections are most common in the first month after transplant. Opportunistic infections, those occurring as a result of immunosuppressive therapy, are rare in the first month after transplant. Further details on these postoperative infections are provided elsewhere in this issue (See Greendyke WG, Pereira MR: Infectious Complications and Vaccinations in the Post-Transplant Population, in this issue).

Through 12-months Posttransplant

Rejection

Acute cellular rejection following liver transplantation has decreased in incidence with the use of potent immunosuppressive agents but it still affects up to 15-30% of liver transplantation recipients.[13,14] It is most common within the first 3 months following LT but can occur at any time. The consequences of acute cellular rejection are variable. Whereas it can predispose to steroid-resistant rejection and graft loss, most episodes do not have long-term adverse effects and are treated with increasing doses of immunosuppression or enforcing medication compliance. Chronic rejection results in fibrosis and disappearance of bile ducts (ductopenia) and this may develop in recipients with uncontrolled acute rejection episodes, resulting in severe biliary obstruction and cholestatic jaundice. Chronic rejection may be treated by increasing immunosuppressive drug levels or the addition of an additional agent, such as sirolimus, but retransplantation should be considered if significant allograft synthetic dysfunction or portal hypertensive complications ensue.[7]

Cytomegalovirus

As discussed earlier, one of the most common causes of acute allograft dysfunction is due to infection in the first few months following LT. The most common opportunistic infection seen is cytomegalovirus (CMV), usually occurring 1 to 4 months post-LT, but can be delayed after prophylaxis with an antiviral agent.[15] This infection may result from reactivation of a remote infection in the recipient, a new infection acquired following LT, or from the allograft itself. Patients at highest risk of CMV infection are CMV-negative before LT and receive a liver from a CMV exposed (positive CMV immunoglobulin [Ig]G) donor. Prophylaxis with antiviral agents such as valganciclovir is common for the first 3 to 6 months, depending on donor and recipient CMV status. Acute CMV disease may manifest with fevers, headaches, myalgias, leukopenia, thrombocytopenia, pneumonitis, nausea, diarrhea, retinitis, and/or hepatitis. Intravenous ganciclovir is the most common treatment but oral valganciclovir and CMV-specific immunoglobulin can also be used in specific cases.[16] CMV infection can also precipitate acute rejection by inflammatory and immune-mediated mechanisms, and can occur in various organs, including the gastrointestinal tract or the liver itself.

Recurrence of primary liver disease

Recurrent primary liver disease is a major concern posttransplant. Most indications for LT carry risk of recurrence, with the exception of fulminant liver failure from a specific medication or toxin that can be completely avoided, or an inherited disease such as alpha-1 antitrypsin deficiency or Wilson disease. Within the first year of LT, 4 underlying diseases, in particular, need to be closely monitored for recurrence: hepatitis C, hepatitis B, alcohol abuse, and hepatocellular carcinoma (HCC).

Hepatitis C virus Hepatitis C virus (HCV) recurrence is universal following LT when a recipient is viremic at the time of transplant. Patients who were treated and achieved sustained virologic response pretransplant do not recur but patients could be at risk of reinfection because there is no persistently protective immunity to hepatitis C after prior infection and treatment or eradication. Rarely, HCV recurrence can be severe in the first year, manifesting as fibrosing cholestatic hepatitis (FCH) in less than 10% of HCV-infected recipients. Donor age greater than 50 years and DCD grafts are risk factors that increase the likelihood of FCH occurring. FCH can lead to rapid allograft dysfunction, graft loss, and death if not identified and treated promptly with antiviral agents. Death within a year of its occurrence was expected in FCH patients before the introduction of new direct-acting antiviral agents (DAAs) to the market in 2011. DAA-based treatment has dramatically improved survival in those who develop FCH. In general, HCV recurrence in the allograft is slowly progressive but progresses much more rapidly than in a native liver, with 30% of patients developing cirrhosis within 5 years of LT, in the absence of antiviral treatment.[17]

Hepatitis B virus recurrence FCH can also occur from hepatitis B virus (HBV) if not treated and, at one point, HBV was not an indication for LT due to risk of FCH. Now, with the use of hepatitis B immune globulin (HBIG) and the availability of multiple antiviral agents (lamivudine, adefovir, entecavir, telbivudine, and tenofovir), severe or even minor recurrence of HBV is negligible.[18] Each transplant program has its own institutional protocol of post-LT hepatitis B prophylaxis, using either nucleoside or nucleotide analog monotherapy, or varying durations of parenteral HBIG in combination with oral antiviral therapy. Routine antiviral treatment before and after LT with these oral agents will prevent clinical recurrence for most patients.

Alcohol abuse Patients transplanted for alcohol-induced cirrhosis are at risk of alcohol recidivism after LT and should be counseled against any alcohol use. Recidivism may occur despite a very thorough pretransplant psychosocial assessment by the social work, transplant psychiatry, and addictions specialist team. Recent data suggest that up to 20% of patients transplanted for alcohol-related liver disease will return to some degree of drinking at some time after LT.[19] Relapse-prevention programs may be appropriate for some patients post-LT. Any abnormal liver test in a patient with previous alcohol abuse should prompt screening for its recurrence.

Hepatocellular carcinoma HCC is the primary indication in 15% to 20% of all adult patients listed for a LT and most often occurs in the setting of underlying HCV- or HBV-related cirrhosis. Patients transplanted with HCC and within Milan criteria (1 lesion<5 cm in diameter, 2 or 3 lesions all <3 cm, and no evidence of vascular involvement or metastasis) have recurrence rates less than 10%. However, patients that are transplanted with HCC outside of Milan criteria have recurrence rates as high as 34%.[20] Those transplanted outside of Milan criteria are generally not recognized to be that advanced at the time of listing but are found to be so on examination of the explanted liver by the pathologist. HCC surveillance posttransplant is recommended for all LT recipients with HCC, particularly within the first few years after transplant, with cross-sectional abdominal imaging and alpha-fetoprotein (AFP) monitoring. For example, the authors' center performs every 3-month MRI abdomen testing and AFP for the first year after transplant, then every 6-month MRI abdomen and AFP for the second year, then both yearly for years 2 to 5 post-LT.

Additionally, in patients transplanted for autoimmune liver diseases, including autoimmune hepatitis, primary biliary cirrhosis, and primary sclerosing cholangitis, the disease recurs in approximately 11% to 22% despite the use of immunosuppressive medications following LT.[21] Fortunately, recurrence is unusual in the first year after transplant and is usually not as severe as primary occurrence and can be medically managed.

Greater than 1 year Posttransplant

Most of the complications that occur during the early posttransplant period can also be seen in the late posttransplant period. However, there are important differences in their relative frequency. Recurrent disease is the most commonly recognized cause of late allograft dysfunction.[22] By contrast, acute and chronic rejection are uncommon at this time and may have different histologic features to those seen in the early posttransplant period.

A substantial proportion of biopsies obtained greater than 1 year post-LT show changes of uncertain cause. Examples include nonspecific portal and/or lobular inflammation, unexplained (idiopathic) chronic hepatitis, and a range of architectural and vascular changes.[23] Transplant patients can also develop de novo liver disease, a term used to describe patients who are transplanted for one type of primary liver disease and subsequently develop features suggesting a different primary liver disease. This applies to viral infection (hepatitis B and C), which may be acquired, autoimmune liver disease, and nonalcoholic fatty liver disease (NAFLD). NAFLD is of particular importance because it is often caused by posttransplant metabolic syndrome and may affect survival in this population.[23] Histologic features are generally similar to those seen in recurrent disease.[24]

EVALUATION, ADJUSTMENT, AND RECURRENCE

Routine monitoring of liver tests, including aminotransferases, alkaline phosphatase, bilirubin, PT or INR, albumin, and platelet count, is recommended after LT. The frequency of monitoring is most intense in the period immediately after LT and lengthens with time from transplant. A suggested monitoring strategy is detailed in **Table 2**.

Any perturbation in these tests should prompt an evaluation for allograft dysfunction. As mentioned in the differential diagnosis section, this evaluation is tailored to the time period in which it occurs posttransplant and to the underlying liver disease. Evaluation usually progresses from least invasive to most invasive in strategy. The less invasive options include additional phlebotomy studies and diagnostic radiology testing, such as ultrasonography with or without color-flow duplex examination. More invasive options include contrast-enhanced imaging, liver biopsy, and ERCP. The type of diagnostic evaluation pursued should correlate to the differential diagnosis of highest probability or concern. Common diagnostic tests associated with their differential diagnosis are highlighted in **Table 3**.

OTHER CONSIDERATIONS DURING EVALUATION

Similar to patients without a transplant, LT recipients are also at risk of drug-induced liver injury. Correlating the onset of allograft dysfunction to the initiation of a new medication or supplement is important to determine because liver biopsy histology may mimic biliary obstruction or viral hepatitis. In particular, drugs metabolized through the cytochrome P450 3A4 pathway (the primary metabolic pathway for many of the LT immunosuppressive agents) may lead to abnormal liver tests. Inducers of 3A4 (eg, rifampin, St. John's Wort) may increase metabolism of immunosuppressive drugs, leading to decreased drug levels precipitating rejection; whereas inhibitors of this pathway (eg, azole antifungals, macrolide antibiotics, certain calcium channel blockers, protease inhibitors) may increase drug levels, precipitating drug toxicity.[25]

Hepatitis E, a virus not considered to cause chronic hepatitis in immunocompetent patients, is another infection to consider in the differential diagnosis of allograft dysfunction. Chronic hepatitis from hepatitis E has been reported in patients after LT and other solid organ transplants, as well as patients infected with human immunodeficiency virus and patients receiving chemotherapy.[26] It is theorized that hepatitis E may become more

Table 2
Routine laboratory monitoring after liver transplant for assessment of allograft function

Time from LT	Frequency	Tests
Day 1–3	2–4/d	CBC, CMP, PT or INR, lactate
Day 4–7	Daily	CBC, CMP, PT or INR, immunosuppressive drug levels
Weeks 2–4	1–2/wk	CBC, CMP, PT or INR, immunosuppressive drug levels
Months 2–6	Monthly	CBC, CMP, PT or INR, immunosuppressive drug levels
Months 7–12	Every 2 mo	CBC, CMP, PT or INR, immunosuppressive drug levels
Years 1–3	Every 3 mo	CBC, CMP, PT or INR, immunosuppressive drug levels
Years 4+	Every 6 mo	CBC, CMP, PT or INR, immunosuppressive drug levels

Abbreviations: CBC, complete blood count; CMP, comprehensive metabolic panel.

Table 3
Diagnostic tests by corresponding differential diagnosis

Differential Diagnosis	Laboratory Tests	Studies
Acute Cellular Rejection	AST, ALT, bilirubin, GGT, alkaline phosphatase, immunosuppressive drug level	Liver biopsy
Bile Leak	CBC, CMP, PT or INR, PTT, ascitic fluid bilirubin level	Nuclear medicine (HIDA) scan, T-tube cholangiography, ERCP
Biliary Obstruction	CBC, AST, ALT, bilirubin, alkaline phosphatase, blood cultures, creatinine	Ultrasound, T-tube cholangiogram, HIDA, CT, MRI or MRCP, ERCP
Chronic Rejection	AST, ALT, bilirubin, GGT, alkaline phosphatase, PT or INR, albumin, platelet count, immunosuppressive drug level	Liver biopsy
CMV Infection	CMV IgM and IgG, CMV DNA quantitative PCR	Endoscopy and colonoscopy, liver biopsy
HAT	AST, ALT, bilirubin, PT or INR, lactate	Duplex liver ultrasound, CT angiogram, angiogram or stent
Hepatitis B	HBV DNA quantitative level, AST, ALT, bilirubin, CBC, creatinine, hepatitis B surface antigen, hepatitis B core Ab IgM or IgG	Liver biopsy
Hepatitis C	HCV RNA quantitative level and genotype, AST, ALT, bilirubin, CBC, creatinine	Liver biopsy, transient elastography
HCC	AFP	Liver ultrasound, CT, MRI, targeted biopsy
NFLD	AST, ALT, bilirubin, lipid panel, hemoglobin A1C	Liver ultrasound
Primary Nonfunction	AST, ALT, bilirubin, PT or INR, albumin, platelet count, lactate, ammonia, creatinine	Duplex liver ultrasound, liver biopsy
Venous Outflow Obstruction	CBC, CMP, PT or INR, PTT	Duplex liver ultrasound, transvenous liver biopsy

Abbreviations: AST, aspartate aminotransferase; ALT, alanine aminotransferase; PTT, partial thromboplastin time; HIDA, hydroxy iminodiacetic acid hepatobiliary scan; MRCP, magnetic resonance cholangiopancreatography; GGT, gamma glutamyl-transferase; CT, computed tomography scan; PCR, polymerase chain reaction.

prevalent after LT in the coming years due to the elimination of interferon and ribavirin-based regimens for the treatment of post-LT HCV recurrence because hepatitis E is often treated with ribavirin and may have been underdiagnosed or incidentally treated in patients treated for HCV.[27] Serum hepatitis E IgM and IgG can be tested through reference laboratories. PCR testing for the virus itself requires sending blood samples to the Centers for Disease Control and Prevention in Atlanta, GA, USA.[28]

MANAGEMENT

The adjustment made to improve allograft dysfunction ultimately depends on the diagnosis. Each cause of liver test abnormalities or allograft dysfunction is managed individually. Common management by differential diagnosis is shown in **Table 4.**

Table 4
Management of allograft dysfunction by differential diagnosis

Differential Diagnosis	Management
Acute Cellular Rejection	1st line: corticosteroids and increase immunosuppressive drug adherence or levels 2nd line: antithymocyte globulin, muronomab
Alcohol Relapse	Abstinence, counseling or therapy, treat or prevent alcohol withdrawal syndrome
Bile Leak	1st line: ERCP and stent placement 2nd line: surgical management
Biliary Obstruction	ERCP with biliary clearance and/or stent placement
Chronic Rejection	Increase immunosuppressive drug adherence or levels Consider retransplantation
CMV Infection	Antivirals
HAT	Interventional radiology intervention: stent, dilation, thrombectomy Urgent retransplantation if early Surgical management and/or endoscopic biliary management
Hepatitis B	Antivirals, HBIG
Hepatitis C	Antivirals, avoid corticosteroid-based immunosuppression
Hepatitis E	Ribavirin
HCC	Locoregional therapy, chemotherapy
NFLD	Weight loss, optimize associated conditions, lower immunosuppression if possible
Primary Nonfunction	Urgent retransplantation; consider molecular adsorbent recirculating system (MARS) as temporary measure before retransplantation
Venous Outflow Obstruction	1st line: venography and endovascular intervention, dilatation, or stent 2nd line: surgical management

Causes of allograft dysfunction can be self-limited, chronic, or relapsing, and some may increase risk of another cause of allograft dysfunction after initial management. Self-limited causes include alcohol relapse, bile leak, biliary obstruction, acute cellular rejection, hepatitis C, and CMV infection. Acute cellular rejection episodes, though self-limited, may predispose a patient to chronic rejection and the treatment of acute cellular rejection or use of steroids in general in a patient with chronic hepatitis C may predispose the patient to more aggressive hepatitis C recurrence.[29] Conversely, treatment of hepatitis C with interferon-based therapy can also increase the risk of chronic rejection.[30] Chronic causes such as hepatitis B, require lifelong treatment with antivirals in a LT recipient and monitoring of viral DNA levels, while assuring medication adherence. Treatment of hepatitis C has advanced significantly in the past few years with the approval of many new DAAs, though it remains slightly less effective than treatment in a native noncirrhotic liver.[31,32] This should greatly improve graft survival in the coming years because hepatitis C is the leading indication for liver transplantation at the current time in the United States. NAFLD, which can recur chronically as primary disease or develop de novo in transplant recipients, also requires lifelong monitoring and optimization of associated conditions such as hypertension, hyperlipidemia, diabetes mellitus, and obesity. New therapies are being investigated for NAFLD but are not yet available.

SUMMARY

LT recipients are living longer than ever today and many will experience some form of allograft dysfunction during their lifespan. Other than the major causes of early allograft dysfunction, such as primary nonfunction and HAT that require urgent retransplantation, most allograft abnormalities are quite manageable with minimally invasive procedures, medications, and lifestyle modification. Collaboration and comanagement of LT recipients between primary care and the transplant hepatologist is essential for optimizing recipient and allograft outcomes.

REFERENCES

1. 2012 OPTN/SRTR Annual Report. Recurrent hepatitis C. Available at: http://optn.transplant.hrsa.gov/ar2012/Chapter_IV_AR_CD.htm?cp=5#3. Accessed July 7, 2015.
2. McCashland TM. Posttransplantation care: role of the primary care physician versus transplant center. Liver Transpl 2001;7:S2.
3. Watt KD, Pedersen RA, Kremers WK, et al. Evolution of causes and risk factors for mortality post-liver transplant: results of the NIDDK long-term follow-up study. Am J Transplant 2010;10(6):1420-7.
4. Deschênes M, Belle SH, Krom RA, et al. Early allograft dysfunction after liver transplantation: a definition and predictors of outcome. National Institute of Diabetes and Digestive and Kidney Diseases Liver Transplantation Database. Transplantation 1998;66:302-10.
5. Olthoff KM, Kulik L, Samstein B, et al. Validation of a current definition of early allograft dysfunction in liver transplant recipients and analysis of risk factors. Liver Transpl 2010;16:943-9.
6. Almusa O, Federle MP. Abdominal imaging and intervention in liver transplantation. Liver Transpl 2006;12:184-93.
7. McGuire BM, Rosenthal P, Brown CC, et al. Long-term management of the liver transplant patient: recommendations for the primary care doctor. Am J Transplant 2009;9(9):1988-2003.
8. Moser M, Wall W. Management of biliary problems after liver transplantation. Liver Transpl 2001;7:S46-52.
9. Sawyer RG, Punch JD. Incidence and management of biliary complications after 291 liver transplants following the introduction of transcystic stenting. Transplantation 1998;66:1201-7.
10. Maheshwari A, Maley W, Li Z, et al. Biliary complications and outcomes of liver transplantation from donors after cardiac death. Liver Transpl 2007;13:1645-53.
11. Thethy S, Thomson BNJ, Pleass H, et al. Management of biliary tract complications after orthotopic liver transplantation. Clin Transplant 2004;18:647-53.
12. Antunes M, Teixeira A, Fortuna P, et al. Infections after liver transplantation: a retrospective, single-center study. Transplant Proc 2015;47(4):1019-24.
13. Maluf DG, Stravitz RT, Cotterell AH, et al. Adult living donor versus deceased donor liver transplantation: a 6-year single center experience. Am J Transplant 2005;5:149.
14. Bhat M, Al-Busafi S, Deschênes M, et al. Care of the liver transplant patient. Can J Gastroenterol Hepatol 2014;28(4):213-9.
15. Sampathkumar P, Paya CV. Management of cytomegalovirus infection after liver transplantation. Liver Transpl 2000;6:144-56.
16. Bruminhent J, Razonable RR. Management of cytomegalovirus infection and disease in liver transplant recipients. World J Hepatol 2014;6(6):370-83.

17. Charlton M. Recurrence of hepatitis C infection: where are we now? Liver Transpl 2005;11(Suppl 2):S57–62.
18. Seehofer D, Berg T. Prevention of hepatitis B recurrence after liver transplantation. Transplantation 2005;80(1 Suppl):S120–4.
19. Lim JK, Keeffe EB. Liver transplantation for alcoholic liver disease: current concepts and length of sobriety. Liver Transpl 2004;10:S31–8.
20. Kim RD, Reed AI, Fujita S, et al. Consensus and controversy in the management of hepatocellular carcinoma. J Am Coll Surg 2007;205:108–23.
21. Gautam M, Cheruvattath R, Balan V. Recurrence of autoimmune liver disease after liver transplantation: a systematic review. Liver Transpl 2006;12:1813–24.
22. Hubscher SG. Recurrent and de-novo disease in the liver allograft. Curr Opin Organ Transplant 2006;11:283–8.
23. Merola J, Liapakis A, Mulligan D, et al. Non-alcoholic fatty liver disease following liver transplantation: a clinical review. Clin Transplant 2015;29(9):728–37.
24. Hübscher SG. What is the long-term outcome of the liver allograft? J Hepatol 2011;55(3):702–17.
25. Parikh ND, Levitsky J. Hepatotoxicity and drug interactions in liver transplant candidates and recipients. Clin Liver Dis 2013;17(4):737–47.
26. Hoofnagle JH, Nelson KE, Purcell RH. Hepatitis E. N Engl J Med 2012;376:1237–44.
27. Koning L, Charlton MR, Pas SD, et al. Prevalence and clinical consequences of Hepatitis E in patients who underwent liver transplantation for chronic Hepatitis C in the United States. BMC Infect Dis 2015;15(1):371.
28. Available at: http://www.cdc.gov/hepatitis/hev/labtestingrequests.htm. Accessed September 4, 2015.
29. Sgourakis G, Radtke A, Fouzas I, et al. Corticosteroid-free immunosuppression in liver transplantation: a meta-analysis and meta-regression of outcomes. Transpl Int 2009;22:892–905.
30. Stanca CM, Fiel MI, Kontorinis N, et al. Chronic ductopenic rejection in patients with recurrent hepatitis C virus treated with pegylated interferon alfa-2a and ribavirin. Transplantation 2007;84(2):180–6.
31. Charlton M, Gane E, Manns MP, et al. Sofosbuvir and ribavirin for treatment of compensated recurrent hepatitis C virus infection after liver transplantation. Gastroenterology 2015;148(1):108–17.
32. Kwo PY, Mantry PS, Coakley E, et al. An interferon-free antiviral regimen for HCV after liver transplantation. N Engl J Med 2014;371(25):2375–82.

Acute and Chronic Allograft Dysfunction in Kidney Transplant Recipients

 CrossMark

Ryan J. Goldberg, MD*, Francis L. Weng, MD, MSCE,
Praveen Kandula, MD, MPH

KEYWORDS

- Kidney transplant • Allograft rejection • Allograft failure • Diagnostic evaluation

KEY POINTS

- Allograft dysfunction after a kidney transplant is often clinically asymptomatic and is usually detected as an increase in serum creatinine level, which corresponds with a decrease in the glomerular filtration rate.
- Kidney allograft dysfunction requires prompt evaluation with tests such as a transplant ultrasonography, radionuclide imaging, and allograft biopsy.
- Early causes of allograft dysfunction that manifest during the first 6 months after transplant include hyperacute rejection, thrombosis, urologic causes (urine leak, ureteral obstruction), and thrombotic microangiopathy.
- Some causes of allograft dysfunction, such as acute rejection, medication toxicity from calcineurin inhibitors, and BK virus nephropathy, can occur early or later after a kidney transplant.
- Other later causes, which usually occur 6 months or more after transplant, include transplant glomerulopathy, recurrent glomerulonephritis, and renal artery stenosis.

INTRODUCTION

Among recipients of kidney transplants, a primary concern of patients and their physicians is the function of the kidney allograft. Transplant nephrologists and surgeons seek to minimize the unwanted, deleterious side effects of transplants (eg, malignancies,[1] infections,[2] and diabetes mellitus[3]) while simultaneously maximizing the function and survival of the allograft (and patient). A well-functioning kidney transplant is ultimately associated with better allograft and patient survival.[4–7] Therefore, allograft dysfunction, whether it occurs early or later in the posttransplant period, is a cause for

Disclosures: The authors have nothing to disclose.
Renal & Pancreas Transplant Division, Saint Barnabas Medical Center, Livingston, NJ, USA
* Corresponding author. Renal & Pancreas Transplant Division, Saint Barnabas Medical Center, East Wing, Suite 305, 94 Old Short Hills Road, Livingston, NJ, 07039
E-mail address: rygoldberg@barnabashealth.org

immediate concern and action. This article reviews the symptoms, testing, differential diagnosis, treatment, and management of allograft dysfunction.

SYMPTOMS

Allograft dysfunction following kidney transplant usually manifests as an increase in the serum creatinine concentration, which corresponds with a decrease in the estimated glomerular filtration rate (eGFR). Other, less common presentations of allograft dysfunction include (1) proteinuria, (2) a sudden reduction in urine output, (3) failure of an expected reduction in creatinine level; or (4) pain over the allograft site (rarely). Causes can be medical or surgical, and a methodical approach almost always leads to a diagnosis. Approaches to categorizing allograft dysfunction include a temporal approach (acute vs chronic, early vs late), immune versus nonimmune causes, or the traditional etiologic approach used in native kidneys (prerenal vs intrinsic vs postrenal). This article categorizes the causes of allograft dysfunction as early versus later (**Box 1**). These causes can also be categorized within the traditional etiologic framework (**Table 1**). This article emphasizes transplant-specific causes of allograft dysfunction, but the traditional causes of acute and chronic kidney disease in native kidneys also occur in kidney transplants.

DIAGNOSTIC TESTING AND IMAGING STUDIES
Assessment of Allograft Function

Function of a kidney allograft is usually measured by the serum creatinine concentration and associated eGFR.[8] The eGFR of a kidney allograft is typically calculated using creatinine-based estimating equations, such as the Modification of Diet in Renal Disease study equations or the Chronic Kidney Disease Epidemiology Collaboration

---

Box 1
Some causes of kidney allograft dysfunction

Early (<6 months posttransplant)

Hyperacute rejection[a]

Thrombosis (of transplant renal artery or renal vein)[a]

Acute rejection

Urinary leak

Obstruction of transplant collecting system

BK polyoma virus infection

Calcineurin inhibitor toxicity

Later (6 months or more posttransplant)

Acute rejection

BK polyoma virus infection

Transplant renal artery stenosis

Calcineurin inhibitor toxicity

Chronic antibody-mediated rejection and transplant glomerulopathy

Recurrent glomerulonephritis

[a] Usually occurs in immediate (<1 week) posttransplant period.

Table 1 Common causes of kidney allograft dysfunction		
Prerenal	**Renal**	**Postrenal**

• Intrarenal vasoconstriction:
  ○ Medications:
    ■ CNI
    ■ ACEI/ARB
    ■ NSAIDs
  ○ Cardiorenal syndrome
  ○ Hypercalcemia (seen from preexisting secondary or tertiary hyperparathyroidism)
• Systemic vasodilatation from sepsis
• Volume depletion
  ○ Blood loss (intraoperative or postoperative)
  ○ Vomiting or diarrhea (medication or infection related)
  ○ Osmotic diuresis from uncontrolled hyperglycemia (steroids/CNIs)
	• Recurrent glomerular diseases (FSGS, membranous, IgA nephropathy)
	• Thrombotic microangiopathy
	• Acute rejection
	• Chronic rejection/transplant glomerulopathy
	• Medications (CNIs, mTORi, sulfamethoxazole-trimethoprim)
	• Infections: BK virus
		• Benign prostatic hypertrophy
		• Bladder detrusor dysfunction from long-standing anuria/oliguria or diabetic neuropathy
		• Ureteral obstruction from edema, necrosis, or stenosis
		• Urinary leak
		• Lymphocele, hematoma, or urinoma

Abbreviations: ACEI, angiotensin-converting enzyme inhibitors; ARB, angiotensin receptor blockers; CNI, calcineurin inhibitors; FSGS, focal segmental glomerulosclerosis; IgA, immunoglobulin A; mTORi, mammalian target of rapamycin inhibitors; NSAIDs, nonsteroidal antiinflammatory drugs.

equation.[9,10] These equations were originally developed to assess eGFR in native kidneys and calculate the eGFR using the serum creatinine level as well as demographic and clinical variables. When providing results of routine metabolic panels, clinical laboratories now often provide the calculated eGFR alongside the creatinine values. A detailed discussion of the merits of each creatinine-based estimating equation as well as other and newer markers of kidney function (eg, cystatin C) is beyond the scope of this article.[8–11] The eGFR is usually measured frequently (up to twice weekly) during the initial posttransplant months and then every 2 to 4 weeks during the rest of the first posttransplant year.[12] After the first posttransplant year, the eGFR should still be estimated every 2 to 3 months.[12]

Most transplant clinicians consider a 15% decrement in eGFR or 0.3-mg/dL increase in serum creatinine level as significant and worthy of further investigation. In native kidneys, a 0.3-mg/dL increase in creatinine level is incorporated into the staging system used by the Acute Kidney Injury Network.[13] Within 3 months of transplant, most kidney transplant recipients have a steady baseline creatinine level and eGFR that can serve as a basis for comparison.

Allograft dysfunction may also be detected using urinalyses and urinary tests. Proteinuria (including albuminuria) is a recognized sign of kidney damage in native kidneys as well as kidney allografts.[14,15] Proteinuria can usually be detected on routine urinalysis and then subsequently quantified, by either 24-hour urine collection or a spot protein/creatinine ratio from a morning urine specimen.[16] Some kidney transplant recipients have pretransplant urine output with proteinuria, which may muddle interpretation of posttransplant urinalyses. However, in most transplant recipients, pretransplant proteinuria from the native kidneys declines rapidly, usually becoming undetectable within 1 to 3 months following the transplant.[17,18] Other urinary abnormalities, such as hematuria or casts, are also useful in detecting and diagnosing allograft dysfunction. Urinalysis and urine protein excretion should be assessed regularly posttransplant; at least every 2 to 3 months during the first posttransplant year and at least annually thereafter.[12]

Radiographic Imaging of the Kidney Allograft

Gray-scale ultrasonography with color Doppler of the kidney allograft is a crucial part of the evaluation of allograft dysfunction and usually the modality of choice for an initial imaging study (**Table 2**).[12,19,20] Ultrasonography is noninvasive, does not subject the patient to any unnecessary radiation, and avoids the potential toxic complications of contrast agents. Ultrasonography is especially useful in the diagnosis and exclusion of (1) urologic and collecting system abnormalities, such as ureteral obstruction from lymphoceles, urinomas (from urine leaks), and other perinephric collections; and (2) vascular causes of allograft dysfunction, such as stenosis of the renal artery or

Table 2
Imaging modalities commonly used in evaluation of kidney allograft dysfunction

Imaging Modality	Causes of Allograft Dysfunction That Can Be Diagnosed	Advantages	Disadvantages
Ultrasonography	Perinephric collections (lymphocele, hematoma, urinoma, abscess) Ureteral obstructions (stones) Bladder dysfunction Subcutaneous collections Renal vessel thrombosis (using color Doppler) Postbiopsy arteriovenous fistulas	Noninvasive No exposure to radiation or contrast dye Can be done at bedside	Operator dependent Bowel gas can impede evaluation Exact delineations of deeper collections may not be clear
Radionuclide imaging (nuclear scan)	Renal vessel thrombosis Ureteral obstruction, urinary leaks Intrinsic kidney dysfunction	Noninvasive Can be useful to diagnose functional obstruction	Time consuming Expensive (?)
CT scan	Perinephric collections (lymphocele, hematoma, urinoma, abscess) Ureteral obstructions (stones) Subcutaneous collections	Noninvasive More specific than ultrasonography	Radiation exposure May need use of contrast dye
MRI	Renal vessel abnormalities	Noninvasive	Expensive May need use of contrast dye

Abbreviation: CT, computed tomography.

thrombosis of the renal artery or vein. Ultrasonography is less useful in the diagnosis of intrinsic, parenchymal causes of allograft dysfunction (eg, acute rejection), which usually require biopsy to diagnose. Ultrasonography can also image the bladder and provide the postvoid residual, if any. Mild hydronephrosis and dilatation may be present within the transplant collecting system and do not necessarily reflect true obstruction.[21] However, increasing hydronephrosis seen on repeated studies may indicate a true obstructive process.

Radionuclide imaging is another noninvasive modality that is especially useful for the diagnosis of some urologic and vascular causes of allograft dysfunction.[20] A radiolabeled tracer, usually either ^{99m}technetium mercaptoacetyltriglycine or ^{99m}technetium diethylenetriamine pentaacetate, is injected into the transplant recipient's venous system. A gamma camera documents any uptake of the tracer by the kidney allograft and excretion of the tracer into the urine and collecting system. In thrombosis of the transplant renal artery, there is no tracer uptake into the allograft. Radionuclide imaging can also help to diagnose urinary obstruction, in which excretion of tracer is delayed, or a urine leak, in which tracer is excreted into the peritransplant space and outside the collecting system. Like ultrasonography, radionuclide imaging is nonspecific and less useful in the diagnosis of intrinsic, parenchymal causes of allograft dysfunction.

Other imaging tests are occasionally used in the evaluation of allograft dysfunction. Computed tomography (CT) scans provide better anatomic detail of peritransplant collections, such as lymphoceles and hematomas. However, CT scans carry the risk of ionizing radiation, and the use of intravenous contrast dye (which is often unnecessary) carries an attendant risk of contrast nephropathy. MRI is occasionally used to diagnose or evaluate allograft dysfunction (eg, to image the transplant vasculature). However, use of gadolinium-based contrast agents with MRI carries the risk of nephrogenic systemic fibrosis in patients with eGFR less than 30 mL/min.[22]

Kidney Allograft Biopsy

The definitive diagnosis of most intrinsic causes of allograft dysfunction (eg, acute rejection, BK virus nephropathy) requires a biopsy of the kidney allograft. Allograft biopsies are usually performed percutaneously under ultrasonography (or sometimes CT) guidance. As an invasive procedure, an allograft biopsy carries a small risk of complications, such as hematuria, perinephric hematoma, and arteriovenous fistula.[23–25] The risk of biopsy-related complications is probably lower in biopsies of transplanted kidney than biopsies of native kidneys.[23]

EARLY POSTTRANSPLANT CAUSES OF ALLOGRAFT DYSFUNCTION (UP TO 6 MONTHS POSTTRANSPLANT)

During the peritransplant and early posttransplant periods, new kidney transplant recipients are usually under the care of the transplant team, which includes surgeons and nephrologists. During the immediate postoperative period, the urine output and serum creatinine level are assessed daily or more frequently, to ensure early detection of any complications. Patients typically spend 3 to 7 days in the hospital recovering from the transplant surgery while the transplant team monitors their allograft function. After the initial hospitalization, kidney transplant recipients are seen regularly by their transplant team for approximately 3 to 6 months, after which they start to return to their local nephrologists and primary care providers.

There are several notable causes of early allograft dysfunction. Some causes tend to occur nearly immediately or in the initial posttransplant hours and days (eg, thrombosis, hyperacute rejection), whereas others occur in the first few weeks and months posttransplant. his article focusses on causes of allograft dysfunction that are specific to kidney transplant recipients. Other causes (eg, prerenal azotemia from diarrhea) are possible and should be entertained. The early posttransplant causes of allograft function typically occur while the transplant recipient is still under the regular care of the transplant team, but primary care providers may encounter allograft dysfunction during the early posttransplant period.

Thrombosis

Thrombosis of either the transplant renal artery or the transplant renal vein is a serious cause of early allograft dysfunction that is associated with high rates of allograft loss. However, thrombosis is rare and is seen in as few as 1% to 3% of transplants.[26]

Transplant renal artery thrombosis (RAT) is painless and presents as a sudden cessation of urine output with either increase in the creatinine level or failure of the creatinine level to decrease as anticipated. RAT can stem from technical reasons, such as intraoperative intimal dissection, kinking, or torsion, and tends to occur in recipients with hypercoagulable states or with allografts that have multiple arteries. Diagnosis can be made using Doppler ultrasonography of transplant vessels or radionuclide imaging.[27,28] Salvage of the allograft requires urgent thrombectomy, but the prolonged duration of ischemia between the occurrence of RAT and its diagnosis usually prevents such salvage. Transplant nephrectomy is usually performed.[29]

Similarly, transplant renal vein thrombosis (RVT) can have technical causes, such as a renal vein that is too short or too long; kinking or clamp injury; extrinsic compression from hematomas or lymphoceles; or other anatomic reasons. Compared with RAT, RVT is more forgiving, with a higher chance of graft survival if the thrombus is removed. Occasionally, patients complain of pain over the allograft, caused by vascular engorgement from venous outflow obstruction. As in RAT, diagnosis is based on ultrasonography of the vessels and radionuclide imaging.[27,28] Contrast venograms are rarely performed, given their invasive nature and requirement for contrast dye. Thrombectomy is the treatment of choice for RVT. If the allograft is not salvageable, then nephrectomy is required, especially given the risk of allograft rupture.[30]

Hyperacute Rejection

As implied by its name, hyperacute rejection occurs when the recipient's immune system immediately rejects the newly transplanted kidney, typically intraoperatively on reperfusion of the allograft. Hyperacute rejection is caused by preexisting antibodies in the recipient that are directed against donor antigens. With widespread use of pretransplant immune-phenotyping and cross-matching techniques, hyperacute rejection is now almost nonexistent, even among immunologically high-risk recipients.[31,32] In hyperacute rejection, the allograft initially perfuses only to turn cyanotic. There is significant tenderness over the kidney allograft, and it becomes firm to palpation. Hyperacute rejection must be distinguished from vascular catastrophes such as RAT and RVT. Doppler ultrasonography or nuclear imaging reveals delayed or absent perfusion. Surgical exploration and, usually, removal of allograft is warranted.

Delayed Allograft Function and Acute Tubular Necrosis

During the first few days and week after a kidney transplant, the transplant may not initially function and may have DGF.[33] DGF is generally defined as the need for dialysis treatment during the first week after transplant. The most common cause of DGF is acute tubular necrosis (ATN), which may already have been present at the time of organ procurement (caused by kidney injury in deceased donors). ATN may also stem from a prolonged time period between the procurement of the donor kidney and the transplant (which includes cold ischemia time and warm ischemia time) or from ischemia-reperfusion injury. ATN can also develop following transplant, caused by hypotension, volume depletion, and nephrotoxic medications. Although a pathologic description, ATN is not always confirmed on biopsy. The general outcomes for ATN are spontaneous, eventual resolution. Dialytic support may be need while awaiting recovery from ATN. To date, no specific therapeutic interventions implemented posttransplant have helped reduce the incidence of, or recovery from, ATN.

Urinary Leaks

Urinary leaks are seen within the first few weeks following kidney transplant.[34] The extravasation of urine outside the urologic collecting system can manifest as persistent drainage from the wound or any surgical drains, decreased urine output, increase in serum creatinine level, allograft incisional tenderness, fever, or pain or swelling of the abdomen or scrotum. Leaks often arise from the site of ureteroneocystostomy. They are unlikely in the presence of ureteral stents, which are routinely placed at the time of the transplant surgery at some centers. Urinary leaks can accumulate around the allograft as collections (urinomas) that can be seen on ultrasonography or CT scan.[28] Common causes for urinary leaks are ischemia to the distal ureter (usually from sacrificing or ligating an artery to the lower pole of the kidney that simultaneously supplies the distal ureter), surgical trauma, or tension from a short ureter. Diagnosis can be made by checking drain fluid or aspirated fluid (in case of urinoma) for its creatinine concentration; if the fluid is from urine, then its creatinine concentration is much higher than in serum creatinine. Confirmation of a urinary leak can be made by radionuclide imaging, voiding cystogram or antegrade nephrostogram, or cystoscopy.[35]

The first step in management of urinary leak is placement of a Foley catheter and a ureteral stent if possible. Small urinary leaks may heal without further intervention,[36] but large or persistent leaks may require operative intervention.[37] Operative treatments of a urinary leak include reimplantation of the transplant ureter into the bladder or ureteroureterostomy, using the native ureter. Occasionally, if this is not possible, the bladder may need to be mobilized and, in rare instances, a ureterostomy may be needed.

Urinary Obstruction

Obstructive uropathy following a transplant can be ureteral or bladder related. Ureteral obstruction can be intrinsic (from ureteral edema, blood clots, stones, or strictures) or extrinsic (caused by compression by urinoma, lymphocele, or hematoma).

Complications with the transplant ureter may be detected with ultrasonography. Confirmation of the obstruction can be made with radionuclide imaging, which assesses excretory function and identifies the location of obstruction. Transplant ureter obstruction is painless because of the absence of innervation in the transplanted kidney, whereas bladder outlet obstruction can be painful.

Ureteral stenosis is reported to occur in 2.4% to 6.5% of kidney transplants.[38] Hydronephrosis or hydroureter without any evidence of a fluid collection or stone may suggest ureteral stenosis. Most ureter complications occur during the first year after the transplant, but cases have been reported years after surgery. Ureteral stenosis is typically thought to be caused by ischemia-induced fibrosis and necrosis of the donor ureter caused by a compromised blood supply.[38] Other triggers for stenosis include recurrent infections, rejection, and BK virus. Relief and correction of most ureteral complications require invasive procedures, such as cystoscopic placement of a ureteral stent, percutaneous placement of a nephrostomy tube, or surgical recon-struction of the transplant ureter.[37,39]

Lymphoceles are another cause of posttransplant urinary obstruction. Lymphoceles develop from surgically disrupted lymphatic vessels and are usually small and asymp-tomatic. Most develop within 2 to 6 weeks after a transplant, but they may also occur and become symptomatic later in the first year posttransplant. Their reported incidence varies widely, ranging up to nearly 20% in some series.[40–42] If large, lymphoceles can cause a mass effect on neighboring structures such as the ureter, causing obstruction. Less commonly, lymphoceles can compress the transplant or native vessels, causing thrombosis, bladder compression with irritation and incontinence, scrotal swelling, or vascular compression resulting lower extremity edema or deep vein thrombosis. The best method to diagnose lymphocele is via ultrasonography, although a CT scan may help to evaluate the collection's size and location if intervention is needed. Aspiration can confirm the lymphocele and exclude abscess or urinoma as the cause of the collec-tion. Small lymphoceles spontaneously resolve, but large ones may require interven-tion, especially if causing symptoms.[43] Percutaneous image-guided aspiration is usually not therapeutic, because the lymphocele often recurs. The standard surgical approach is creation of a peritoneal window either by laparoscopic or open technique. Injecting a sclerosing agent after inserting a drainage catheter is an option but is asso-ciated with risk of infection and recurrence and is not common.

Kidney transplant urolithiasis may also be diagnosed during the evaluation of possible postrenal kidney injury. It is an uncommon complication, occurring in approx-imately 1% or less of transplant recipients.[44] Treatment protocols include both percu-taneous nephrolithotripsy and shockwave lithotripsy.[44]

Bladder dysfunction (commonly seen in diabetics) or benign prostatic hypertrophy (especially in older men who have been oligoanuric for a long period before the trans-plant) can manifest as obstruction following removal of the Foley catheter. Ultrasonog-raphy is a reasonably sensitive diagnostic tool revealing hydronephrosis.

Acute Rejection

Early acute rejection can be mediated by T cells (acute cellular rejection) or antibodies (acute antibody-mediated rejection). Acute cellular rejection (ACR) usually manifests beyond 1 week of the transplant. Donor tissue antigens are presented to the recipi-ent's immune system via antigen-presenting cells such as macrophages, Langerhans cells, or B cells, which leads to a proliferation of donor-specific sensitized T cells (cyto-toxic CD8 T cells) in the regional lymph nodes that infiltrate the allograft and mediate cell damage. Acute rejection manifests as a reduction in urine output, increase in creatinine level, or plateauing of a decreasing creatinine level. The classic findings of pain and fever seen with hyperacute rejection are usually not seen with ACR. How-ever, allograft dysfunction and associated oliguria can lead to volume overload, hyper-tension, and electrolyte abnormalities.

The incidence of ACR during the first year posttransplant has decreased to 10% or less.[45] This low rate of ACR likely stems from the widespread use of induction immu-nosuppression at the time of transplant, especially T cell–depleting agents such as rabbit antithymocyte globulin. ACR is a pathologic diagnosis and requires a kidney allograft biopsy to confirm the diagnosis. The severity of ACR is graded using a peri-odically upgraded grading system known as the Banff Criteria.[46,47] Most early ACRs can be treated effectively with several days of either high-dose intravenous corticoste-roids or rabbit antithymocyte globulin.

Antibody-mediated rejection (AMR) can be acute or chronic. Early AMR usually oc-curs when the recipient harbors preexisting antibodies, which can be seen in ABO blood group or human leukocyte antigen (HLA)–incompatible transplants. In HLA-incompatible transplants, the recipients are sensitized and have preexisting anti-HLA antibodies, which can arise from previous blood transfusions, pregnancies, transplants, or infections. Anti-HLA antibodies mediate their effects via activation of the complement system. Clinical manifestations of AMR are similar to those of ACR but can be differentiated on allograft biopsy. A cornerstone of diagnosis of AMR is the presence of C4d (a complement activation remnant) that is seen in the endothelia of peritubular capillaries. Like ACR, AMR is gauged using the Banff Criteria.[48–51]

Treatment of AMR usually involves some combination of steroids, plasmapheresis, and intravenous immunoglobulin. Rituximab,[52] bortezomib,[53] eculizumab, and splenectomy[54] may also have a role. Treatment and management of AMR almost always require the expertise of the transplant center. The outcomes of early AMR are usually better than the outcomes of late-onset acute AMR.[55]

BK Virus Nephropathy

BK virus is a polyomavirus that causes disease primarily in immunocompromised hosts. After primary infection, the virus remains latent in genitourinary cells. In immunosuppressed kidney transplant recipients, the virus can reactivate and cause tubulointerstitial nephritis and, in late cases, ureteral stenosis. Patients are asymptomatic with active infection. BK virus infection in transplant recipients is usually seen in the first year. BK virus screening is done either in urine or blood at regular intervals. When BK viremia develops, the mainstay of treatment is reduction in immunosuppression, with close monitoring of allograft function.[56] Allograft biopsy can confirm BK virus nephropathy but, in many instances (given the medullary location of the virus), biopsy can be falsely negative. In general, a serum viral load of more than 10,000 copies/mL is suggestive of BK virus nephropathy.[57]

Thrombotic Microangiopathy

Thrombotic microangiopathy (TMA) can be a serious complication following a transplant.[58] It is particularly common among patients with a preexisting history of thrombotic thrombocytopenic purpura or atypical hemolytic ureic syndrome (aHUS). However, TMA can also be seen with calcineurin inhibitor (CNI) toxicity or as a manifestation of AMR. Rarely, patients with antiphospholipid antibody syndrome also have TMA. A common underlying mechanism in all these conditions is endothelial injury. Diagnosis is based on biopsy. Treatment may vary from removal of the causative agent (eg, changing CNIs to mammalian target of rapamycin inhibitors [mTORi]), aggressive plasmapheresis with AMR, or use of complement blockers such as eculizumab with aHUS.

Medication-associated Acute Allograft Dysfunction

The CNIs tacrolimus and cyclosporine are used in more than 90% of immunosuppression regimens for kidney transplants.[45] Although they are effective in preventing acute rejection, they can also be associated with nephrotoxicity. CNIs can cause a dose-related afferent arteriolar vasoconstriction that can reduce the glomerular filtration pressure and rate, thereby causing an increased creatinine level. Vasoconstriction can be mediated via an alteration in arachidonic acid metabolism (increase thromboxane and endothelin levels) or via altered NO pathway. These effects could be reversed with dose reduction. CNI toxicity can also manifest directly on tubules and is seen on transplant biopsy as isometric vacuolization. As mentioned earlier, CNIs are also associated with TMA.[59]

Patients on CNIs require monitoring of their trough drug concentrations to make sure that they are maintained at the appropriate level. This therapeutic drug monitoring is usually performed by the transplant center or general nephrologist. The CNIs are metabolized by the hepatic enzyme system cytochrome P-450 3A4, which is also responsible for the metabolism of numerous drugs. Many transplant patients are burdened by the necessity for polypharmacy, which increases the potential for drug interactions. Many medications (eg, antifungal, antibacterial, and antiretroviral agents) have the potential to interact with the CNIs (**Table 3**). These interactions can cause acute allograft dysfunction by either increasing the serum concentrations of the CNI (leading to nephrotoxicity) or decreasing the concentrations of the CNI (leading to sub-therapeutic levels and an increase chance of acute rejection). To minimize the chances of medication-induced acute allograft dysfunction, health care providers should remain in close communication with the transplant team and check for drug-drug interactions when prescribing new medications to transplant recipients.

Sulfamethoxazole-trimethoprim (SMP-TMP) is prescribed in transplant recipients as prophylaxis against pneumocystis infection. SMP-TMP can cause an increase in creatinine level by causing either an interstitial nephritis or by reducing creatinine secretion in the renal tubules. It can cause significant hyperkalemia, especially in the presence of other medications with similar side effects. Atovaquone and dapsone are alternatives if the patient is intolerant to SMP-TMP.

LATER CAUSES OF ALLOGRAFT DYSFUNCTION

After the immediate and early posttransplant period, the causes of allograft dysfunction are less often surgical and more often require confirmation via a kidney transplant biopsy. Stable patients greater than 1 year posttransplant are generally able to minimize the intensity of their clinic follow-up visits. Despite its limitations, the serum creatinine concentration is still the most widely used and most available biomarker to monitor allograft function and should still be followed several times a year.

Despite declines in acute rejection rates and improvement in short-term (0–6 month) and medium-term (1, 3, and 5 years) allograft survival, long-term allograft survival has failed to improve and continues to be a problem.[60] By 10 years after transplant, almost a third of all transplants have failed. Approximately 15% of the patients awaiting kidney transplants have a failed prior transplant,[45] making prior transplant failure one of the most common causes of end-stage kidney disease in the United States.

Acute Rejection

Although acute rejection most often occurs during the first few months posttransplant, it can still occur at any time. Nonadherence with transplant immunosuppressive

Table 3	
Common drugs that can interact with the CNIs cyclosporine and tacrolimus	
Antifungals	Azole antifungals decrease the clearance of CNIs
Antibiotics	Macrolide antibiotics decrease the clearance of CNIs
Antihypertensives	Nondihydropyridine calcium channel blockers decrease the clearance of CNIs
Antiretrovirals	Protease inhibitors greatly decrease the clearance of CNIs
Grapefruit juice	Decreases the clearance of CNIs
Antiepileptics	Phenytoin, carbamazepine, and phenobarbital may increase the clearance of CNIs

medications is an especially common, important, and frustrating cause of later acute rejection.[61] Treatment of later acute rejection is similar to the treatment of early acute rejection, but the outcomes of later acute rejection are suboptimal.[62]

Chronic Antibody-mediated Rejection

Chronic AMR is an increasingly common occurrence. Chronic AMR typically leads to transplant glomerulopathy, a chronic condition marked by significant glomerular changes that occurs most commonly in patients with humoral rejection. Transplant glomerulopathy is a challenging lesion to treat and often is a predictor of a poor prognosis.

Transplant kidney biopsies may also show chronic changes, including interstitial fibrosis and tubular atrophy. As previously mentioned, CNIs were blamed for much of the chronicity seen in late biopsies. However, other immune-mediated mechanisms are now being implicated as the pathophysiologic processes that need to be targeted to prevent later failure of kidney transplants.[63]

Transplant Renal Artery Stenosis

Transplant renal artery stenosis (TRAS) is associated with allograft dysfunction. The reported incidence of TRAS varies from 1% to 25%, but recent series have an incidence closer to 2% to 5%.[64,65] TRAS usually occurs between 3 months and 2 years after a transplant. Risk factors include technical issues with either the procurement or implantation of the donor kidney, older recipient age, marginal donor kidneys, delayed graft function, prolonged cold ischemia time, acute rejection, and cytomegalovirus infection. The stenosis can occur at any point along the renal transplant artery but is frequently near the surgical anastomosis between the donor's renal artery and recipient's artery, which is typically the external iliac artery.

Patient's with TRAS typically present with allograft dysfunction, worsening or refractory hypertension, and fluid retention. This constellation of symptoms is a direct result of the pathophysiology of TRAS. The stenosis decreases kidney perfusion, resulting in the activation of the renin-angiotensin system causing sodium retention and volume expansion.

The diagnosis of TRAS is made by imaging the renal artery. Invasive angiography makes the definitive diagnosis; however, it has the risk of various complications. Doppler ultrasonography, magnetic resonance angiography, and spiral CT angiography are also all well described as suitable diagnostic choices.[66] Ultrasonography is often used as the initial modality, because it does not require administration of a contrast agent and can therefore be performed at any degree of kidney dysfunction. TRAS is usually diagnosed when acceleration time in the transplant renal and intrarenal arteries is greater than or equal to 0.1 second, peak systolic velocity in the transplant renal artery is greater than 200 cm/s, or a ratio of peak systolic velocity in the transplant renal artery/external iliac artery is greater than 1.8.[67]

The allograft dysfunction caused by TRAS is potentially reversible with timely diagnosis and treatment. Endovascular intervention with percutaneous transluminal angioplasty with or without a bare-metal stent is usually the first-line therapy.[68,69] Surgical repair is reserved for cases in which angioplasty is unsuccessful.

Recurrent Glomerulonephritis and Native Kidney Disease

Glomerulonephritis (GN) constitutes one of the most common reasons for kidney failure and the need for transplant, but its incidence may be imprecise because a specific diagnosis is not made frequently before a transplant. Most forms of GN have an immunologic basis, so the standard use of immunosuppression in kidney transplantation makes recurrence less likely. Nevertheless, recurrence of GN following a kidney transplant affects between 10% and 20% of patients and accounts for 8% to 41% of graft failures at 10 years[70–73] (**Table 4**).

Rates of recurrence vary depending on the type of GN. Histologic recurrence (without significant clinical impact on serum creatinine level) is very common with immunoglobulin A nephropathy (40%–60%).[74] Primary focal segmental glomerulosclerosis (FSGS) is highly likely to recur, especially in the presence of an earlier failed transplant from recurrence, with recurrence rates reported up to 50%.[75,76] Recurrent FSGS is also common among recipients whose kidney disease was diagnosed at a very early age or who had rapid progression to dialysis following the transplant. Primary membranous nephropathy can recur very early (within the first year of transplant) and is associated with a high rate of graft loss. More recently, the identification of the pathogenic role of anti–phospholipase A2 receptor antibodies may help in identifying patients at risk for recurrence of membranous disease.[77–79] Atypical hemolytic uremic syndrome, membranoproliferative GN, and C3 glomerulopathy have recurrence rates as high as 40% in some studies.[80–82] When a specific GN diagnosis is confirmed to be present before a transplant, recurrence should always be in the differential of acute allograft dysfunction. Allograft biopsy is the gold standard for diagnosis.

Chronic Toxicity from Calcineurin Inhibitors and Other Medications

Almost since their introduction, CNIs have also been blamed for chronic allograft dysfunction. The search for immunosuppressive medications that allow the reduction or elimination of CNIs without sacrificing acute rejection rates has been a major research focus for decades. In the 1990s, the histologic lesion describing progressive fibrosis and vascular injury, termed chronic allograft nephropathy (CAN), was identified to be a major cause of graft loss. CNIs were known to cause fibrosis, so it was hypothesized that CAN was a consequence of long-term CNI use. In 2007, the revised Banff classification system renamed CAN to interstitial fibrosis and tubular atrophy (IF/TA) without any specific cause, with the expectation that a more specific cause could one day be identified.[83] More recently, there has been more debate on the theory that CNIs themselves are the sole cause of IF/TA. Investigators argue that the CNI-associated lesion is a diagnosis of exclusion made in clinical situations in which no other explanation can be identified.

Table 4
Frequency of clinically relevant GN recurrence after kidney transplant

Cause	Frequency (%)
Atypical hemolytic uremic syndrome	>50
Membranoproliferative GN	
Type 1 (immune-complex mediated)	20–50
Type 2 (complement mediated)	>50
Focal segmental glomerulosclerosis	20–40
IgA nephropathy	10–25
Membranous nephropathy	5–30
Antineutrophil cytoplasmic antibody–associated GN	15–20
Systemic lupus erythematosus–associated GN	5–30
Antiglomerular basement membrane antibody	<5

From Floege J, Regel H, Gesualdo L. The ERA-EDTA database on recurrent glomerulonephritis following renal transplantation. Nephrol Dial Transplant 2014;29(1):15–21; with permission.

The mTORi sirolimus and everolimus are a group of antimetabolite immunosuppressive agents that are used either together with or as an alternative to the CNIs. The mTORi have been associated with development of de novo or worsening proteinuria, nephrotic syndrome, and FSGS.[84-86] mTORi have also been implicated in delaying wound healing and recovery from ATN. As a result, mTORi are not commonly used among the initial immunosuppressive agents. Instead, patients are sometimes converted from their CNIs to an mTORi, whether because of side effects attributed to their CNIs or for other reasons.

SUMMARY

Acute and chronic allograft dysfunction can occur early or later after a kidney transplant. Allograft dysfunction is often clinically asymptomatic and is usually detected as an increase in serum creatinine level and decrease in glomerular filtration rate. The diagnostic evaluation may include bloodwork, urinalysis, transplant ultrasonography, radionuclide imaging, and allograft biopsy. Whether it occurs early or later after transplant, allograft dysfunction requires prompt evaluation to determine its cause and subsequent management. Early causes of dysfunction can be immediate, in the first hours and days after transplant, or they can occur during the initial 6 months after transplant. Early causes of allograft dysfunction include hyperacute rejection, thrombosis, urologic causes (urine leak, ureteral obstruction), and thrombotic microangiopathy. Acute rejection, medication toxicity from CNIs, and BK virus nephropathy can occur early or later. Other later causes, which usually occur 6 or more months after transplant, include transplant glomerulopathy, recurrent GN, and renal artery stenosis.

REFERENCES

1. Engels EA, Pfeiffer RM, Fraumeni JF Jr, et al. Spectrum of cancer risk among US solid organ transplant recipients. JAMA 2011;306:1891–901.
2. Fishman JA. Infection in solid-organ transplant recipients. N Engl J Med 2007; 357:2601–14.
3. Bloom RD, Crutchlow MF. New-onset diabetes mellitus in the kidney recipient: diagnosis and management strategies. Clin J Am Soc Nephrol 2008;3(Suppl 2):S38–48.
4. Heaphy EL, Poggio ED, Flechner SM, et al. Risk factors for retransplant kidney recipients: relisting and outcomes from patients' primary transplant. Am J Transplant 2014;14:1356–67.
5. Schnitzler MA, Lentine KL, Axelrod D, et al. Use of 12-month renal function and baseline clinical factors to predict long-term graft survival: application to BENEFIT and BENEFIT-EXT trials. Transplantation 2012;93:172–81.
6. Woo YM, Jardine AG, Clark AF, et al. Early graft function and patient survival following cadaveric renal transplantation. Kidney Int 1999;55:692–9.
7. Hariharan S, McBride MA, Cherikh WS, et al. Post-transplant renal function in the first year predicts long-term kidney transplant survival. Kidney Int 2002;62:311–8.
8. Stevens LA, Coresh J, Greene T, et al. Assessing kidney function–measured and estimated glomerular filtration rate. N Engl J Med 2006;354:2473–83.
9. Earley A, Miskulin D, Lamb EJ, et al. Estimating equations for glomerular filtration rate in the era of creatinine standardization: a systematic review. Ann Intern Med 2012;156:785–95.
10. Levey AS, Stevens LA, Schmid CH, et al. A new equation to estimate glomerular filtration rate. Ann Intern Med 2009;150:604–12.

11. Buron F, Hadj-Aissa A, Dubourg L, et al. Estimating glomerular filtration rate in kidney transplant recipients: performance over time of four creatinine-based formulas. Transplantation 2011;92:1005–11.

12. Kidney Disease: Improving Global Outcomes (KDIGO) Transplant Work Group. KDIGO clinical practice guideline for the care of kidney transplant recipients. Am J Transplant 2009;9(Suppl 3):S1–155.

13. Mehta RL, Kellum JA, Shah SV, et al. Acute kidney injury network: report of an initiative to improve outcomes in acute kidney injury. Crit Care 2007;11:R31.

14. Amer H, Fidler ME, Myslak M, et al. Proteinuria after kidney transplantation, relationship to allograft histology and survival. Am J Transplant 2007;7:2748–56.

15. Amer H, Cosio FG. Significance and management of proteinuria in kidney transplant recipients. J Am Soc Nephrol 2009;20:2490–2.

16. Steinhauslin F, Wauters JP. Quantitation of proteinuria in kidney transplant patients: accuracy of the urinary protein/creatinine ratio. Clin Nephrol 1995;43: 110–5.

17. D'Cunha PT, Parasuraman R, Venkat KK. Rapid resolution of proteinuria of native kidney origin following live donor renal transplantation. Am J Transplant 2005;5: 351–5.

18. Myslak M, Amer H, Morales P, et al. Interpreting post-transplant proteinuria in patients with proteinuria pre-transplant. Am J Transplant 2006;6:1660–5.

19. Rodgers SK, Sereni CP, Horrow MM. Ultrasonographic evaluation of the renal transplant. Radiol Clin North Am 2014;52:1307–24.

20. Sharfuddin A. Renal relevant radiology: imaging in kidney transplantation. Clin J Am Soc Nephrol 2014;9:416–29.

21. Kashi SH, Lodge JP, Giles GR, et al. Ultrasonography of renal allografts: collecting system dilatation and its clinical significance. Nephrol Dial Transplant 1991;6: 358–62.

22. Lemy AA, del Marmol V, Kolivras A, et al. Revisiting nephrogenic systemic fibrosis in 6 kidney transplant recipients: a single-center experience. J Am Acad Dermatol 2010;63:389–99.

23. Preda A, Van Dijk LC, Van Oostaijen JA, et al. Complication rate and diagnostic yield of 515 consecutive ultrasound-guided biopsies of renal allografts and native kidneys using a 14-gauge Biopty gun. Eur Radiol 2003;13:527–30.

24. Schwarz A, Gwinner W, Hiss M, et al. Safety and adequacy of renal transplant protocol biopsies. Am J Transplant 2005;5:1992–6.

25. Wilczek HE. Percutaneous needle biopsy of the renal allograft. A clinical safety evaluation of 1129 biopsies. Transplantation 1990;50:790–7.

26. Matas AJ, Humar A, Gillingham KJ, et al. Five preventable causes of kidney graft loss in the 1990s: a single-center analysis. Kidney Int 2002;62:704–14.

27. Gao J, Ng A, Shih G, et al. Intrarenal color duplex ultrasonography: a window to vascular complications of renal transplants. J Ultrasound Med 2007;26:1403–18.

28. Brown ED, Chen MY, Wolfman NT, et al. Complications of renal transplantation: evaluation with US and radionuclide imaging. Radiographics 2000;20:607–22.

29. Ponticelli C, Moia M, Montagnino G. Renal allograft thrombosis. Nephrol Dial Transplant 2009;24:1388–93.

30. Richardson AJ, Higgins RM, Jaskowski AJ, et al. Spontaneous rupture of renal allografts: the importance of renal vein thrombosis in the cyclosporin era. Br J Surg 1990;77:558–60.

31. Montgomery RA, Locke JE, King KE, et al. ABO incompatible renal transplantation: a paradigm ready for broad implementation. Transplantation 2009;87: 1246–55.

32. Riella LV, Safa K, Yagan J, et al. Long-term outcomes of kidney transplantation across a positive complement-dependent cytotoxicity crossmatch. Transplantation 2014;97:1247–52.
33. Siedlecki A, Irish W, Brennan DC. Delayed graft function in the kidney transplant. Am J Transplant 2011;11:2279–96.
34. Di Carlo HN, Darras FS. Urologic considerations and complications in kidney transplant recipients. Adv Chronic Kidney Dis 2015;22:306–11.
35. Titton RL, Gervais DA, Hahn PF, et al. Urine leaks and urinomas: diagnosis and imaging-guided intervention. Radiographics 2003;23:1133–47.
36. Matalon TA, Thompson MJ, Patel SK, et al. Percutaneous treatment of urine leaks in renal transplantation patients. Radiology 1990;174:1049–51.
37. Berli JU, Montgomery JR, Segev DL, et al. Surgical management of early and late ureteral complications after renal transplantation: techniques and outcomes. Clin Transplant 2015;29:26–33.
38. Dreikorn K. Problems of the distal ureter in renal transplantation. Urol Int 1992;49: 76–89.
39. Giessing M. Transplant ureter stricture following renal transplantation: surgical options. Transplant Proc 2011;43:383–6.
40. Pengel LH, Liu LQ, Morris PJ. Do wound complications or lymphoceles occur more often in solid organ transplant recipients on mTOR inhibitors? a systematic review of randomized controlled trials. Transpl Int 2011;24:1216–30.
41. Derweesh IH, Ismail HR, Goldfarb DA, et al. Intraoperative placing of drains decreases the incidence of lymphocele and deep vein thrombosis after renal transplantation. BJU Int 2008;101:1415–9.
42. Cooper M, Wiseman AC, Zibari G, et al. Wound events in kidney transplant patients receiving de novo everolimus: a pooled analysis of three randomized controlled trials. Clin Transplant 2013;27:E625–35.
43. Lucewicz A, Wong G, Lam VW, et al. Management of primary symptomatic lymphocele after kidney transplantation: a systematic review. Transplantation 2011; 92:663–73.
44. Challacombe B, Dasgupta P, Tiptaft R, et al. Multimodal management of urolithiasis in renal transplantation. BJU Int 2005;96:385–9.
45. Department of Health and Human Services, Health Resources and Services Administration. Organ Procurement and Transplantation Network (OPTN) and Scientific Registry of Transplant Recipients (SRTR). OPTN/SRTR 2012 annual data report. Rockville (MD): 2014.
46. Racusen LC, Solez K, Colvin RB, et al. The Banff 97 working classification of renal allograft pathology. Kidney Int 1999;55:713–23.
47. Solez K, Colvin RB, Racusen LC, et al. Banff 07 classification of renal allograft pathology: updates and future directions. Am J Transplant 2008;8:753–60.
48. Racusen LC, Colvin RB, Solez K, et al. Antibody-mediated rejection criteria - an addition to the Banff 97 classification of renal allograft rejection. Am J Transplant 2003;3:708–14.
49. Sis B, Mengel M, Haas M, et al. Banff '09 meeting report: antibody mediated graft deterioration and implementation of Banff working groups. Am J Transplant 2010; 10:464–71.
50. Mengel M, Sis B, Haas M, et al. Banff 2011 meeting report: new concepts in antibody-mediated rejection. Am J Transplant 2012;12:563–70.
51. Haas M, Sis B, Racusen LC, et al. Banff 2013 meeting report: inclusion of c4d-negative antibody-mediated rejection and antibody-associated arterial lesions. Am J Transplant 2014;14:272–83.

52. Becker YT, Becker BN, Pirsch JD, et al. Rituximab as treatment for refractory kidney transplant rejection. Am J Transplant 2004;4:996–1001.
53. Everly MJ, Everly JJ, Susskind B, et al. Bortezomib provides effective therapy for antibody- and cell-mediated acute rejection. Transplantation 2008;86:1754–61.
54. Locke JE, Zachary AA, Haas M, et al. The utility of splenectomy as rescue treatment for severe acute antibody mediated rejection. Am J Transplant 2007;7: 842–6.
55. Dorje C, Midtvedt K, Holdaas H, et al. Early versus late acute antibody-mediated rejection in renal transplant recipients. Transplantation 2013;96:79–84.
56. Hardinger KL, Koch MJ, Bohl DJ, et al. BK-virus and the impact of pre-emptive immunosuppression reduction: 5-year results. Am J Transplant 2010;10:407–15.
57. Sawinski D, Goral S. BK virus infection: an update on diagnosis and treatment. Nephrol Dial Transplant 2015;30:209–17.
58. Nadasdy T. Thrombotic microangiopathy in renal allografts: the diagnostic challenge. Curr Opin Organ Transplant 2014;19:283–92.
59. Naesens M, Kuypers DR, Sarwal M. Calcineurin inhibitor nephrotoxicity. Clin J Am Soc Nephrol 2009;4:481–508.
60. Stegall MD, Gaston RS, Cosio FG, et al. Through a glass darkly: seeking clarity in preventing late kidney transplant failure. J Am Soc Nephrol 2015;26:20–9.
61. Butler JA, Roderick P, Mullee M, et al. Frequency and impact of nonadherence to immunosuppressants after renal transplantation: a systematic review. Transplantation 2004;77:769–76.
62. Wu K, Budde K, Schmidt D, et al. Pathologic characteristics of early or late acute cellular rejection and outcome after kidney transplant. Exp Clin Transplant 2014; 12:314–22.
63. Gaston RS. Chronic calcineurin inhibitor nephrotoxicity: reflections on an evolving paradigm. Clin J Am Soc Nephrol 2009;4:2029–34.
64. Hurst FP, Abbott KC, Neff RT, et al. Incidence, predictors and outcomes of transplant renal artery stenosis after kidney transplantation: analysis of USRDS. Am J Nephrol 2009;30:459–67.
65. Hernandez D, Rufino M, Armas S, et al. Retrospective analysis of surgical complications following cadaveric kidney transplantation in the modern transplant era. Nephrol Dial Transplant 2006;21:2908–15.
66. Browne RF, Tuite DJ. Imaging of the renal transplant: comparison of MRI with duplex sonography. Abdom Imaging 2006;31:461–82.
67. de Morais RH, Muglia VF, Mamere AE, et al. Duplex Doppler sonography of transplant renal artery stenosis. J Clin Ultrasound 2003;31:135–41.
68. Biederman DM, Fischman AM, Titano JJ, et al. Tailoring the endovascular management of transplant renal artery stenosis. Am J Transplant 2015;15:1039–49.
69. Touma J, Costanzo A, Boura B, et al. Endovascular management of transplant renal artery stenosis. J Vasc Surg 2014;59:1058–65.
70. Morozumi K, Takeda A, Otsuka Y, et al. Recurrent glomerular disease after kidney transplantation: an update of selected areas and the impact of protocol biopsy. Nephrology (Carlton) 2014;19(Suppl 3):6–10.
71. Briganti EM, Russ GR, McNeil JJ, et al. Risk of renal allograft loss from recurrent glomerulonephritis. N Engl J Med 2002;347:103–9.
72. Golgert WA, Appel GB, Hariharan S. Recurrent glomerulonephritis after renal transplantation: an unsolved problem. Clin J Am Soc Nephrol 2008;3:800–7.
73. Floege J, Regele H, Gesualdo L. The ERA-EDTA database on recurrent glomerulonephritis following renal transplantation. Nephrol Dial Transplant 2014;29: 15–21.

74. Odum J, Peh CA, Clarkson AR, et al. Recurrent mesangial IgA nephritis following renal transplantation. Nephrol Dial Transplant 1994;9:309–12.
75. Ponticelli C. Recurrence of focal segmental glomerular sclerosis (FSGS) after renal transplantation. Nephrol Dial Transplant 2010;25:25–31.
76. Cravedi P, Kopp JB, Remuzzi G. Recent progress in the pathophysiology and treatment of FSGS recurrence. Am J Transplant 2013;13:266–74.
77. Seitz-Polski B, Payre C, Ambrosetti D, et al. Prediction of membranous nephropathy recurrence after transplantation by monitoring of anti-PLA2R1 (M-type phospholipase A2 receptor) autoantibodies: a case series of 15 patients. Nephrol Dial Transplant 2014;29:2334–42.
78. Quintana LF, Blasco M, Seras M, et al. Antiphospholipase A2 receptor antibody levels predict the risk of posttransplantation recurrence of membranous nephropathy. Transplantation 2015;99(8):1709–14.
79. Kattah A, Ayalon R, Beck LH Jr, et al. Anti-phospholipase A(2) receptor antibodies in recurrent membranous nephropathy. Am J Transplant 2015;15: 1349–59.
80. Zuber J, Le Quintrec M, Morris H, et al. Targeted strategies in the prevention and management of atypical HUS recurrence after kidney transplantation. Transplant Rev (Orlando) 2013;27:117–25.
81. Green H, Rahamimov R, Rozen-Zvi B, et al. Recurrent membranoproliferative glomerulonephritis type I after kidney transplantation: a 17-year single-center experience. Transplantation 2015;99:1172–7.
82. Barbour S, Gill JS. Advances in the understanding of complement mediated glomerular disease: implications for recurrence in the transplant setting. Am J Transplant 2015;15:312–9.
83. Solez K, Colvin RB, Racusen LC, et al. Banff '05 meeting report: differential diagnosis of chronic allograft injury and elimination of chronic allograft nephropathy ('CAN'). Am J Transplant 2007;7:518–26.
84. Wiseman AC, McCague K, Kim Y, et al. The effect of everolimus versus mycophenolate upon proteinuria following kidney transplant and relationship to graft outcomes. Am J Transplant 2013;13:442–9.
85. Murakami N, Riella LV, Funakoshi T. Risk of metabolic complications in kidney transplantation after conversion to mTOR inhibitor: a systematic review and meta-analysis. Am J Transplant 2014;14:2317–27.
86. Izzedine H, Brocheriou I, Frances C. Post-transplantation proteinuria and sirolimus. N Engl J Med 2005;353:2088–9.

The ABCs of Immunosuppression
A Primer for Primary Care Physicians

Gregory Malat, PharmD, BCPS[a],*, Christine Culkin, DNP, FNP-BC[b]

KEYWORDS

• Transplant • Immunosuppression • Primary care • Medication interactions

KEY POINTS

• Explain basic pharmacology of commonly prescribed immunosuppression.
• Summarize key comorbidities that occur with chronic immunosuppression.
• Provide general guidance for selecting medication therapies to treat such comorbidities.

EARLY TRANSPLANTATION

The idea of allograft transplantation started much earlier than the practice of immunosuppressive therapy was instituted. Both Emerich Ullmann and Mathieu Jaboulay described the act of kidney xenotransplantation as far back as the early twentieth century.[1–3] Through these procedures the current surgical technique of vascular anastomosis was described by a practitioner working with M. Jaboulay, named Alexis Carrel. It was Alexis Carrel who lectured to medical students that the surgical technique of transplantation had been solved. However, until a therapy can effectively inhibit the recognition of foreign proteins, the routine practice of transplantation could not be successful. This warning referred to the not-yet-discovered use of exogenous substances to inhibit the immune system, namely immunosuppressants. Another landmark finding, describing the essential need for immunosuppression, followed Emile Holman's work with skin grafting in pediatric burn patients. Because grafting required repeating, E. Holman noted that the skin graft's survival time was shortened, reflecting recognition of the foreign proteins through repeated exposure.

Disclosures: The authors have no disclosures.
[a] Solid Organ Transplantation, Hahnemann University Hospital, Drexel University College of Medicine, 216 North Broad Street, MS 417, 5th Floor Feinstein Building, Philadelphia, PA 19102, USA; [b] Solid Organ Transplantation, Hahnemann University Hospital, Philadelphia, PA, USA
* Corresponding author.
E-mail address: gregory.malat@tenethealth.com

EARLY IMMUNOSUPPRESSION

In 1954, the first successful kidney transplant between identical twins was performed by a team in Boston led by Dr Joseph Murray. The kidney allograft recipient survived for approximately 9 years, providing proof that transplantation could be a successful modality used to treat end-stage kidney disease. Iterations of immunosuppression protocols following that successful case led to the initial use of total body irradiation and cortisone as immunosuppression.[1,2] However, this method resulted in early patient demise, most commonly from radiation toxicity. Burroughs Wellcome funded research to identify a better-tolerated, but still immunosuppressive, agent similar to the already-used chemotherapeutic agent 6-mercaptopurine. Gertrude Elion and George Hitchings ultimately discovered azathioprine, which, when combined with corticosteroids and antilymphocyte globulin, significantly improved 1-year patient and graft survival.

ENTER THE CALCINEURIN ERA

Jean Borel discovered the compound cyclosporine, and, less than a decade later, the medication was approved by the US Food and Drug Administration (FDA) for use in organ transplantation. The medication alone moved transplantation into the now highly successful so-called calcineurin era, resulting in survival consistently around 90%.[4] Since the approval of cyclosporine, many other immunosuppression medications have been approved for organ transplantation (**Table 1**), all of which are reviewed later in this article.

CURRENT IMMUNOSUPPRESSION

The approach to immunosuppression management reflects the idea that the immune system is redundant. Redundancy enables immune system activation and recognition through numerous pathways. Adapted immune cellular recognition requires 4 major stepwise signals that move lymphocytes, namely T cells, from a resting G0 phase to active mitotic M phase.

Immune activation starts with antigen presentation from antigen-presenting cells to T-helper cells, by binding/interacting with the T-cell receptor. In an attempt to prevent a false response, costimulatory receptor binding is necessary for the reaction to

Table 1 Immunosuppression timeline	
1990–1994	Cyclosporine (modified) Tacrolimus Mycophenolate (mofetil)
1995–1999	Sirolimus Antithymocyte globulin Daclizumab (no longer available) Basiliximab
2000–2005	—
2005–2010	Mycophenolate (sodium) Everolimus
2010–2015	Belatacept Tacrolimus (extended-release capsules) Tacrolimus (extended-release tablets)

initiate T-helper cell activation. Following binding of both receptor pathways, there is a conformational change in the membrane of the T-helper cell allowing influx of key mediators. One such mediator is calcium, which, along with calmodulin, activates calcineurin. Calcineurin is a key phosphatase that phosphorylates the nuclear factor of activated T cells (NfAT). Following phosphorylation, NfAT translocates into the nucleus, stimulating the transcription of certain cytokines, specifically interleukin 2 (IL-2).

With the release of IL-2 from the lymphocyte, IL-2 acts as a ligand for CD25, which is the IL-2 receptor, ultimately leading to proliferation and multiplication of other T-helper cells. IL-2 receptor binding sets off a chain reaction pathway that goes through the mammalian target of rapamycin (mTOR) kinase. The mTOR kinase is the gatekeeper for the synthesizing of key proteins and factors required to move the lymphocyte into preparation for the S phase of the cell cycle. One key component required for S phase is nucleotide synthesis, which is required for mitosis (**Fig. 1**).

Immunosuppression therapy generally consists of 3 phases following successful organ transplantation. First is the induction phase, in which the recipient receives potent immunosuppressive agents to either inhibit immune recognition or lyse immunoactive lymphocytes. The rejection phase/therapy often uses many of the induction agents. However, this therapy is initiated when immune recognition has already occurred and potent immunosuppressive agents are used to remove lymphocytes from the allograft. The maintenance phase targets specific receptors to maintain immunosuppression and prevent stimulation of the immune system. The maintenance phase immunosuppressants are often not as potent as induction or rejection therapy, and use an assortment of agents to block the immune system at multiple sites.

IMMUNOSUPPRESSION WITHIN THE IMMUNE SYSTEM

Many of the commonly used immunosuppressants focus on inhibiting T-helper cells from being stimulated and activated, as well as from proliferating. Each of the immunosuppression classes, namely calcineurin inhibitors, antiproliferatives, corticosteroids, mTOR inhibitors, and antibodies, are discussed later.

Calcineurin Inhibitors

As their name suggests, calcineurin inhibitors block calcineurin phosphatase, thus inhibiting the translocation of NfAT to the nucleus, and ultimately preventing the transcription of IL-2, which acts to mute T-cell responses. Calcineurin inhibitors are considered the backbone of most current immunosuppression protocols. As mentioned earlier, cyclosporine was the first available calcineurin inhibitor. About 10 years later a more potent calcineurin inhibitor, tacrolimus, was approved for organ transplant rejection prevention and is now the most widely used inhibitor.

Both of these calcineurin inhibitors are similar in their side effects and drug interactions. Because of the marked toxicities and narrow therapeutic window, virtually all patients experience some side effects from these potent agents, so an integral part of the care of transplant patients is monitoring and adjusting these medications. One of the most common and serious side effects is nephrotoxicity. Nephrotoxicity can be thought as both acute, secondary to drug-induced vasoconstriction, and chronic, related to long-term upregulation of fibrosis mediators in the allograft. Cyclosporine is thought to have slightly more metabolic side effects, including hypertension, hypercholesterolemia, and hyperuricemia, although each of these is seen with both agents. Tacrolimus is considered to be more diabetogenic and neurotoxic.

Drug interactions are common and cumbersome with the concurrent use of calcineurin inhibitors. The frequency of drug interactions with calcineurin inhibitors stems

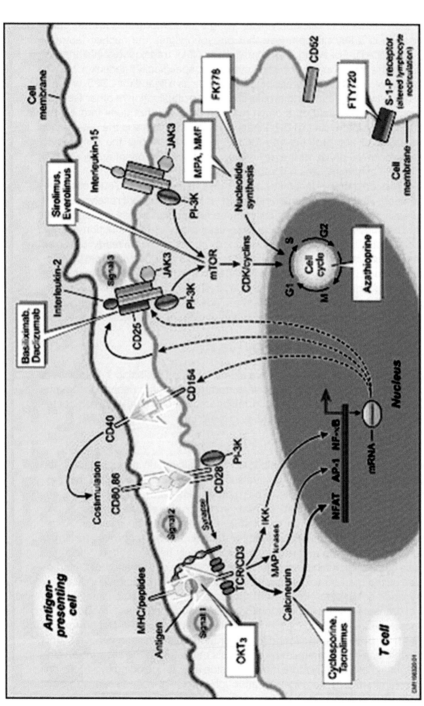

Fig. 1. Immunosuppression in liver transplantation. The activation of a T lymphocyte (via 3-signal pathway) by an antigen-presenting cell. Specific sites targeted by the calcineurin inhibitors (tacrolimus and cyclosporine A) are included, showing inhibition of interleukin 2 (IL-2) production. Monoclonal antibodies (basiliximab, daclizumab) target the IL-2 receptor, whereas OKT3 targets the T-cell receptor. Sirolimus, mycophenolic acid, mycophenolate mofetil, azathioprine, and FK778 interfere with the proliferative phase in the cell cycle. Novel agent FTY720 alters lymphocyte trafficking/homing patterns through modulation of cell surface adhesion receptors, inducing a lymphopenic effect. (*From* Post DJ, Douglas DD, Mulligan DC. Immunosuppression in liver transplantation. Liver Transplant 2005;11(11):1308; with permission.)

from their metabolism through the cytochrome P450 system and p-glycoprotein efflux system. **Tables 2** and **3** identify common medications that can increase or decrease exposure to calcineurin inhibitors. By inhibiting cytochrome P450 (CYP450) metabolism, levels of these agents increase, so there is an increased chance of calcineurin inhibitor toxicity. Alternatively, induction of CYP450 metabolism decreases the efficacy of calcineurin inhibitors, increasing the likelihood of allograft rejection.

Antiproliferative Agents

Antiproliferative agents prevent lymphocytes from progressing through the cell cycle following stimulation of the T-cell receptor. Antiproliferatives can be thought of as antimetabolites or mTOR inhibitors.

Antimetabolites

One of the earliest available immunosuppressant agents that showed promise was azathioprine, which was derived from the original compound, 6-mercaptopurine. Although azathioprine is still used, it has largely been supplanted by a more potent antimetabolite, mycophenolate. Both compounds inhibit DNA purine base pair production, through different enzymatic pathways. Azathioprine is metabolized to 6-mercaptopurine and inhibits DNA purine nucleoside synthesis. Mycophenolate similarly inhibits DNA purine nucleoside synthesis by blocking the enzyme inosine monophosphate dehydrogenase. Mycophenolate has been marketed as 2 different products, differing by the salt attached to the compound. Once absorbed through the gastrointestinal wall, both products are converted to the active moiety, mycophenolic acid. Because of the salt differences, the dosing is different between the two compounds. The original product, mycophenolate mofetil 1000 mg, is equimolar with mycophenolate sodium 720 mg.

A risk evaluation/mitigation strategy was imposed by the FDA on any use of mycophenolate products, which stems from the teratogenic risk associated with such

Table 2
Metabolic interactions that increase calcineurin inhibitor exposure/drug level

Mediation Class	Examples
Calcium channel blockers	Verapamil Diltiazem Nicardipine
Antifungal agents	Ketoconazole Fluconazole Itraconazole Voriconazole Posaconazole
Immunosuppression	Sirolimus
Antibiotics	Erythromycin Clarithromycin Nafcillin Ciprofloxacin
HIV medications	Ritonavir
Foods	Grapefruit juice Grapefruits
Miscellaneous	Octreotide Nefazodone

Abbreviation: HIV, human immunodeficiency virus.

Table 3
Metabolic interactions that decrease calcineurin inhibitor exposure/drug level

Medication Class	Examples
Antituberculosis medications	Rifampin
	Rifabutin
	Isoniazid
Anticonvulsants	Barbiturates
	Phenytoin
	Carbamazepine
HIV medications	Efavirenz
	Nevirapine
Herbal medications	St. John's Wort

products. Practitioners are required to inform female recipients of the potential risk, as well as to request female patients to use a double contraceptive method. Female patients are encouraged to discuss with their physicians changing immunosuppression regimens before attempting to get pregnant.

The side effects of the antimetabolites are largely hematologic. Profound or resistant cytopenias are possible with either agent and may dictate the dosing of these agents. Erythropoietin-stimulating agents may be necessary to counter the subtle anemia that may be encountered following the use of these agents. Azathioprine causes a macrocytic anemia, which should be monitored and can be used as a clue to verify compliance. Mycophenolate has prominent gastrointestinal side effects (ie, nausea, vomiting, and diarrhea), so dosing has to be balanced against these side effects. The mycophenolate sodium product is enteric coated, and thus may be better tolerated on an individual basis, although this has not been confirmed in formal studies.[5]

Drug interactions with the antimetabolites are not as concerning as with calcineurin inhibitors, because of the lack of CYP450 metabolism. Allopurinol use inhibits azathioprine metabolism, leading to an accumulation of toxic metabolites and significant side effects. Mycophenolate has the potential to be chelated by divalent cations, and thus dosing should be separated throughout the day. In addition, drug interactions secondary to concurrent side effects may be compounded. These combinations should be avoided or the complete blood count should be monitored closely when using other hematologic toxic medications.

Mammalian target of rapamycin inhibitors

The original mTOR inhibitor approved for immunosuppression was sirolimus. Sirolimus inhibits the mTOR kinase, which inhibits the downstream production of certain key proteins or factors necessary for lymphocytes to progress through the cell cycle. mTOR inhibitors are extremely potent antiinflammatory and immunosuppressive agents. Everolimus is the other commonly used mTOR inhibitor, with a similar mode of action and side effect profile, but associated with a shorter half-life.

The profound antiproliferative actions of mTOR inhibitors result in decreased wound healing, which can be expected following procedures. Fast-growing cells may be influenced by the mTOR inhibitors, as noted by the potential for aphthous ulcers, diarrhea, and leukopenia. Because of the effects on wound healing, the use of these agents should be suspended before a planned procedure, because wound dehiscence is a serious concern. Addition of mTOR inhibitors to patients with chronic kidney disease also worsens nephropathy. Inhibition of tubular epithelial cell healing further impairs cell function, often leading to proteinuria. Other side effects have been noted with use of these products, including pneumonitis, hypertriglyceridemia, and thrombocytopenia. Sirolimus carries with it a black box warning for use in liver transplantation within 30 days. Early de novo experience with sirolimus after liver transplant resulted in an increased frequency of hepatic artery thrombosis.

Drug interactions are expected with mTOR inhibitors, secondary to their metabolism by the CYP450 system, similar to the calcineurin inhibitors. One drug interaction of particular note is the mTOR and calcineurin inhibitor interaction. mTOR inhibitors inhibit the metabolism of calcineurin inhibitors, leading to increased toxicity associated with calcineurin inhibitors. It is recommended to decrease doses of both agents to limit the toxicities associated with this particular drug interaction.

Corticosteroids

Corticosteroids were recognized from the onset of successful organ transplantation as potent antiinflammatory agents. The mechanism of action includes binding to a cytoplasmic ligand that inhibits the translocation of nuclear factor kappa B into the nucleus. Corticosteroids' ease of use and pleiotropic effects support these agents' place in induction, maintenance, and rejection therapy.

The side effects of corticosteroids are well known and are mostly metabolic. Long-term chronic use may lead to increased risk of diabetes, hypertension, hypercholesterolemia, and osteoporosis. Short-term, high doses may lead to hyperglycemia, edema, moon-face appearance, and steroid psychosis. Mostly because of the untoward side effects, some transplant programs avoid corticosteroids, minimize long-term high-dose exposure, or taper off corticosteroids over time.

Drug interactions are clinically minimal, and may be related to the additive toxicities of other agents that exacerbate the side effects of corticosteroids.

Costimulation Blockade

Costimulation blockade is one of the newest classes of immunosuppressive agents available for solid organ transplantation. Costimulation is required along with the cognate T-cell receptor–antigen-presenting cell interaction to precipitate a positive immune response. One of the principal costimulatory systems for T cells is the interaction with B7-1/B7-2 with either CD-28, which elicits a positive response, or cytotoxic T-lymphocyte 4 (CTLA-4), which elicits an immune-dampening response. Belatacept, which mimics a soluble CTLA-4, competitively binds to B7-1/B7-2, blocking these molecules' ability to positively interact with CD-28, thus providing a negative inhibition on the potential immune response. In many instances in which belatacept is used, it allows avoidance or minimization of calcineurin inhibitor use, which may limit toxicity and perhaps increase allograft survival in the right circumstances. Belatacept is administered intravenously on a monthly basis in the outpatient setting.

Side effects that patients commonly experience with belatacept are minimal; however, there are a few reported potential toxicities that are concerning. In the initial studies of belatacept, cellular rejection rates were increased compared with the control arm.[6] Also more common was the incidence of posttransplant lymphoproliferative disorder (PTLD), specifically central nervous system PTLD. After further investigation, it was noted that many of the PTLD cases were in patients seronegative for the Epstein-Barr virus (EBV). In addition, an increased risk of progressive multileukoencephalopathy was described with the use of belatacept.

For these reasons, the FDA mandated a Risk Evaluation and Mitigation Strategy program for ongoing clinical use of belatacept. Practitioners are required to confirm the EBV serostatus of recipients before initiation of belatacept therapy, and to perform a neurologic checklist before each infusion.

Drug interactions are not expected with the use of belatacept.

Antibodies

Synthetic antibodies seek to target physiologic receptors/ligands located on or used by lymphocytes. Antibodies are defined by the number of sites the medication targets. Polyclonal antibodies target multiple epitopes, whereas monoclonal antibodies are synthesized to target only 1 receptor/ligand. Because antibodies cause a profound immunosuppressant effect, the use of antibodies is most commonly restricted to rejection and induction therapy.

The most common polyclonal antibody used in organ transplantation is antithymocyte globulin. Historically, antilymphocyte globulins have been used to prevent allograft rejection since almost the beginning of organ transplantation. The current agent being used is an antibody derived from rabbit sera targeting the many ligands/receptors found on T cells.

Monoclonal antibodies are specific for 1 antigen. Traditionally, antibodies are murine derived, which raises the possibility of a recipient foreign antimurine immune recognition during repeated clinical exposure, leading to neutralization of the medication. One way to circumvent this issue is to alter the antibody structure. Antibodies are made up of a variable region (Fab) and a constant region (Fc). The variable region is essential for epitope recognition and binding. The constant region is used for isotype stratification of the antibodies (eg, immunoglobulin [Ig] G, IgA, and IgM) and complement signaling and activation. For this reason, often all or some of the variable region remains murine, but the constant region is cleaved and replaced with a human constant region. This process decreases the immunogenicity of the medication and thus decreases the likelihood of neutralization.

Basiliximab is a commonly used monoclonal antibody that targets CD25, which is an essential component of the IL-2 receptor required for continuing the initial signal for T-cell proliferation. Basiliximab is not lymphocyte depleting, and simply blocks IL-2 from binding to its ligand. Therefore, basiliximab is primarily used during the induction phase.

Rituximab was developed for use in lymphomas because of its potential to target and lyse B cells by binding to CD20. B cells are essential as antigen-presenting cells to T cells. In addition, B cells produce endogenous antibodies capable of allograft recognition, leading to a severe, often immunosuppressant-resistant, form of rejection.

Alemtuzumab is also a recognized chemotherapy agent, adapted for use in organ transplantation. Alemtuzumab targets CD52, which is a receptor located on many immune cells, including natural killer cells, B and T lymphocytes, and macrophages. Alemtuzumab can be used for either induction or rejection therapy.

Drug interactions are unlikely with concurrent use of antibody therapy, and are mostly related to additive toxicities of antibodies. Side effects often center on the antibodies' ability to lyse lymphocytes and produce profound immunosuppression. Often lymphocyte epitopes targeted by antibodies are shared by other blood cell lines, leading to destruction of unintended targets. Use of antibodies can sometimes lead to neutropenia and thrombocytopenia. In addition, because of the intense immunosuppressive effects, antibody therapy has been associated with posttransplant infections and malignancies.

PHARMACOKINETICS

Narrow therapeutic index medications are those medications with a small window of efficacy. Many standard-of-care immunosuppression agents have a narrow therapeutic index and rely on therapeutic drug monitoring. Immunosuppressants included in this list of narrow therapeutic index medications are tacrolimus, cyclosporine, everolimus, and sirolimus. Subtherapeutic dosing of these medications leads to decreased efficacy, and, in the case of transplantation, increased risk of rejection. Supratherapeutic dosing of these mediations leads to toxicity. With the exception of sirolimus, which is a once-daily drug, the other immunosuppressants are commonly dosed every 12 hours. A timed 12-hour trough is used to monitor these medications. Ideally, a 12-hour trough is collected before the next dose, approximately 12 hours after the last dose. In the case of sirolimus, the trough is collected approximately 24 hours after the last dose. Transplant teams evaluate these troughs in the context of individualized, expected goals. Transplant teams set immunosuppressant goals based on a multitude of patient-specific factors, which include, but are not limited to, the type of organ transplanted, time from transplant, patient age, and rejection/infection/malignancy history since transplant.

COMMONLY PRESCRIBED ADJUNCT AGENTS

The increase in organ transplantation has led to primary care physicians assuming a greater role in the provision of health care.[7] These patients are frequently on many medications with unique interactions, so they present a challenge to health care providers. As the following describes, they require health maintenance follow-up along with more extensive preventive testing and vaccinations than the general population.

Antibiotics and Antifungals

Medications used to treat common bacterial infections can have a multitude of interactions with transplant immunosuppression. Medications to avoid include ciprofloxacin, macrolide antibiotics, and azole antifungals. Most antibiotics need dose adjustments based on the patient's current renal and hepatic function. When possible, cultures for streptococcus pharyngitis and influenza can help guide treatment. It is no longer a recommendation to give antibiotic prophylaxis before minor dental procedures and colonoscopy.[8]

Antihypertensives

When treating hypertensive disease, it is important to maximize the patient's blood pressure control to help extend the life of the allograft. Angiotensin receptor blockers, angiotensin-converting enzyme inhibitors, and direct renin inhibitors should be carefully considered because of the risk of hyperkalemia and acute renal failure following initiation. Therefore, collaboration with the patient's transplant program before initiation of these medications is warranted.

Preferred agents for treatment of hypertension in the transplant population are the calcium channel blockers (CCB), β-blockers, thiazide diuretics, and α-blockers. The exceptions to this rule are diltiazem and verapamil, which affect the metabolism of the patient's immunosuppression, through inhibition of CYP450 metabolic inhibition. The downside to using CCBs in this population is the risk of development of lower extremity edema. β-Blockerscan increase the patient's fatigue and dizziness. While on thiazide diuretics, electrolyte levels need to be monitored after initiation.

Hyperlipidemia

Treatment of dyslipidemia in transplant patient should be aggressive to aid in halting the development of cardiovascular disease. When lifestyle changes through diet and exercise fail to control lipids, medication needs to be initiated. Dosing of statins needs to be adjusted for renal and hepatic function. Simvastatin or lovastatin should not be used in transplant patients currently taking calcineurin inhibitor therapy. Preferred agents include rosuvastatin and pravastatin, which have less risk of rhabdomyolysis induced by drug-drug interaction.

Mental Health

Depression and anxiety disorders appear during the transplant process because of psychological stressors, medications, and physiologic disturbances.[9] Counseling with the addition of medications to treat depression and anxiety may be necessary. Most of the medications need to be adjusted for renal and hepatic function. Selective serotonin reuptake inhibitors are generally well tolerated, with citalopram and escitalopram seeming to have the least severe drug-drug interactions. For short-term management of anxiety, benzodiazepines are useful but should be discontinued as soon as possible to avoid dependency.

Over-the-counter Preparations and Herbals

For seasonal allergies, loratadine, cetirizine, and fexofenadine are all acceptable choices, whereas pseudoephedrine-containing products should be avoided. For the common cold, guaifenesin, dextromethorphan, and diphenhydramine help to alleviate symptoms, again avoiding pseudoephedrine. For treatment of acid reflux, famotidine may help to prevent the symptoms. For pain relief, acetaminophen is an acceptable choice, but nonsteroidal antiinflammatory drugs should be avoided because of the risk for renal failure.

Most herbal medications are not recommended in transplant patients. The FDA does not regulate herbal supplements for dose, content, or pureness. Herbal supplements may interact with prescription medicines to either decrease or increase the medicine's effect. St. John's wort, valerian, *Echinacea*, and kava are a few popular herbals to be avoided. Grapefruit and grapefruit juice affect the metabolism of many medications secondary to its influence on the cytochrome P450 metabolism.

Vaccinations and Preventive Health Care

Vaccine-preventable diseases remain a major source of morbidity and mortality in transplant recipients. Transplant patients may not benefit from immunizations within the first 3 months after transplant, following potent induction immunosuppression therapy. Posttransplant patients should not receive any live vaccines, such as the live nasal flu vaccine; measles, mumps, rubella; varicella; or zoster.[10]

Recommended vaccines include:

- A 1-time booster of Tdap (tetanus, diphtheria, and pertussis)
- Pneumococcal vaccine
- Pneumococcal 7-valent vaccine
- Yearly influenza shot
- Hepatitis A
- Hepatitis B series

COMPLICATIONS ASSOCIATED WITH CHRONIC USE OF IMMUNOSUPPRESSION

As with any medical therapy in clinical use, there is a trade-off between efficacy and toxicity. Too little immunosuppression leads to decreased efficacy, which can result in an increased risk of allograft rejection. Too much immunosuppression leads to toxicity, often in the forms of infections and malignancy. Selected side effects of immunosuppression, either manifested by overdosing or just through chronic exposure, are reviewed here. **Table 4** provides a synopsis of commonly experienced side effects seen in maintenance immunosuppression.

Nephrotoxicity

One adverse effect of immunosuppression that has affected the long-term benefit of organ transplants is nephrotoxicity. Nephrotoxicity is a side effect of exposure to calcineurin inhibitors, and can occur in kidney transplant recipients, as well as extrarenal allograft recipients. The acute nephrotoxicity associated with calcineurin inhibitors can be managed with therapeutic drug monitoring and avoidance of supratherapeutic drug levels. However, the more concerning cause of nephrotoxicity is associated with chronic exposure to calcineurin inhibitors, which leads to an insidious decline of renal function.

Conversion immunosuppression is one promising area that may have a lasting effect on long-term nephrotoxicity. Agents being researched include mTOR inhibitors and belatacept. Studies are underway to describe the outcomes of such conversion to these nonnephrotoxic immunosuppressants. Of note, much of the research has sought to institute conversion in patients with good, stable renal function as opposed to declining function. For that reason, one question that remains unanswered is the appropriate time for conversion. Such time should minimize the risk of allograft rejection by continuing calcineurin inhibitors for a sufficient time posttransplant, but not so long that the effects of calcineurin inhibitor exposure are already underway.

New-onset Diabetes Mellitus after Transplant

Diabetes mellitus continues to be major cause of kidney morbidity, as well as cardiovascular morbidity and mortality. However, even recipients who have no documented history of diabetes can develop the untoward complications of hyperglycemia. This form of diabetes has been termed new-onset diabetes mellitus after transplant (NODAT). The incidence rates of NODAT vary by organ transplanted and posttransplant interval. The estimated rates at 12 months posttransplant are 20% to 50% for kidney transplants and 9% to 21% for liver transplants.[11] Certain recipient demographics/characteristics, coupled with concurrent diabetogenic immunosuppressants, namely tacrolimus and corticosteroids, place recipients at risk of developing NODAT.

Treatment of NODAT is similar to treatment of diabetes mellitus type 2. Sulfonylureas, metformin, DPP-4 inhibitors, GLP-1 agonists, and insulin can be used in treatment, but, when there is impaired kidney or hepatic function, special precautions are necessary.[12] Oral hypoglycemic agents are usually a mainstay of therapy and may be coupled with adjunctive agents, such as DPP-4 inhibitors. Ultimately, patients with NODAT may progress to insulin dependence. Metformin is an agent that could be considered for treatment of NODAT, depending on the level of renal dysfunction.

Cardiovascular Morbidity/Mortality

Cardiovascular demise continues to be a major concern following organ transplant. This outcome may be related to irreversible damage secondary to the underlying

Table 4
Side effects of commonly prescribed medications

Toxicity	CNS	Kidney	Hematologic	Diabetogenic	Cardiovascular	Gastrointestinal
Cyclosporine	+	+++	+	+	+++	+
Tacrolimus	+++	+++	+	+++	++	+
Corticosteroids	+	−	−	+++	+	−
Azathioprine	−	−	++	−	−	−
Mycophenolate	−	−	++	−	−	+++
Sirolimus	−	++ (indirect; proteinuria)	+++	+	+	−
Everolimus	−	++ (indirect; proteinuric)	+++	+	+	−
Belatacept	+++	−	−	−	−	−

Abbreviation: CNS, central nervous system.
Data from Zand M. Immunosuppression and immune monitoring after renal transplantation. Semin Dial 2005;18(6):511–9.

disease (eg, diabetes) and/or the adverse effects associated with long-term, chronic exposure to immunosuppression (eg, NODAT, hypercholesterolemia, hypertension).

The tool that assists the population in estimating cardiovascular risk, the Framingham Risk Score, may underestimate the cardiovascular risk imposed on organ transplant recipients.[13,14] Longitudinal follow-up of transplant recipients resulted in a calculated observed/predicted event ratio score of 1.64. In addition, the risk factors associated with cardiovascular risk in transplant recipients differ from the traditional risk factors. Those risk factors identified in the transplant population included estimated glomerular filtration rate, older age, prior cardiovascular disease, diabetes, smoking, and systolic blood pressure.

Malignancy

Similar to cardiovascular morbidity/mortality, malignancy is mostly considered an unpreventable outcome associated with long-term exposure to immunosuppression. Although the estimated risk of malignancy following the first year after transplant is estimated to be 10%, the risk jumps to 87% more than 15 years after transplant.[15] Almost a third of the documented malignancies in transplant recipients are from skin cancer. This finding emphasizes the point that skin protection and skin surveillance are essential hallmarks of good posttransplant care.

SUMMARY

With the improvement in allograft recognition/rejection prophylaxis, coupled with improved long-term patient survival, chronic health care issues are at the forefront of outpatient care for organ transplant recipients. Careful monitoring for morbidities following organ transplant is warranted. However, medical therapy must be chosen carefully and monitored closely to prevent iatrogenic complications. Such complications may be a result of misunderstanding the recipients' immunosuppression regimens and/or potential drug interactions. Understanding immunosuppression medications will better equip practitioners to make safer decisions when treating chronic comorbidities, and will benefit allograft and patient survival.

REFERENCES

1. Morris PJ. Transplantation–a medical miracle of the 20th century. N Engl J Med 2004;351(26):2678–80.
2. Sayegh MH, Carpenter CB. Transplantation 50 years later–progress, challenges, and promises. N Engl J Med 2004;351(26):2761–6.
3. Watson CJE, Dark JH. Organ transplantation: historical perspective and current practice. Br J Anaesth 2012;108(Suppl 1):i29–42.
4. Linden PK. History of solid organ transplantation and organ donation. Crit Care Clin 2009;25(1):165–84.
5. Pietruck F, Budde K, Salvadori M, et al. Efficacy and safety of enteric-coated mycophenolate sodium in renal transplant patients with diabetes mellitus: post hoc analyses from three clinical trials. Clin Transplant 2007;21(1):117–25.
6. Vincenti F, Charpentier B, Vanrenterghem Y, et al. A phase III study of belatacept-based immunosuppression regimens versus cyclosporine in renal transplant recipients (BENEFIT study). Am J Transplant 2010;10(3):535–46.
7. Tannock LR, Reynolds LR. Management of dyslipidemia in patients after solid organ transplantation. Postgrad Med 2008;120(1):43–9.
8. Wilson W, Taubert KA, Gewitz M, et al. Prevention of infective endocarditis: guidelines from the American Heart Association: a guideline from the American Heart

Association Rheumatic Fever, Endocarditis, and Kawasaki Disease Committee, Council on Cardiovascular Disease in the Young, and the Council on Clinical Cardiology, Council on Cardiovascular Surgery and Anesthesia, and the Quality of Care and Outcomes Research Interdisciplinary Working Group. Circulation 2007;116(15):1736–54.

9. Crone CC, Gabriel GM. Treatment of anxiety and depression in transplant patients: pharmacokinetic considerations. Clin Pharmacokinet 2004;43(6):361–94.

10. Avery RK, Michaels M. Update on immunizations in solid organ transplant recipients: what clinicians need to know. Am J Transplant 2008;8(1):9–14.

11. Lane JT, Dagogo-Jack S. Approach to the patient with new-onset diabetes after transplant (NODAT). J Clin Endocrinol Metab 2011;96(11):3289–97.

12. Therasse A, Wallia A, Molitch ME. Management of post-transplant diabetes. Curr Diab Rep 2013;13(1):121–9.

13. Kiberd B, Panek R. Cardiovascular outcomes in the outpatient kidney transplant clinic: the Framingham Risk Score revisited. Clin J Am Soc Nephrol 2008;3(3):822–8.

14. Weiner DE, Carpenter MA, Levey AS, et al. Kidney function and risk of cardiovascular disease and mortality in kidney transplant recipients: the FAVORIT trial. Am J Transplant 2012;12(9):2437–45.

15. Apel H, Walschburger-Zorn K, Häberle L, et al. De novo malignancies in renal transplant recipients: experience at a single center with 1882 transplant patients over 39 yr. Clin Transplant 2013;27(1):E30–6.

Managing Cardiovascular Risk in the Post Solid Organ Transplant Recipient

Mrudula R. Munagala, MD[a],*, Anita Phancao, MD[b]

KEYWORDS

- Solid organ transplant • Cardiovascular disease • Risk factors
- Immunosuppression • Survival

KEY POINTS

- Overall mortality among solid organ transplant recipients has improved owing to advances in surgical techniques and immunosuppressive therapy.
- Although short-term survival rates have improved significantly, long-term survival rates are suffering secondary to enhanced cardiovascular mortality.
- Identifying comorbidities that contribute to enhanced cardiovascular risk and modifying these risks while awaiting transplantation and after transplantation are imperative to improve long-term graft and patient survivals.

INTRODUCTION

Solid organ transplantation has become the standard of care for patients with end-stage liver, kidney, lung, and heart diseases and has significantly improved the survival and quality of life for successful recipients. A mean of 4.3 life years per solid organ transplant recipient (SOTR) are saved based on retrospective analysis of data from the United Network for Organ Sharing for solid organ transplants over a 25-year period by Rana and colleagues.[1] Despite improvements in overall graft and patient survival rates that have followed the major advances in the management of transplant recipients and improvements in cardiovascular health that follow successful transplantation, cardiovascular disease (CVD) remains the leading cause of posttransplant mortality.[2–5] The prevalence of CVD is high among kidney and liver transplant recipients compared with the general population, which has been attributed to metabolic and systemic derangements that are associated with end-stage organ disease processes and exacerbations of these processes with immunosuppression, as well as

[a] Department of Cardiology, Newark Beth Israel Medical Center, 201 Lyons Avenue, Suite # L4, Newark, NJ 07112, USA; [b] Integris Baptist Medical Center, 3400 Northwest Expressway, Building C, Suite 200, Oklahoma City, OK 73112, USA
* Corresponding author.
E-mail address: mrudula@munagala.net

Med Clin N Am 100 (2016) 519–533
http://dx.doi.org/10.1016/j.mcna.2016.01.004
medical.theclinics.com
0025-7125/16/$ – see front matter © 2016 Elsevier Inc. All rights reserved.

the added risks of infection and rejection with transplantation. CVD in SOTR can be categorized primarily into atherosclerotic heart disease/ischemic heart disease, which manifests secondary to abnormality in cardiac perfusion, disorders of cardiac function (left ventricular hypertrophy, left ventricular systolic and diastolic dysfunction), which typically present as congestive heart failure and cardiac arrhythmias. Despite the high prevalence and mortality associated with CVD in SOTRs, there is limited evidence available for management of risk factors and prevention. CVD is the most frequent cause of death with functioning graft in kidney transplant recipients (KTRs) and thus the leading cause of graft loss. This review summarizes the risk factors contributing to cardiovascular mortality and therapeutic strategies to address these risk factors in SOTRs. In this review, we discuss CVD risk factors in KTRs that can then be extrapolated to other SOTRs.

EPIDEMIOLOGY OF CARDIOVASCULAR DISEASE IN SOLID ORGAN TRANSPLANT RECIPIENTS

SOTRs are at increased risk for premature CVD and cardiovascular mortality. Although the risk of CVD improves after kidney transplantation when compared with patients with end-stage kidney disease awaiting transplantation, CVD risk remains significantly greater in KTRs when weighed against the age- and sex-matched general population.[6,7] Several variables contribute to the CVD risk in SOTRs including recipient's pretransplant disease process, traditional and nontraditional risk factors and transplant related risk factors such as exposure to immunosuppression.[8] **Fig. 1** depicts the various risk factors contributing to CVD risk in SOTRs. There are also organ-related risk factors, such as pretransplant uremic cardiomyopathy and dialysis vintage in KTRs, and pulmonary hypertension (HTN) and cirrhotic cardiomyopathy[9] in liver transplant recipients. Detailed discussion of organ-specific and donor-specific cardiovascular risk factors is beyond the scope of this article.

The United States Renal Data System 2014 annual data report system revealed that mortality from CVD among KTRs is approximately twice as frequent when compared

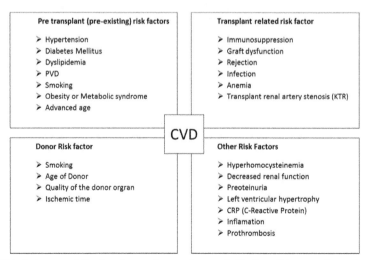

Fig. 1. Risk factors contributing to cardiovascular mortality in solid organ transplant recipients. CVD, cardiovascular disease; KTR, kidney transplant recipient; PVD, peripheral vascular disease.

with malignancy and infection.[10] Many of the end-stage organ disease patients would have been exposed to various risk factors for CVD and may have covert disease and pretransplant cardiovascular event is a strong predictor of posttransplant cardiac events.[11] Hence, the risk factor modification should begin before transplantation.

Striking rates of acute myocardial infarction were noted early after kidney transplantation by Kasiske and colleagues[12] in an observational study. Lentine and colleagues[13] concluded that approximately 11.1% of KTRs experience myocardial infarction by 3 years posttransplantation. The magnitude of CVD in SOTRs may be difficult to capture accurately owing to the significant number of nonfatal events. Congestive heart failure is associated with a poor prognosis in patients with end-stage renal disease and improvement of left ventricular systolic function after transplantation is noted in some studies. However, congestive heart failure is one of the frequent causes of hospitalization in KTRs and de novo congestive heart failure is noted to be a potent predictor of subsequent mortality in KTRs.[14]

TRADITIONAL AND NONTRADITIONAL RISK FACTORS

Conventional risk factors for coronary artery disease (CAD) include advanced age, HTN, elevated low-density lipoprotein cholesterol, low high-density lipoprotein cholesterol, diabetes mellitus (DM) and smoking,[15,16] and presence of peripheral vascular disease is considered to be CAD equivalent. Various risk factors for CAD have been identified both in the general population and SOTRs.[4,7,17,18] Many clinical and laboratory parameters have been described as predictors of CAD, but the clinical usefulness and cost effectiveness of screening to recommend their routine use is insufficient at this time. Both traditional and nontraditional risk factors are more prevalent in the transplant population compared with the general population even after adjusting for age and sex. This high prevalence of cardiovascular risk factors in SOTRs is attributed to frequent association of these risk factors in patients with end-stage organ disease along with exacerbation of preexisting systemic and metabolic conditions after transplantation owing to use of immunosuppression therapy. Some of these risk factors are modifiable with lifestyle changes and pharmacotherapy (**Table 1**).

Hypertension

HTN is a strong predictor of CVD in SOTRs. HTN is a risk factor for CVD and also is an independent risk for graft failure in KTRs.[19–21] HTN is associated with left ventricular hypertrophy before and after transplantation, and left ventricular hypertrophy is an independent risk factor for cardiovascular mortality.[22,23] HTN in renal transplant

Table 1 Risk factors for cardiovascular diseases	
Modifiable	**Nonmodifiable**
HTN	Age (men >45 y and women >55 y)
Diabetes mellitus	Gender
Dyslipidemia (low HDL and high LDL cholesterol level)	Race/ethnic factors
Smoking	Family history of premature CAD (<55 y of age in male first-degree relative or <65 in female first-degree relative)
Obesity (BMI ≥30 kg/m^2) or the metabolic syndrome	
Elevated HDL ≥60 mg/dL (positive risk factor)	

Abbreviations: BMI, body mass index; CAD, coronary artery disease; HDL, high-density lipoprotein; LDL, low-density lipoprotein.

recipients is defined as a blood pressure (BP) of greater than 130/80 mm Hg by Kidney Disease Improving Global Outcome (KDIGO) guidelines. HTN in SOTRs is usually multifactorial, including preexisting disease process, donor factors, and effects of immunosuppression. Exposure to immunosuppression is a major contributor to post-transplant HTN and effects are dose dependent. Steroids cause fluid retention and calcineurin inhibitors (CNIs) cause HTN through vasoconstrictive and nephrotoxic effects.

BP control in SOTRs is challenging. KDIGO guidelines recommended achieving a goal BP of less than 130/80 mm Hg regardless of proteinuria in KTRs. The Collaborative Transplant Study, an observational study, showed that achieving lower systolic BPs even within the normal ranges has incremental benefit. Patients with systolic BPs in the range of 120 mm Hg have better outcomes than the group with 130 mm Hg.[20,24] Opelz and Dohler[25] stated that approximately 55% of KTRs with HTN did not attain their goal BP in the examined group. This study also demonstrated that even delayed control of HTN as late as 3 years after the transplantation could still contribute to improved outcomes and mortality. Ambulatory BP monitoring is suggested to uncover HTN and assist in the management of HTN.[26] **Fig. 2** summarizes the HTN evaluation and monitoring in SOTRs.

Although there are reported advantages with lower BP targets[20,24] in the past, Eighth Joint National Committee recommended a goal systolic BP of less than 140 mm Hg and diastolic BP of less than 90 mm Hg for all age patients with CKD.[27] There is insufficient evidence to assert any additional cardiovascular, cerebrovascular, or mortality benefit with lower BP targets, but lower BP (<130/80 mm Hg) goals are recommended for CKD patients with proteinuria. Goal BP in SOTRs is a topic of

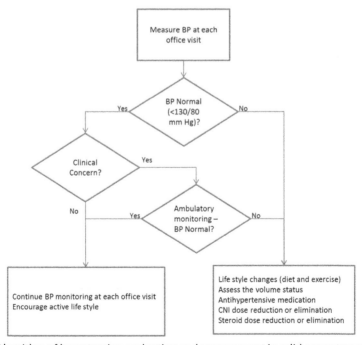

Fig. 2. Algorithm of hypertension evaluation and management in solid organ transplant recipients. BP, blood pressure; CNI, calcineurin inhibitor.

debate and until further concrete evidence is available, following current KDIGO guideline recommendations is prudent.

Lifestyle modification, including smoking cessation and weight loss, and management of coexisting diseases, such as treating DM, are the initial steps in the management of HTN in SOTRs. Reviewing medication lists, including over-the-counter medications and herbal supplements, and discontinuing any potential offending agents is recommended. BP can also be improved by changes in immunosuppression; however, most patients typically require pharmacotherapy and may require more than 1 agent for optimal BP control. There is no conclusive evidence at this time to recommend use of one class of agents over the other. CNIs cause HTN through vasoconstriction and the use of calcium channel blockers (CCB) is preferred owing to their vasodilator effects. Cross and colleagues[28] showed that institution of CCB in KTRs is associated with lesser decline in glomerular filtration rate and angiotensin-converting enzyme inhibitors (ACEi) have beneficial effects on proteinuria. The use of an ACEi is associated with more anemia and hyperkalemia when compared with CCB. A subsequent randomized controlled trial by Paoletti and colleagues[29] demonstrated that long-term use of ACEi has favorable outcomes from cardiac stand point without any significant deleterious effect on graft function.

Corticosteroids are part of routine immunosuppressive regimen and cause HTN via mineralocorticoid-induced sodium retention, enhance the sensitivity to vasoconstrictors, and reduce the production of vasodilators. A thiazide or loop diuretic can be considered based on volume assessment and renal function. Diuretics are also favored in the setting of hyperkalemia; however, close monitoring of volume status and electrolytes is recommended. Choice of antihypertensive agents depends on coexisting medical conditions, the side effect profile, and the severity of HTN.[24,30] An ACEi is an appropriate choice when there is concurrent proteinuria or posttransplant erythrocytosis. Although CCBs are well-tolerated, nondihydropyridine CCBs such as verapamil and diliazem increase plasma levels of CNIs by inhibiting hepatic P-450 enzymes. **Table 2** summarizes commonly used antihypertensive agents in SOTRs, clinical variables favoring the use, and common adverse effects.

Diabetes Mellitus

DM is a common comorbidity among SOTRs and is strongly associated with adverse cardiovascular events. For a detailed review on posttransplant DM management, please review the article (See Wallia A, Illuri V, Molitch ME: Diabetes Care after Transplant: Definitions, Risk Factors, and Clinical Management, in this issue). When examining United States Renal Data System data of KTRs who died with functioning grafts, Ojo and colleagues[5] noted that mortality from CVD was most marked in the diabetic group and nearly 2-fold higher compared with other groups. The prevalence of DM is higher in SOTRs compared with general population owing to the additive burden of immunosuppression. Posttransplant DM is a strong independent predictor of graft failure CVD and mortality.[33] Among posttransplant patients, DM can be a preexisting condition before transplant or they may have new-onset diabetes mellitus after transplant (NODAT). **Table 3** describes various risk factors for NODAT including pretransplant, donor, and posttransplant risk factors.[33–39]

NODAT and preexisting DM patients have comparable outcomes of graft survival, but survival rates are worse when compared with nondiabetic group in a single-center experience.[40] The International Consensus Guidelines on new-onset diabetes after transplantation were published initially in 2003 and focused predominantly in KTRs, and later extended to other SOTRs. Diagnoses of diabetes and glucose intolerance are made when serum testing meets the criteria described in **Table 4**.

Table 2
Common coexisting conditions and routinely used antihypertensive agents in solid organ transplant recipients

Medication	Clinical Variable that Favors the Use of this Medication	Adverse Effects
Diuretics (thiazide or loop diuretics)	Volume overloaded Hyperkalemia	Monitor electrolytes
Nondihydropyridine CCB (diltiazem, verapamil etc) Dihydropyridine CCBs (amlodipine, nifedipine, etc)	CNI-induced HTN HTN associated with advanced CKD or significantly reduced GFR LVH[31] Proteinuria	CNI drug toxicity Bradycardia Peripheral edema
ACEI/ARB	DM LVH[31,32] Proteinuria Erythrocytosis	Kidney dysfunction (monitor creatinine and potassium) Anemia
Beta blockers	Known CAD or IHD	Bradycardia Erectile dysfunction Dyslipidemia
Doxazosin	BPH	Orthostatic hypotension
Clonidine	DM associated with autonomic dysfunction	Redound HTN Fatigue Bradycardia
Minoxidil	Refractory HTN	Hirsutism Edema Reflex tachycardia
Hydralazine	—	Lupus

Abbreviations: ACEI, angiotensin-converting enzyme inhibitor; ARB, angiotensin receptor blocker; BPH, benign prostatic hypertrophy; CAD, coronary artery disease; CCB, calcium channel blocker; CKD, chronic kidney disease; CNI, calcineurin inhibitor; DM, diabetes mellitus; GFR, glomerular filtration rate; HTN, hypertension; IHD, ischemic heart disease; LVH, left ventricular hypertrophy.

Early detection and management of NODAT and good glycemic control of preexisting DM are essential in posttransplant management of SOTRs. Pretransplant screening should be performed to identify patients who are at risk to develop NODAT and modifying the risks while on transplant waiting list minimizes the risk of CVD subsequently. Lifestyle modification, adjusting immunosuppression, and pharmacotherapy are to be initiated with intent to achieve sustained glycemic control.[41] Alterations to immunosuppressive regimen including dose reduction, withdrawal of CNI, dose reduction of corticosteroids, or steroid-sparing regimens can be considered if clinically acceptable and need to be weighed carefully against the risk of rejection (**Box 1**). The use of CNIs is associated with increased incidence of NODAT and tacrolimus is considered to be more diabetogenic than cyclosporine (CsA).[42,43]

Hyperlipidemia or Dyslipidemia

Dyslipidemia is a frequent complication after solid organ transplantation. Similar to HTN and DM, dyslipidemia may be either preexisting or of new onset in these patients. Routine immunosuppression used in the posttransplant care is a major risk factor for developing lipid abnormalities in this population. Dyslipidemia is association with poor cardiovascular outcomes and is a major risk factor for CAD. Commonly seen lipid

Table 3
Risk factors for new-onset DM after transplant

Factors	High-Risk Factors	Positive Factors
Pretransplant	Impaired glucose tolerance History of stress related DM African American or Hispanic race Advanced age (>40 y) Male gender Family history of DM Obesity Hepatitis C infection	Higher education Glomerulonephritis is etiology of renal failure
Donor	Male gender Cadaveric donor HLA mismatches	
Posttransplant	Immunosuppression Corticosteroids CNIs (Tac > CsA) mTORi (sirolimus) Early glucose intolerance History of acute rejection	Use of mycophenolate mofetil Use of azathioprine

Abbreviations: CNIs, calcineurin inhibitors; CsA, cyclosporine; DM, diabetes mellitus; mTORi, mammalian target of rapamycin inhibitors; Tac, tacrolimus.
   Data from Refs.[33–36]

abnormalities in transplant population are elevated serum levels of total cholesterol, low-density lipoprotein cholesterol, high-density lipoprotein cholesterol, and triglycerides. Several clinical variables influence the lipid profile in posttransplant patients, including age, obesity, pretransplant dyslipidemia, DM, proteinuria, and regimen of immunosuppression.[44] Corticosteroids, CNIs and the mTORis sirolimus and everolimus have unfavorable effects on serum lipids. The mTORis are associated with the most negative effects on lipid profile and almost always necessitate the concomitant use of lipid-lowering agents when used. Total cholesterol was found be an independent predictor of ischemic heart disease in KTRs.[18] Transplant patients with increased concentrations of total cholesterol and triglycerides are nearly twice at risk for developing ischemic heart disease after the first year.[6]

Although lifestyle modification and reduction in immunosuppression may improve dyslipidemia, implementation of statin therapy has become an essential component

Table 4
Criteria for diabetes mellitus and impaired glucose tolerance

Plasma Glucose	2-H OGTT	Diagnosis
FPG <100 mg/dL	Not indicated	Normal
FPG is ≥110 mg/dL and <126 mg/DL	<140 mg/dL ≥140 mg/dL and <200 mg/dL ≥200 mg/dL	— IGT Diabetes mellitus
FPG ≥126 mg/dL	Not indicated	Diabetes mellitus
RPG ≥200 mg/dL	Not indicated	Diabetes mellitus

Abbreviations: 2-H OGTT, 2-hour oral glucose tolerance test (this is performed by administering 75 g of glucose and measure plasma glucose after 2 hours); FPG, fasting plasma glucose; IGT, impaired glucose tolerance; RPG, random plasma glucose.

Box 1

Clinical management and follow-up recommendations for patients with diabetes mellitus in solid organ transplants

- Hemoglobin A1C less than 6.5% every 3 months
- Lipid profile monitoring with intent to achieve target lipids (low-density lipoprotein cholesterol <100 mg/dL, high-density lipoprotein cholesterol >50 mg/dL for women and >40 mg/dL for men and triglycerides <200 mg/dL)
- Blood pressure <130/80 mm Hg
- Weight loss
- Microalbuminuria screening
- Prophylactic aspirin (65–100 mg) is suggested
- Annual eye examination
- Feet examination

---

of transplant management in SOTRs. Beneficial effects of statin institution have been reported in KTRs and heart transplant recipients and a large, randomized, controlled trial is initiated to confirm the effects of statin in KTRs. Despite not attaining statistical significance in primary composite endpoints (cardiac death, nonfatal myocardial infarction, or coronary intervention), the Assessment of Lescol in Renal Transplantation (ALERT) trial demonstrated a downward trend of cardiovascular events in statin arm.[45] Post hoc analyses of the ALERT study suggested that earlier institution of statin therapy has greater benefit.[19,46] Long-term use of statins in the transplant population needs periodic monitoring of creatinine kinase and lipid profile because there is an enhanced risk of myositis and rhabdomyolysis. However, the long-term use of fluvastatin was well-tolerated by those in the treatment arm.

CsA and several statins are metabolized via hepatic P-450 enzyme pathway and simultaneous use of these medications may result in higher incidence of adverse events such as myositis, rhabdomyolysis, and hepatotoxicity.[47,48] Although KDIGO guidelines do not state any preferred statin, pravastatin is more commonly used in SOTRs because it is metabolized primarily via non–CYP isozymes and has better safety profile.[49] Rosuvastatin also has desirable safety profile and it does not significantly interact with CYP isozymes. Approximately 10% of rosuvastatin is metabolized in the liver and most potent inhibition is noted for CYP2C9 isozyme.[50] Fluvastatin is also favorable because it metabolized predominantly via CYP2C9 and has less potential for toxicity compared with atorvastatin and simvastatin, which are metabolized via CYP3A4 isozyme. In 2011, the US Food and Drug Administration issued a communication that stated the use of simvastatin is contraindicated in patients who are on CsA.[47] It is reasonable to initiate statin at a lower dose and uptitrate slowly while monitoring creatinine kinase and liver function tests to avert toxicity.

Tobacco Use

Tobacco use is associated with increased cardiovascular mortality and decreased graft survival after solid organ transplantation. Smoking is one of the major preventable risk factors contributing to CVD and mortality in SOTRs. Smoking history of greater than 25 pack-years at the time of transplantation is a strong predictor of graft failure and increased CVD in renal transplant recipients.[51] Quitting smoking for more than 5 years reduced the overall mortality burden and graft failure in renal transplant recipients.[51] A successful strategy for smoking cessation involves behavioral modification and drug therapy.[52]

Obesity and the Metabolic Syndrome

Obesity and the metabolic syndrome have been increasing and are a global health concern in the general population. Similar trends are noted in the transplant population. SOTRs are additionally at greater risk for obesity and the metabolic syndrome secondary to corticosteroid administration and improvement in their appetite secondary to general improvement in their health. Obesity is an independent risk factor for HTN, hyperlipidemia, diabetes, and CVD in the general population and observational studies in SOTRs have demonstrated similar associations.[53–55]

NONTRADITIONAL RISK FACTORS

Several nontraditional risk factors that contribute to elevated CVD risk have been described in the literature both in the general population and SOTRs.[7] Decreased renal function (elevated serum creatinine or reduced glomerular filtration rate) is considered to be an independent risk factor for CVD.[19,56–58] A multivariate analysis of the placebo arm of ALERT trial demonstrated increased serum creatinine as an independent risk factor for cardiac death, noncardiovascular death, and all-cause mortality. Proteinuria is also considered to be an important risk factor for CVD and mortality.[58,59] mTORi discontinuation and institution of ACEi can be considered, if clinically appropriate. Posttransplant anemia at 1 year is noted to be associated with poor outcomes[60] and use of erythropoietin is controversial owing to increased mortality noted in KTRs.[61,62] Enhanced cardiovascular mortality is reported with low physical activity,[63,64] and increased serum levels of C-reactive protein[65] and homocysteine.[61] Treatment with vitamin B_6, B_{12}, or with high- or low-dose folic acid failed to show any mortality benefit.[66] Endothelial dysfunction, inflammation, oxidative stress, and prothrombotic factors are associated with increased cardiovascular mortality.[8] Further research is required to understand the clinical usefulness of modifying these novel risk factors.

TRANSPLANT-RELATED RISK FACTORS
Immunosuppression

The combination of corticosteroids, CNIs, antiproliferative agents, and mTORis is routinely instituted in posttransplant care of transplant recipients for immunosuppression. They contribute to CVD risk by worsening of preexisting metabolic and systemic risk factors. Their use is associated with increased rates of HTN, NODAT, hyperlipidemia, nephrotoxicity, and weight gain/obesity.

Corticosteroids are used widely for induction and maintenance immunosuppression and for the treatment of acute rejection in SOTRs. Given the undesired adverse risk profile, rapid weaning of steroid protocol and steroid-sparing immunosuppressive regimens have been developed.[67,68] A metaanalysis by Knight and Morris[69] demonstrated similar graft and patient survival with steroid avoidance when compared with standard protocols despite increased incidence of acute rejection. The introduction of CsA revolutionized the management of transplant recipients. However, the pronounced nephrotoxic and negative metabolic effects of CsA spurred a search for alternative, less harmful agents. Tacrolimus is another CNI that has enjoyed greater clinical use owing to a better side effect profile compared with CsA.[42,70] Although tacrolimus causes HTN and dyslipidemia to a lesser degree, the occurrence of NODAT is significantly high in patients treated with tacrolimus when compared with CsA,

Table 5
Commonly used immunosuppressive agents

Medication	HTN	NODAT	Dyslipidemia	Weight Gain	↓ GFR
Steroids	++	++	++	++	—
CsA	++	+	++	—	+
Tacrolimus	+	++	+	—	+
mTORi (sirolimus, everolimus)	—	+	+++	—	Proteinuria +

Abbreviations: CsA, cyclosporine A; GFR, glomerular filtration rate; HTN, hypertension; mTORi, mammalian target of rapamycin inhibitors; NODAT, new-onset diabetes after transplantation.

especially in those patients infected with hepatitis C. Short-term outcomes have significantly improved with introduction of these agents; however, metabolic complications and nephrotoxicity became a major concern. Sirolimus was believed to be less nephrotoxic and was favored over CNIs and several studies were performed testing the concept of CNI minimization and switching to mTORis or supplementing with mTORis.[71–73] Although there is some benefit noticed with kidney function, a higher trend of late acute rejection is noted.[72] It also has a profound effect on lipid metabolism and worsens proteinuria. **Table 5** summarized the effects of commonly used immunosuppressive agents.

When immunosuppression is being modified, diligent monitoring of graft function and laboratory parameters is warranted. Drug interactions are a major concern and

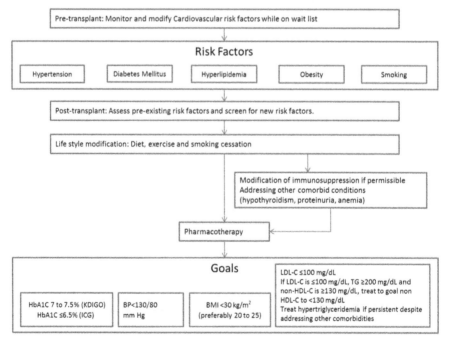

Fig. 3. Risk factors and goals. BMI, body mass index; BP, blood pressure; HbA1c, hemoglobin A1c; HDL-C, high-density lipoprotein cholesterol; ICG, International Consensus Guidelines; KDIGO, Kidney Disease; Improving Global Outcome; LDL-C, low-density lipoprotein cholesterol; TG, triglycerides.

several medications that are commonly used in posttransplant patients interact with one another. Interactions between CNIs and nondihydropyridine CCBs, statins, and azole class drugs are notable. Careful review of the medication list at each office visit, including over-the-counter medications, is necessary to avoid toxicity. Graft dysfunction, history of rejection and cytomegalovirus infections are also associated with enhanced cardiovascular risk and mortality[74–76] (**Fig. 3**).

SUMMARY

This review focused predominantly on the recognition and management of CVD risk factors in kidney and liver transplant recipients, but much of what was discussed can be extrapolated to other SOTRs. The incidence and prevalence of these risk factors may vary based on the transplanted organ, but general principles of CVD risk factors, risk association, and management of the risk factors are similar. Therapeutic goals of management are derived predominantly from the general population, because available data regarding CV risk management in SOTRs is limited to a modest number of observational and randomized, controlled trials. Because of the great amount of risk and clear associations with CV disease and worse posttransplant graft and patient survival, we recommend that the management of cardiovascular risk factors should begin before transplantation with aggressive screening and risk modification and then continue as a top priority of care in the posttransplant period. Optimal management requires a detailed knowledge of the available strategies and their potential interactions with the immunosuppressive regimens and demands an individualized approach that balances the competing risks of rejection, infection, medication toxicity, metabolic derangements, and cardiovascular complications.

REFERENCES

1. Rana A, Gruessner A, Agopian VG, et al. Survival benefit of solid-organ transplant in the United States. JAMA Surg 2015;150(3):252–9.
2. Wolfe RA, Ashby VB, Milford EL, et al. Comparison of mortality in all patients on dialysis, patients on dialysis awaiting transplantation, and recipients of a first cadaveric transplant. N Engl J Med 1999;341:1725–30.
3. Arend SM, Mallat MJ, Westendorp RJ, et al. Patient survival after renal transplantation; more than 25 years follow-up. Nephrol Dial Transplant 1997;12:1672–9.
4. Briggs JD. Causes of death after renal transplantation. Nephrol Dial Transplant 2001;16:1545–9.
5. Ojo AO, Hanson JA, Wolfe RA, et al. Long-term survival in renal transplant recipients with graft function. Kidney Int 2000;57:307–13.
6. Kasiske BL, Chakkera HA, Roel J. Explained and unexplained ischemic heart disease risk after renal transplantation. J Am Soc Nephrol 2000;11:1735–43.
7. Ducloux D, Kazory A, Chalopin JM. Predicting coronary heart disease in renal transplant recipients: a prospective study. Kidney Int 2004;66:441–7.
8. Ojo AO. Cardiovascular complications after renal transplantation and their prevention. Transplantation 2006;82(5):603–11.
9. Myers RP, Lee SS. Cirrhotic cardiomyopathy and liver transplantation. Liver Transpl 2000;6(Suppl 1):S44–52.
10. Saran R, Li Y, Robinson B, et al. US renal data system 2014 annual data report: epidemiology of kidney disease in the United States. Am J Kidney Dis 2015;66(1): S1–306.

11. de Mattos AM, Prather J, Olyaei AJ, et al. Cardiovascular events following renal transplantation: role of traditional and transplant specific risk factors. Kidney Int 2006;70:757–64.

12. Kasiske BL, Maclean JR, Snyder JJ. Acute myocardial infarction and kidney transplantation. J Am Soc Nephrol 2006;17:900.

13. Lentine KL, Brennan DC, Schnitzler MA. Incidence and predictors of myocardial infarction after kidney transplantation. J Am Soc Nephrol 2005;16:496.

14. Lentine KL, Schnitzler MA, Abbott KC, et al. De novo congestive heart failure after kidney transplantation: a common condition with poor prognostic implications. Am J Kidney Dis 2005;46:720–33.

15. Gurundy SM, Pasternak R, Greenland P, et al. Assessment of cardiovascular risk by use of multiple-risk-factor assessment equations. J Am Coll Cardiol 1999;34: 1348–59.

16. Vanrenterghem YF, Claes K, Montagnino G, et al. Risk factors for cardiovascular events after successful renal transplantation. Transplantation 2008;85:209–16.

17. Lentine KL, Salvatore P, Costa MD, et al. Cardiac disease evaluation and management among kidney and liver transplantation candidates. AHA/ACCF statement. Circulation 2012;126:617–63.

18. Aker S, Ivens K, Grabensee B, et al. Cardiovascular risk factors and diseases after renal transplantation. Int Urol Nephrol 1998;30:777–88.

19. Jardine AG, Fellstrom B, Logan JO, et al. Cardiovascular risk and renal transplantation: post hoc analyses of the Assessment of Lescol in Renal Transplantation (ALERT) study. Am J Kidney Dis 2005;46:529–36.

20. Opelz G, Wujciak T, Ritz E. Association of chronic kidney graft failure with recipient blood pressure. Collaborative Transplant Study. Kidney Int 1998;53:217–22.

21. Hillebrand U, Suwelack BM, Loley K, et al. Blood pressure, antihypertensive treatment, and graft survival in kidney transplant patients. Transpl Int 2009;22: 1073–80.

22. Rigatto C, Parfrey P, Foley R, et al. Congestive heart failure in renal transplant recipients: risk factors, outcomes, and relationship with ischemic heart disease. J Am Soc Nephrol 2002;13:1084–90.

23. Israni A, Snyder J, Skeans M, et al. Predicting coronary heart disease after kidney transplantation: Patient Outcomes in Renal Transplantation (PORT) study. Am J Transplant 2010;10:338–53.

24. Midtvedt K, Neumayer HH. Management strategies for posttransplant hypertension. Transplantation 2000;70(Suppl 11):SS64–9.

25. Opelz G, Dohler B. Improved long-term outcomes after renal transplantation associated with blood pressure control. Am J Transplant 2005;5:2725–31.

26. Ramesh Prasad GV. Ambulatory blood pressure monitoring in solid organ transplantation. Clin Transplant 2012;26:185–91.

27. James PA, Oparil S, Carter BL, et al. 2014 evidence-based guideline for the management of high blood pressure in adults. Report from panel members appointed to the Eighth Joint National Committee (JNC 8). JAMA 2014;311(5):507–20.

28. Cross NB, Webster AC, Masson P, et al. Antihypertensives for kidney transplant recipients: systematic review and meta-analysis of randomized controlled trials. Transplantation 2009;88:7.

29. Paoletti E, Bellino D, Marsano L, et al. Effects of ACE inhibitors on long-term outcome of renal transplant recipients: a randomized controlled trial. Transplantation 2013;95:889.

30. Weir MR. Blood pressure management in the kidney transplant recipient. Adv Chronic Kidney Dis 2004;11:172–83.

31. Midtvedt K, Ihlen H, Hartmann A, et al. Reduction of left ventricular mass by lisinopril and nifedipine in hypertensive renal transplant recipients: a prospective randomized double-blind study. Transplantation 2001;72:107–11.
32. Paoletti E, Cassottana P, Amidone M, et al. ACE inhibitors and persistent left ventricular hypertrophy after renal transplantation: a randomized clinical trial. Am J Kidney Dis 2007;50:133.
33. Kasiske BL, Snyder JJ, Gilbertson D, et al. Diabetes mellitus after kidney transplantation in the united states. Am J Transplant 2003;3:178–85.
34. Baid S, Cosimi AB, Farrell ML, et al. Post-transplant diabetes mellitus in liver transplant recipients: risk factors, temporal relationship with hepatitis C virus allograft hepatitis, and impact on mortality. Transplantation 2001;72:1066–72.
35. Pham PT, Pham PC, Lipshutz GS, et al. New onset diabetes mellitus after solid organ transplantation. Endocrinol Metab Clin North Am 2007;36:873–90.
36. Rakel A, Karelis AD. New-onset diabetes after transplantation: risk factors and clinical impact. Diabetes Metab 2011;37:1–14.
37. KDIGO 2012 clinical practice guideline for the evaluation and management of chronic kidney disease. 2013;3(1). Available at: www.kidney-international.org.
38. Wilkinson A, Davidson J, Dotta F, et al. Guidelines for the treatment and management of new-onset diabetes after transplantation. Clin Transplant 2005;19:291–8.
39. Roodnat JI, Mulder PG, Zietse R, et al. Cholesterol as an independent predictor of outcome after renal transplantation. Transplantation 2000;69:1704–10.
40. Revanur VK, Jardine AG, Kingsmore DB, et al. Influence of diabetes mellitus on patient and graft survival in recipients of kidney transplantation. Clin Transplant 2001;15:89.
41. Davidson J, Wilkinson A, Dantal J, et al. New-onset diabetes after transplantation: 2003 International Consensus Guidelines. Transplantation 2003;7:SS3–S24.
42. Henry ML. Cyclosporine and tacrolimus (FK506): a comparison of efficacy and safety profiles. Clin Transplant 1999;13:209–20.
43. Weiner DE, Carpenter MA, Levey AS, et al. Kidney function and risk of cardiovascular disease and mortality in kidney transplant recipients: the FAVORIT trial. Am J Transplant 2012;12:2437–45.
44. Massy ZA, Kasiske BL. Post-transplant hyperlipidemia: mechanisms and management. J Am Soc Nephrol 1996;7:971–7.
45. Holdaas H, Fellstrom B, Jardine AG, et al. Assessment of LEscol in Renal Transplantation (ALERT) study investigators: effect of fluvastatin on cardiac outcomes in renal transplant recipients: a multicentre, randomised, placebo-controlled trial. Lancet 2003;361:2024–31.
46. Holdaas H, Fellstrom B, Cole E, et al. Long-term cardiac outcomes in renal transplant recipients receiving fluvastatin: the ALERT extension study. Am J Transplant 2005;5(12):2929–36 [Erratum appears in Am J Transplant 2006;5(12):2929].
47. U.S. Food and Drug Administration (FDA). FDA drug safety communication: new restrictions, contraindications, and dose limitations for Zocor (simvastatin) to reduce the risk of muscle injury. Available at: www.fda.gov/Drugs/DrugSafety/ucm256581.htm. Accessed June 8, 2011.
48. Shirali AC, Bia MJ. Management of cardiovascular disease in renal transplant recipients. Clin J Am Soc Nephrol 2008;3:491–504.
49. McKenny JM, Pharm D. Pharmacologic characteristics of statins. Clin Cardiol 2003;26(Suppl III):32–8.
50. Olsson AG, Mc Taggart F, Raza A. Rosuvastatin: a highly effective new HMG-CoA reductase inhibitor. Cardiovasc Drug Rev 2002;20(4):303–28.

51. Kasiske BL, Klinger D. Cigarette smoking in renal transplant recipients. J Am Soc Nephrol 2000;11:753–9.
52. Anthonisen NR, Skeans MA, Wise RA, et al. The effects of a smoking cessation intervention on 14.5-year mortality: a randomized clinical trial. Ann Intern Med 2005;142:233–9.
53. Nicoletto BB, Fonseca NK, Manfro RC, et al. Effects of obesity on kidney transplantation outcomes: a systematic review and meta-analysis. Transplantation 2014;98:167–76.
54. Meier-Kriesche HU, Arndorfer JA, Kaplan B. The impact of body mass index on renal transplant outcomes: A significant independent risk factor for graft failure and patient death. Transplantation 2002;73:70–4.
55. Lodhi SA, Lamb KE, Meier-Kriesche HU. Solid organ allograft survival improvement in the United States: the long-term does not mirror the dramatic short-term success. Am J Transplant 2011;11:1226–35.
56. Fellstrom B, Jardineb AG, Soveria I, et al. Renal dysfunction is a strong and independent risk factor for mortality and cardiovascular complications in renal transplantation. Am J Transplant 2005;5:1986–91.
57. Ojo AO. Renal disease in recipients of nonrenal solid organ transplantation. Semin Nephrol 2007;27:498.
58. Meier-Kriesche HU, Baliga R, Kaplan B. Decreased renal function is a strong risk factor for cardiovascular death after renal transplantation. Transplantation 2003; 75:1291–5.
59. Hernández D, Pérez G, Marrero D, et al. Early association of low-grade albuminuria and allograft dysfunction predicts renal transplant outcomes. Transplantation 2012;93:297–303.
60. Kamar N, Rostaing L. Negative impact of one-year anemia on long-term patient and graft survival in kidney transplant patients receiving calcineurin inhibitors and mycophenolate mofetil. Transplantation 2008;85:1120.
61. Ducloux D, Motte G, Challier B, et al. Serum total homocysteine and cardiovascular disease occurrence in chronic, stable renal transplant recipients: a prospective study. J Am Soc Nephrol 2000;11:134.
62. Heinze G, Kainz A, Hörl WH, et al. Mortality in renal transplant recipients given erythropoietins to increase haemoglobin concentration: cohort study. BMJ 2009;339:b4018.
63. Zelle DM, Corpeleijn E, Stolk RP, et al. Low physical activity and risk of cardiovascular and all-cause mortality in renal transplant recipients. Clin J Am Soc Nephrol 2011;6:898.
64. Abedini S, Holme I, Marz W, et al. Inflammation in renal transplantation. Clin J Am Soc Nephrol 2009;4:1246.
65. Varagunam M, Finney H, Trevitt R, et al. Pretransplantation levels of C-reactive protein predict all-cause and cardiovascular mortality, but not graft outcome, in kidney transplant recipients. Am J Kidney Dis 2004;43:502.
66. Bostom AG, Carpenter MA, Kusek JW, et al. Homocysteine-lowering and cardiovascular disease outcomes in kidney transplant recipients: primary results from the folic acid for vascular outcome reduction in transplantation trial. Circulation 2011;123:1763.
67. Vincenti F, Schena FP, Paraskevas S, et al. A randomized, multicenter study of steroid avoidance, early steroid withdrawal or standard steroid therapy in kidney transplant recipients. Am J Transplant 2008;8:307.
68. Pascual J, Zamora J, Galeano C, et al. Steroid avoidance or withdrawal for kidney transplant recipients. Cochrane Database Syst Rev 2009;(1):CD005632.

69. Knight SR, Morris PJ. Steroid sparing protocols following nonrenal transplants; the evidence is not there. A systematic review and meta-analysis. Transpl Int 2011;24(12):1198–207.
70. Webster AC, Woodroffe RC, Taylor RS, et al. Tacrolimus versus cyclosporin as primary immunosuppression for kidney transplant recipients: meta-analysis and meta-regression of randomised trial data. BMJ 2005;331:810–21.
71. Paoletti E, Ratto E, Bellino D, et al. Effect of early conversion from CNI to sirolimus on outcomes in kidney transplant recipients with allograft dysfunction. J Nephrol 2012;25:709–18.
72. Schena FP, Pascoe MD, Alberu J, et al. Conversion from calcineurin inhibitors to sirolimus maintenance therapy in renal allograft recipients: 24-month efficacy and safety results from the CONVERT trial. Transplantation 2009;87:233–42.
73. Flechner SM, Goldfarb D, Solez K, et al. Kidney transplantation with sirolimus and mycophenolate mofetil-based immunosuppression: 5-year results of a randomized prospective trial compared to calcineurin inhibitor drugs. Transplantation 2007;83:883.
74. Sarnak MJ, Levey AS. Cardiovascular disease and chronic renal disease: a new paradigm. Am J Kidney Dis 2000;35(Suppl 1):S117–31.
75. Humar A, Gillingham K, Payne WD, et al. Increased incidence of cardiac complications in kidney transplant recipients with cytomegalovirus disease. Transplantation 2000;70:310–3.
76. Kalil RS, Hudson SL, Gaston RS. Determinants of cardiovascular mortality after renal transplantation: a role for cytomegalovirus? Am J Transplant 2003;3:79–81.

Diabetes Care After Transplant

Definitions, Risk Factors, and Clinical Management

Amisha Wallia, MD, MS, Vidhya Illuri, MD, Mark E. Molitch, MD*

KEYWORDS

- Diabetes • NODAT • Transplant • Transplantation • Kidney • Liver
- Immunosuppression • Insulin

KEY POINTS

- Transplant patients may have preexisting diabetes mellitus, develop new-onset diabetes after transplantation, or have transient postoperative hyperglycemia.
- Although insulin is the usual inpatient treatment, following discharge the usual diabetes oral and parenteral medications can be used.
- Immunosuppression medications may impair kidney function and dose adjustments of diabetes medications are often needed for this.
- Medications interacting with the CYP3A4 enzyme pathway may interact with immunosuppressive drug metabolism and dose adjustments may be needed.
- Glycemic goals should be individualized for patients with significant comorbidities.

INTRODUCTION

Patients who undergo solid organ transplantation may have preexisting diabetes mellitus (DM), which puts them at increased risk from any surgery.[1] It is important to evaluate the glycemic status of each patient before transplantation, when possible. This includes an evaluation of their current diabetes status, including level of control, medication use, and known complications of DM (nephropathy, retinopathy, neuropathy, cardiovascular disease). Obtaining an A1c level before transplantation can be helpful in determining the existence of previously undiagnosed DM, but a normal level does not exclude the existence of DM.

Disclosure Statement: Dr A. Wallia receives research support from Merck, Abbvie and Novartis. Dr V. Illuri has no disclosures. Dr M.E. Molitch receives research support from Novartis, Novo Nordisk, Bayer, and Abbvie and has consulted for Lilly, Novo Nordisk, Novartis, Merck, Pfizer, Bristol Myers Squibb, Janssen, and AstraZeneca.
Division of Endocrinology, Metabolism and Molecular Medicine, Northwestern University Feinberg School of Medicine, Chicago, IL 60611, USA
* Corresponding author. 645 North Michigan Avenue, Suite 530, Chicago, IL 60611.
E-mail address: molitch@northwestern.edu

Regardless of previous DM status, transplant patients are at risk for postoperative hyperglycemia due to the stress of surgery and use of high-dose corticosteroids given for induction.[2,3] For those without a previous history of DM and who have a normal A1c, the risk factors for new-onset diabetes after transplantation (NODAT) (see later in this article) should be ascertained. However, given that end-stage kidney and liver disease can confer changes to insulin resistance, glucose metabolism, and DM status, it is important to take an expanded history of pre-DM/DM status that includes a time before the patient's organ failure.

INPATIENT MANAGEMENT OF HYPERGLYCEMIA AFTER TRANSPLANTATION

Intensive glycemic control with the use of insulin therapy can have beneficial short-term and long-term effects. Intensive insulin therapy with glucose goals of 80 to 100 mg/dL in a general surgical intensive care unit (ICU) setting has been demonstrated to reduce morbidity and mortality.[4] However, hypoglycemia can be a limiting factor in achieving such benefits, as seen in studies in mixed or medical ICUs.[5,6]

Previous data suggest that transplant patients with lower glucose levels immediately after transplantation may have lower rates of rejection, infection, posttransplant diabetes, and rehospitalization in most,[7–10] but not all studies.[11,12] Preexisting DM is associated with higher glucose values after surgery and increased rejection rates; implementation of a dedicated Glucose Management Service as part of an inpatient transplant team improves glycemic control (without increasing hypoglycemic events) and decreases infection rates after liver transplantation.[13]

At our transplant center, we use insulin drips in the inpatient period with a glucose goal of 110 to 140 mg/dL in the ICU for transplant patients without an increased risk of hypoglycemia. If an experienced team is not available, then the increased risk of death associated with hypoglycemia[14] would make 140 to 180 mg/dL a safer target, as outlined by the 2009 American Diabetes Association (ADA) guidelines.[15] Our team uses a basal/bolus insulin strategy following the transition from the ICU to the inpatient floor, regardless of DM status, with a continued preprandial glucose goal of 110 to 140 mg/dL and random glucose goal of less than 180 mg/dL. Generally, we calculate the insulin drip rate for the last 6 hours in the ICU, extrapolate that out to a 24-hour rate (ie, multiply $\times$ 4) and give a dose of long-acting insulin (eg, glargine insulin) as a percentage of that total amount (usually between 40% and 80%, depending on renal function, steroid dose, and time away from surgery). Ten percent of that basal dose is then given as a bridging dose of rapid-acting insulin together with the long-acting insulin and the insulin drip is then turned off. Ten percent to 15% of that basal dose is also used as the prandial bolus dose of rapid-acting insulin. Insulin doses need continued attention, as conditions change in these labile patients. We generally recommend holding all oral medications for glycemic control while in the hospital and use only insulin. Currently the use of other oral medications, such as dipeptidyl peptidase-4 (DPP-4) inhibitors and glucagonlike peptide 1 (GLP-1) receptor agonists, are being studied in inpatients and future use may be considered pending results.

TRANSITION FROM INPATIENT TO OUTPATIENT CARE

Patients are often discharged within a few days of surgery and the transition from inpatient to outpatient care is complex and is known to be prone to errors.[16] For patients without a previous history of DM who are still requiring insulin therapy on the day of discharge, the health care team must decide whether to send the patient home on insulin therapy, on an oral hypoglycemic medication, or on no diabetic medication. Stress of surgery, high-dose corticosteroid taper, and fluctuating levels of kidney function contribute to the unpredictability of glycemic excursions during the first weeks after discharge. It is important to discharge the patient on a flexible regimen that can be changed as the clinical status changes. For this reason, we recommend basal/bolus insulin therapy if the total daily dosage of insulin on discharge day is greater than approximately 0.25 units/kg. If the total daily dosage of insulin is less than 0.25 units/kg, one could consider basal insulin alone with a correction scale given for glucose levels greater than 200 mg/dL or possibly an oral agent. Basal/bolus insulin therapy can be precisely titrated, in contrast to oral hypoglycemic therapy, and this is critical given the variability of clinical course.[17]

Patients who require outpatient treatment need to have DM education before leaving the hospital if they have no history of DM or have a step-up in regimen (eg, oral hypoglycemic agents to insulin). Ideally, an introduction of DM concepts should be done during pretransplant education. Patients are often still experiencing postoperative pain requiring sedating medications, and it may be difficult to retain DM education during inpatient hospitalization. Therefore, such education generally has to be limited to instruction on survival skills, specifically insulin/medication dosing and administration, glucose meter use, and understanding glucose goals. Caregivers who will be involved in posttransplant care should be involved in training, when possible. The discharge instructions should include a complete list and administration instructions of all DM medications/supplies.

EVALUATION AND TREATMENT AFTER HOSPITAL DISCHARGE

Patients who are hyperglycemic following hospital discharge after solid organ transplantation comprise 3 groups: (1) those with preexisting DM, whether diagnosed before transplantation or not; (2) those with hyperglycemia related to stress of the surgery in whom the hyperglycemia usually resolves over several days following surgery; and (3) those with NODAT following resolution of the initial posttransplant hyperglycemia. The management aspects of the 3 groups are discussed below. However, NODAT is a type of DM that is specifically related to transplantation and therefore deserves more explanation as to its cause and importance.

New-Onset Diabetes After Transplantation: Definition and Diagnosis

Patients who develop NODAT have increased rates of acute rejection and infection, diminished long-term survival, and increased health care costs.[2,18–21] The International Consensus Guidelines for the diagnosis of NODAT used the ADA criteria then in place for the diagnosis of DM.[3] A recent international consensus conference[22] suggested that the term "posttransplant diabetes mellitus" be used instead of NODAT so as to capture those patients who had previously undiagnosed DM and use the same criteria for diagnosis; however, here we are discussing truly new-onset DM and will continue to use the term NODAT. The ADA criteria include fasting plasma glucose $\geq$126 mg/dL, symptoms of polyuria, polydipsia, or unexplained weight loss and a random plasma glucose concentration of $\geq$200 mg/dL, or a 2-hour plasma glucose level of $\geq$200 mg/dL on an oral glucose tolerance test (OGTT). The ADA added an A1c value $\geq$6.5% as a criterion for the diagnosis of DM in 2010.[23] In practice, we recommend using A1c values greater than 6.5% in addition to the previously mentioned criteria to diagnose NODAT, but with the understanding that anemia, a history of recent blood transfusion, and renal failure may affect these values.[22]

The timing of actual screening to make a diagnosis of NODAT is important. Almost all patients will have hyperglycemia postoperatively due to the stress of surgery and administration of high-dose steroids. Immunosuppression protocols for kidney transplants are now often free of glucocorticoids after the first few days following transplantation, but most other solid organ transplant regimens include a steroid taper for several weeks, and cases of acute rejection are almost always treated with high-dose steroids. As glucocorticoids are known to cause hyperglycemia,[24] it may be difficult to diagnose patients with DM while they are still on high doses of glucocorticoids. We recommend waiting until the patient is on a stable glucocorticoid dose equivalent to 10 mg per day or less of prednisone before making the diagnosis of NODAT, based on our clinical experience.

Risk Factors for New-Onset Diabetes After Transplantation

Risk factors for the development of NODAT are similar to those for the development of DM in general, and include glucose intolerance before transplantation, immediate posttransplant hyperglycemia, older age, being of African American or Hispanic origin, increased body weight, a family history of DM, and hepatitis C.[25–28] In liver transplant patients, those receiving living donor livers have a lower risk of NODAT than those receiving deceased donor livers.[29] Other more transplant-related risk factors for NODAT include polycystic kidney disease, cytomegalovirus infection, hypomagnesemia, and HLA mismatch.[25]

Effect of Immunosuppressive Drugs on New-Onset Diabetes After Transplantation

In a systematic review of the literature, Montori and colleagues[2] estimated that the immunosuppressive regimen explains 74% of the risk of NODAT.

Corticosteroids

Corticosteroids are used as induction therapy, for maintenance, and for treatment of rejection. Although there are some steroid-free maintenance regimens for kidney transplants, even these use high-dose steroids for induction and treatment of rejection. Suggested mechanisms for hyperglycemia include increased insulin resistance, increased hepatic gluconeogenesis, and decreased insulin secretion.[24] The risk of NODAT increases with both the dose and duration of corticosteroid therapy. In kidney transplant patients, incremental dose increases of 0.1 mg/kg prednisolone per day correlated with a 5% increased risk of NODAT and a 4% increased risk of impaired glucose tolerance.[30]

Antiproliferative agents

The antiproliferative agents, azathioprine and mycophenolate mofetil/mycophenolic acid, do not cause hyperglycemia.

Calcineurin inhibitors

The calcineurin inhibitors, tacrolimus and cyclosporine, are commonly the cornerstone of the immunosuppression used after solid organ transplantation. Calcineurin inhibitors impair insulin secretion and sensitivity, inhibit insulin gene transcription, and cause direct damage to pancreatic islet cells.[26,31] Tacrolimus use is associated with a much higher risk of NODAT when compared with cyclosporine.[32] At 36 months after kidney transplantation, 31.8% of tacrolimus users had developed NODAT compared with 21.9% of patients who had received cyclosporin.[33] One retrospective study showed that this differential effect of tacrolimus versus cyclosporine was seen only in patients who were hepatitis C positive,[28] but the prospective, randomized DIRECT study showed this increased risk with tacrolimus even in hepatitis C–negative patients.[34] There is evidence for higher incidence of NODAT with tacrolimus compared with cyclosporine use in liver transplants as well.[35] Converting patients from tacrolimus to cyclosporine after transplantation lowers the risk of NODAT.[36]

Mammalian target of rapamycin inhibitors

The use of sirolimus, a mammalian target of rapamycin (mTOR) inhibitor, has decreased in recent years but is still used in some circumstances. Sirolimus also has been shown to have islet cell toxicity.[37] A retrospective analysis in kidney transplant patients receiving cyclosporine, tacrolimus, or sirolimus in addition to glucocorticoids did not find a statistically significant difference in NODAT development among the 3 groups.[38] Everolimus is another mTOR inhibitor and early studies suggest that it also increases the risk for NODAT.[39]

Belatacept

Belatacept, a cytotoxic T-lymphocyte–associated antigen 4-immunoglobulin fusion protein that selectively inhibits T-cell activation,[40] was introduced into clinical practice in 2011, and is given intravenously once monthly instead of calcineurin inhibitors or mTOR inhibitors.[41] Studies show no increased risk for NODAT with belatacept in kidney transplant recipients.[41] Belatacept is less effective for prevention of liver transplant rejection[42] and is not currently approved for liver transplantation.

MANAGEMENT STRATEGIES FOLLOWING DISCHARGE

Patients with preexisting DM could go back on their pretransplant regimen, if they were in good control before transplantation, once their immediate stress/transplant-related hyperglycemia resolves and if steroids are not currently being taken at doses that may cause excess hyperglycemia. If they were in poor control, then the hospitalization and immediate posthospital care period may serve as a good opportunity to intensify their treatment.[43–45] However, some changes also may be needed because there are certain drug-drug interactions as well as kidney function–related changes that may be needed, which are reviewed below.

The patient without a previous history of diabetes may have persistent hyperglycemia after discharge and may have had preexisting DM that had not been discovered before transplantation. Such patients should continue on their insulin regimen with frequent testing so as to determine when insulin dose reductions may be needed and when they might ultimately be able to convert to an oral agent regimen.

Patients without a prior history of DM and who return to normal glucose levels after transplantation should be counseled regarding the risk of NODAT. Lifestyle changes that can decrease this risk should be reviewed with the patient and instituted following stability of their clinical condition after transplantation.[46] Given the multiple care providers involved in their care, including primary care providers, subspecialists, transplant subspecialists, and various midlevel providers, patient-centered education should be used when possible.[44,45]

The use and doses of immunosuppressive medications are directed by the transplant team and are based on the immunosuppression needs of the patients. *The health of the transplanted organ is of primary importance and, in our opinion, altering the type of immunosuppression simply to reduce the risk of NODAT[47] should not be done. The hyperglycemia of NODAT is manageable but losing a transplanted organ is a medical catastrophe.* We are in agreement with the recent international consensus conference in this regard.[22] Therefore, the clinician managing the hyperglycemia just needs to understand that immunosuppressive medications can cause hyperglycemia and NODAT and needs to be prepared to adjust insulin or other medications as needed if immunosuppressive drugs and/or doses change. It is important for the providers managing the hyperglycemia to be an integral part of the transplant team from shortly after discharge, so that changes in glycemic management can occur whenever there are changes in the immunosuppression regimen or changes in kidney function.

A regular review of glucose levels, both fasting and random by the providers managing the hyperglycemia, should occur. Blood chemistries are routinely ordered by the transplant team twice weekly for the first 2 months, then monthly for 2 years, and then quarterly following transplant. These may be fasting or randomly collected, so attention must be paid to the time of collection when assessing the glucose levels. We recommend testing HbA1c every 3 to 6 months starting 3 to 4 months posttransplant. One study demonstrated that at 1 year after kidney transplantation, an A1c of 6.5% was an accurate measure for diagnosing diabetes that had been diagnosed by OGTT criteria.[48]

GLYCEMIC MANAGEMENT OF HYPERGLYCEMIC TRANSPLANT PATIENTS

Glycemic management should follow general treatment guidelines currently in place for diabetes, whether the patient has preexisting diabetes or NODAT.[23,44,45] However, it is important to assess the risks and benefits of adhering to glycemic goals in a given patient. Many patients undergoing solid organ transplantation have multiple comorbidities, so that an A1c goal of 7.5% to 8.0% may be reasonable compared with less than 7.0% for healthy individuals with an anticipated long life span.[44,45]

Obviously, for patients with type 1 diabetes, continued insulin management will be required. In contrast, the first step of glycemic management for most patients with type 2 DM or NODAT is the initiation of lifestyle modifications. If this fails to bring the A1c to goal after a short trial, oral agent monotherapy is initiated.[44,45] There are no studies determining which oral agents are safest or most efficacious in posttransplant patients. The choice of agent is usually made based on the side-effect profile of the medication and possible interactions with the patient's immunosuppression regimen (which are metabolized by cytochrome P450 family 3 subfamily A [CYP3A]) and other drugs commonly used in transplant patients, such as imidazole antifungal agents, which inhibit CYP3A (**Table 1**). Drug dose adjustment may be required because of decreases in the glomerular filtration rate (GFR), a relatively common complication in transplant patients from kidney transplant rejection, calcineurin inhibitor nephrotoxicity,[49] or other kidney injury (see **Table 1**).

Metformin

Metformin is generally preferred as the initial oral agent in patients with type 2 DM.[23,44,45] Metformin increases insulin sensitivity and decreases hepatic gluconeogenesis; it does not cause hypoglycemia. Metformin is not metabolized by CYP3A4 and therefore has no drug-drug interactions with immunosuppressive agents or imidazoles. However, metformin is renally cleared.[50] As many patients have impaired kidney function after transplantation, which has been thought to increase the risk of lactic acidosis,[51] it has not been advocated as a first-line drug in such patients.[3] The Food and Drug Administration recommends that metformin should not be used in men with a serum creatinine of $\geq$1.5 mg/dL or women with a serum creatinine of $\geq$1.4 mg/dL. However, in studies of patients continuing to receive metformin with GFR levels in the 30 to 60 mL/min/1.73 m^2 range, lactic acidosis is still exceedingly rare.[51] Metformin use in transplant patients has been advocated[52] and 2 studies showed it to be safe and effective in kidney transplant patients who had estimated GFR (eGFR) levels down to 30 mL/min/1.73 m^2.[53,54] Given the marked clinical benefit of metformin, we agree with the recent recommendation[51] that metformin be used without dose

Table 1
Dose adjustments for insulin and other medications used to treat diabetes

Medication Class	CKD Stages 3–5	Use in Liver/Kidney Transplant
Insulin		
Glargine, detemir, NPH, regular, aspart, lispro, glulisine	No specific dose adjustment. Decrease doses depending on patient responses	All acceptable
Sulfonylureas		
Glipizide	eGFR <30[a]: use with caution	Acceptable, interaction with cotrimoxazole
Glimepiride	eGFR <60: use with caution, <30 avoid use	Acceptable, tolerated well
Glyburide	eGFR <60: avoid use	Avoid use
Glinides		
Repaglinide	eGFR <30: use with caution eGFR <60: avoid use (can use if dialysis)	Metabolized by CYP3A4; reduce dose if cyclosporine/tacrolimus used but does not affect cyclosporine/tacrolimus levels
Nateglinide		
Biguanide		
Metformin	*Per FDA*: do not use if creatinine ≥1.5 mg/dL in men and ≥1.4 mg/dL in women *Consider* (controversial, not FDA approved): eGFR 45–59: use caution, follow renal function every 3–6 mo eGFR 30–44: maximum dose 1000 mg/d, follow renal function every 3–6 mo. Do not start as new therapy eGFR <30: avoid use	GI side effects Lactose acidosis very rare with impaired kidney function
Thiazolidinediones		
Pioglitazone, rosiglitazone	No dose adjustment needed	Well tolerated. Concern regarding fluid retention, CHF, and bone fractures. Both have been used in transplantation
Alpha-glucosidase inhibitors		
Acarbose, Miglitol	Serum creatinine >2 mg/dL: avoid use	No experience reported in transplantation GI side effects may be limiting
DPP-4 inhibitors		
Sitagliptin	eGFR ≥50: 100 mg daily eGFR 30–49: 50 mg daily eGFR <30: 25 mg daily	Several small studies show that it is well tolerated in transplant patients.

(*continued on next page*)

		Use in Liver/Kidney
Medication Class	**CKD Stages 3–5**	**Transplant**
Saxagliptin	eGFR >50: 2.5 or 5 mg daily eGFR ≤50: 2.5 mg daily.	Metabolized by CYP3A4; reduce dose if cyclosporine/tacrolimus used but does not affect cyclosporine/tacrolimus levels Concern for CHF
Alogliptin	eGFR >60: 25 mg daily eGFR 30–59: 12.5 mg daily eGFR <30: 6.25 mg daily	—
Linagliptin	No dose adjustment needed	Has been used in transplant patients
SGLT2 inhibitors		
Canagliflozin	eGFR 45–60: maximum dose 100 mg daily eGFR <45: avoid use	No interaction with cyclosporine dosing
Dapagliflozin	eGFR <60: avoid use	
Empagliflozin	eGFR <45: avoid use	
GLP-1 receptor agonists		
Exenatide	eGFR <30: avoid use	No interaction with
Liraglutide, dulaglutide, albiglutide	No dose adjustments needed	cyclosporine or tacrolimus in small studies (primarily pancreas transplants)

Table 1
(*continued*)

Abbreviations: CHF, congestive heart failure; CKD, chronic kidney disease; eGFR, estimated glomerular filtration rate; FDA, Food and Drug Administration; GI, gastrointestinal; GLP-1, glucagonlike peptide 1; NPH, neutral protamine hagedorn; SGLT2, sodium-glucose cotransporter 2.
[a] For all eGFR values, the units are mL/min/1.73 m^2.

reduction down to an eGFR of 45 mL/min/1.73 m^2, with a reduction to a maximum of 1000 mg daily if the eGFR is ≥30 to 44 mL/min/1.73 m^2 and stopped with an eGFR less than 30 mL/min/1.73 m^2 or in situations associated with hypoxia or an acute decline in kidney function, such as sepsis/shock, hypotension, and use of radiographic contrast or other nephrotoxic agents. In addition, the gastrointestinal side effects might also be limiting in view of similar side effects from mycophenolate mofetil/mycophenolic acid.

Sulfonylureas and Glinides

Sulfonylureas and glinides increase insulin secretion and can cause hypoglycemia. Sulfonylureas and their metabolites are renally cleared, leading to an increased risk of hypoglycemia as GFR declines.[55–57] Glyburide should be avoided with an eGFR less than 60 mL/min/1.73 m^2.[58] Glimepiride should be used with caution if the eGFR is less than 60 mL/min/1.73 m^2 and not be used with eGFR less than 30 mL/min/1.73 m^2.[59] Less than 10% of glipizide is cleared renally but it should still be used with caution with an eGFR less than 30 mL/min/1.73 m^2.[60,61] Glyburide and glimepiride interfere with cyclosporine metabolism, resulting in significant increases in cyclosporine levels,[62,63] but glipizide has no such effect.[64] Cotrimoxazole is often given to transplant patients for *Pneumocystis carinii* prophylaxis and it can impair the metabolism of glipizide, resulting in hypoglycemia so that caution with dosing should be used in this setting.[65]

Nateglinide and repaglinide result in a rapid and short duration of insulin release and should be taken before meals. The active metabolite of nateglinide accumulates in chronic kidney disease (CKD); nateglinide should not be used with an eGFR less than 60 mL/min/1.73 m^2.[66] Repaglinide appears safe to use in CKD[67] and it has been used successfully in patients with NODAT following kidney transplantation.[68] However, because repaglinide is metabolized by CYP3A4, cyclosporine and itraconazole can increase its levels, increasing the risk of hypoglycemia[69]; conversely, however, repaglinide use does not alter the levels of cyclosporine, tacrolimus, or sirolimus levels.[68] These agents are less efficacious than other oral medications.

Alpha-glucosidase Inhibitors

Acarbose and miglitol decrease the breakdown of oligosaccharides in the small intestine delaying absorption of glucose after a meal and do not cause hypoglycemia. Neither has been studied long-term in patients with a creatinine greater than 2 mg/dL, so their use should be avoided in these patients. There are no data regarding their use in patients following transplantation, and the gastrointestinal side-effect profile may add to that of the immunosuppressive drugs, particularly mycophenolate mofetil/mycophenolic acid.

Thiazolidinediones

Pioglitazone and rosiglitazone increase insulin sensitivity and do not cause hypoglycemia. They are hepatically metabolized and can be used in CKD without dose adjustment. However, fluid retention is a major adverse effect that may worsen heart failure, which limits their use in patients with significant liver or kidney disease.[70] They are associated with increased fracture rates and bone loss in women[71]; thus, use in patients with underlying bone disease (such as renal or hepatic osteodystrophy) potentially could be problematic. Both drugs have been used successfully in patients with liver and kidney transplants without problems[72–75] and they do not alter the metabolism of cyclosporine or tacrolimus.[73,74]

Dipeptidyl Peptidase-4 Inhibitors

DPP-4 inhibitors increase incretin levels, inhibit glucagon secretion, increase insulin release, and do not cause hypoglycemia.[76] Sitagliptin, saxagliptin, and alogliptin require dose reductions in patients with CKD, whereas linagliptin does not and all can be used safely in patients with moderate liver disease.[77,78] Saxagliptin, but not the other DPP-4 inhibitors, is metabolized by the CYP3A4 pathway and the dose needs to be reduced when CYP3A4 inhibitors such as cyclosporine and itraconazole are used.[77] On the other hand, saxagliptin does not inhibit or induce CYP3A4, so it will not affect calcineurin inhibitor dosing.[79] Several small studies have now documented the efficacy and safety with no effect on cyclosporine, tacrolimus, or sirolimus blood levels in renal transplant patients with NODAT treated with sitagliptin[54,80–82] and linagliptin.[83]

Some but not all studies have shown an association of DPP-4 use with pancreatitis but a meta-analysis has concluded there is no risk.[84] A slight increase in hospitalization for congestive heart failure (CHF) but not other cardiac outcomes has been shown with saxagliptin.[85,86]

Glucagon-like peptide 1 receptor agonists

Exenatide, liraglutide, dulaglutide, and albiglutide are injectable GLP-1 receptor agonists, leading to increased insulin release, delayed glucagon secretion, delayed gastric emptying, and appetite suppression with weight loss and do not cause hypoglycemia.[76] Clearance of exenatide decreases with declines in GFR.[87] Cases of acute kidney injury associated with exenatide use have been reported and it should not be used if the GFR is less than 30 mL/min/1.73 m². [88] Liraglutide is not metabolized by the kidney and no dose adjustment is indicated in those with renal impairment, including end-stage renal disease, although data in this population are limited. [89] No dose changes are needed for dulaglutide or albiglutide with worsening renal function. Nausea is a common side effect of all drugs in this class. Although their use has been associated with pancreatitis in some patients, the overall frequency of pancreatitis with their use is not greater than in diabetic patients using other agents. [90]

There are minimal data on GLP-1 agonist use in transplantation. One study has shown no problems with liraglutide use in 5 patients with kidney transplantation using tacrolimus [91] and other studies have shown no problems with exenatide in patients with islet cell transplantation [92,93] or liraglutide in patients with whole-pancreas transplantation. [94]

Sodium-glucose Cotransporter 2 Inhibitors

Sodium-glucose cotransporter 2 (SGLT2) inhibitors reduce glucose reabsorption in the proximal tubule, leading to an increase in glucose excretion, a reduction in A1c of approximately 0.8%, and weight loss and do not cause hypoglycemia. Because of a small increase in adverse events related to intravascular volume contraction, no more than 100 mg once daily of canagliflozin should be used in patients with an eGFR of 45 to less than 60 mL/min/1.73 m². [95] Canagliflozin and empagliflozin should be stopped if the eGFR is less than 45 mL/min/1.73 m² and dapagliflozin stopped at 60 mL/min/1.73 m², primarily because of a decrease in efficacy. In addition, there have been recent reports of "euglycemic" diabetic ketoacidosis, primarily in those with type 1 diabetes but also in some with type 2 diabetes. [96] There are no data available with their use in transplant patients but one pharmacokinetic study showed no clinically meaningful interactions with canagliflozin or cyclosporine. [97]

Insulin

All insulin preparations can be used in transplant patients with CKD and liver dysfunction, and there are no specific reductions in dosing for patients. However, reduced kidney function results in a prolongation of insulin half-life and a decrease in insulin requirements [98] and patients are at increased risk for hypoglycemia. [98,99] An inpatient study randomizing weight-based basal and bolus insulin in patients with eGFR less than 45 mL/min to 0.5 units/kg body weight versus 0.25 units/kg showed similar glycemic control but significantly less hypoglycemia in the group with the lower weight-based dose. [100] Therefore, it is imperative that patients being treated with insulin monitor their glucose levels closely and reduce their doses as needed to avoid hypoglycemia.

Additional Considerations

Table 1 gives a summary of the recommendations for use of oral hypoglycemic agents in patients after transplantation with specific remarks if CKD develops. If oral agent monotherapy fails, then combination therapy with 2 or more oral agents or a GLP-1 agonist is typically attempted. If combination therapy is insufficient, initiation of basal insulin is the next step. In most practices, glipizide has generally been the initial drug used because of concern about use of metformin with developing CKD. However, the recent emphasis on the safety of metformin even with stage 3 CKD would make it a very reasonable first-line drug. Subsequently DPP-4 inhibitors, pioglitazone, or GLP-1 agonists could be added, all with side-effect profiles that must be weighed against the patient's comorbidities and immunosuppression regimen. A single dose of basal insulin can be added to patients who are still uncontrolled on a regimen of 2 or more oral medications, as with any patient with type 2 DM.[17] Those not controlled on such a regimen may require more aggressive management with basal-bolus insulin therapy.[17,44,45]

SUMMARY

Although it is known that NODAT leads to worse outcomes, there are, as yet, no data that demonstrate prevention of these complications with improved glycemic control. However, there are short-term risks of hyperglycemia contributing to rejection and infection. Much more data are needed regarding the types of treatment and their implementation, given the complexity of care in this population. Glycemic control also must be carried out without excessive hypoglycemia, which may be tolerated poorly in patients with impaired kidney and liver function. Close communication among the transplant team, the primary provider, the diabetes care provider, and the patient is critical in maintaining improved short-term and long-term outcomes. The recent report that 5-year mortality after kidney transplantation is the same for subjects with and without pretransplant diabetes in recent years concluded that management of patients both before and after transplantation has been critical in this regard.[101]

REFERENCES

1. Yeh C-C, Yang H-R, Liao C-C, et al. Adverse outcomes after noncardiac surgery in patients with diabetes: a nation-wide population-based retrospective study. Diabetes Care 2013;36(10):3216–21.
2. Montori VM, Basu A, Erwin PJ, et al. Posttransplantation diabetes: a systematic review of the literature. Diabetes Care 2002;25(3):583–92.
3. Davidson J, Wilkinson A, Dantal J, et al. New-onset diabetes after transplantation: 2003 international consensus guidelines. Proceedings of an international expert panel meeting. Barcelona, Spain, 19 February 2003. Transplantation 2003;75(10 Suppl):SS3–S24.
4. Van den Berghe G, Wouters P, Weekers F, et al. Intensive insulin therapy in the critically ill patients. N Engl J Med 2001;345(19):1359–67.
5. Finfer S, Chittock DR, Su SY, et al. Intensive versus conventional glucose control in critically ill patients. N Engl J Med 2009;360(13):1283–97.
6. Preiser JC, Devos P, Ruiz-Santana S, et al. Prospective randomised multi-centre controlled trial on tight glucose control by intensive insulin therapy in adult intensive care units: the Glucontrol study. Intensive Care Med 2009;35:1738–48.
7. Ammori JB, Sigakis M, Englesbe MJ, et al. Effect of intraoperative hyperglycemia during liver transplantation. J Surg Res 2007;140(2):227–33.
8. Thomas MC, Mathew TH, Russ GR, et al. Early peri-operative glycaemic control and allograft rejection in patients with diabetes mellitus: a pilot study. Transplantation 2001;72(7):1321–4.
9. Thomas MC, Moran J, Mathew TH, et al. Early peri-operative hyperglycaemia and renal allograft rejection in patients without diabetes. BMC Nephrol 2000; 1:1.
10. Wallia A, Parikh ND, Molitch ME, et al. Posttransplant hyperglycemia is associated with increased risk of liver allograft rejection. Transplantation 2010;89(2): 222–6.

11. Hermayer KL, Egidi MF, Finch NJ, et al. A randomized controlled trial to evaluate the effect of glycemic control on renal transplantation outcomes. J Clin Endocrinol Metab 2012;97(12):4399–406.

12. Ramirez SC, Maaske J, Kim Y, et al. The association between glycemic control and clinical outcomes after kidney transplantation. Endocr Pract 2014;20(9): 894–900.

13. Wallia A, Parikh ND, O'Shea-Mahler E, et al. Glycemic control by a glucose management service and infection rates following liver transplantation. Endocr Pract 2011;17(4):546–51.

14. Finfer S, Liu B, Chittock DR, et al. Hypoglycemia and risk of death in critically ill patients. N Engl J Med 2012;367(12):1108–18.

15. Moghissi ES, Korytkowski MT, DiNardo M, et al. American Association of Clinical Endocrinologists and American Diabetes Association Consensus statement on inpatient glycemic control. Diabetes Care 2009;32(6):1119–31.

16. Ong MS, Coiera E. A systematic review of failures in handoff communication during intrahospital transfers. Jt Comm J Qual Patient Saf 2011;37(6):274–84.

17. Wallia A, Molitch ME. Insulin therapy for type 2 diabetes mellitus. JAMA 2014; 311:2315–25.

18. Ganji MR, Charkhchian M, Hakemi M, et al. Association of hyperglycemia on allograft function in the early period after renal transplantation. Transplant Proc 2007;39(4):852–4.

19. Hosseini MS, Nemati E, Pourfarziani V, et al. Early hyperglycemia after allogenic kidney transplantation: does it induce infections. Ann Transplant 2007;12(4): 23–6.

20. Cosio FG, Pesavento TE, Kim S, et al. Patient survival after renal transplantation: IV. Impact of post-transplant diabetes. Kidney Int 2002;62(4):1440–6.

21. Woodward RS, Schnitzler MA, Baty J, et al. Incidence and cost of new onset diabetes mellitus among U.S. wait-listed and transplanted renal allograft recipients. Am J Transplant 2003;3(5):590–8.

22. Sharif A, Hecking A, deVries APJ, et al. Proceedings from an international consensus meeting on posttransplantation diabetes mellitus: recommendations and future directions. Am J Transplant 2014;14:1992–2000.

23. American Diabetes Association. Standards of medical care in diabetes–2016. Diabetes Care 2016;39(Suppl 1):S1–112.

24. Van Raalte DH, Ouwens DM, Diamant M. Novel insights into glucocorticoid-mediated diabetogenic effects: towards expansion of therapeutic options? Eur J Clin Invest 2009;39(2):81–93.

25. Hecking M, Werzowa J, Haidinger M, et al, for the European-New-Onset Diabetes after Transplantation Working Group. Novel views on new-onset diabetes after transplantation: development, prevention and treatment. Nephrol Dial Transplant 2013;28:550–66.

26. Markell M. New-onset diabetes mellitus in transplant patients: pathogenesis, complications, and management. Am J Kidney Dis 2004;43(6):953–65.

27. Baid S, Cosimi AB, Farrell ML, et al. Posttransplant diabetes mellitus in liver transplant recipients: risk factors, temporal relationship with hepatitis C virus allograft hepatitis, and impact on mortality. Transplantation 2001;72(6):1066–72.

28. Bloom RD, Rao V, Weng F, et al. Association of hepatitis C with posttransplant diabetes in renal transplant patients on tacrolimus. J Am Soc Nephrol 2002; 13(5):1374–80.

29. Yadav AD, Chang Y-U, Aqel BA, et al. New onset diabetes mellitus in living donor versus deceased donor liver transplant recipients: analysis of the UNOS/OPTN Database. J Transplant 2013;2013:269096.
30. Hjelmesaeth J, Hartmann A, Kofstad J, et al. Glucose intolerance after renal transplantation depends upon prednisolone dose and recipient age. Transplantation 1997;64(7):979–83.
31. Rostambeigi N, Lanza IR, Dzeja PP, et al. Unique cellular and mitochondrial defects mediate FK506-induced islet beta-cell dysfunction. Transplantation 2011; 91(6):615–23.
32. Heisel O, Heisel R, Balshaw R, et al. New onset diabetes mellitus in patients receiving calcineurin inhibitors: a systematic review and meta-analysis. Am J Transplant 2004;4(4):583–95.
33. Vincenti F, Jensik SC, Filo RS, et al. A long-term comparison of tacrolimus (FK506) and cyclosporine in kidney transplantation: evidence for improved allograft survival at five years. Transplantation 2002;73(5):775–82.
34. Vincenti F, Friman S, Scheuermann E, et al, on the behalf of the DIRECT (Diabetes Incidence after Renal Transplantation: Neoral C2 Monitoring Versus Tacrolimus) Investigators. Results of an international, randomized trial comparing glucose metabolism disorders and outcome with cyclosporine versus tacrolimus. Am J Transplant 2007;7:1506–14.
35. Xu X, Ling Q, He ZL, et al. Post-transplant diabetes mellitus in liver transplantation: Hangzhou experience. Hepatobiliary Pancreat Dis Int 2008;7(5):465–70.
36. Ghisdal L, Bouchta NB, Broeders N, et al. Conversion from tacrolimus to cyclosporine A for new-onset diabetes after transplantation: a single-centre experience in renal transplanted patients and review of the literature. Transpl Int 2008;21(2):146–51.
37. Barlow AD, Nicholson ML, Herbert TP. Evidence for rapamycin toxicity in pancreatic β-cells and a review of the underlying molecular mechanisms. Diabetes 2013;62(8):2674–82.
38. Araki M, Flechner SM, Ismail HR, et al. Posttransplant diabetes mellitus in kidney transplant recipients receiving calcineurin or mTOR inhibitor drugs. Transplantation 2006;81(3):335–41.
39. Murakami N, Riella LV, Funakoshi T. Risk of metabolic complications in kidney transplantation after conversion to mTOR inhibitor: a systematic review and meta-analysis. Am J Transplant 2014;14:2317–27.
40. Su VC, Harrison J, Rogers C, et al. Belatacept: a new biologic and its role in kidney transplantation. Ann Pharmacother 2012;46(1):57–67.
41. Masson P, Henderson L, Chapman JR, et al. Belatacept for kidney transplant recipients. Cochrane Database Syst Rev 2014;(11):CD010699.
42. Klintmalm GB, Feng S, Lake JR, et al. Belatacept-based immunosuppression in de novo liver transplant recipients: 1-year experience from a phase II randomized Study. Am J Transplant 2014;14:1817–27.
43. Umpierrez GE, Reyes D, Smiley D, et al. Hospital discharge algorithm based on admission HbA1c for the management of patients with type 2 diabetes. Diabetes Care 2014;37(11):2934–9.
44. Inzucchi SE, Bergenstal RM, Buse JB, et al. Management of hyperglycemia in type 2 diabetes: a patient-centered approach: position statement of the American Diabetes Association (ADA) and the European Association for the Study of Diabetes (EASD). Diabetes Care 2012;35(6):1364–79.
45. Inzucchi SE, Bergenstal RM, Buse JB, et al. Management of hyperglycemia in type 2 diabetes 2015: a patient centered approach. Update to a position

statement of the American Diabetes Association and the European Association for the Study of Diabetes. Diabetes Care 2015;38:140–9.

46. Chakkera HA, Pomeroy J, Weil EJ, et al. Can new-onset diabetes after kidney transplant be prevented? Diabetes Care 2013;36:1406–12.

47. Ghisdal L, Vanholder R, Van Laecke S, et al. New-onset diabetes after renal transplantation. Risk assessment and management. Diabetes Care 2012;35:181–8.

48. Shabir S, Jham S, Harper L, et al. Validity of glycated haemoglobin to diagnose new onset diabetes after transplantation. Transpl Int 2013;26:315–21.

49. Chapman JR. Chronic calcineurin inhibitor nephrotoxicity–lest we forget. Am J Transplant 2011;11:693–7.

50. Sambol NC, Chiang J, Lin ET, et al. Kidney function and age are both predictors of pharmacokinetics of metformin. J Clin Pharmacol 1995;35(11):1094–102.

51. Inzucchi SE, Lipska KJ, Mayo H, et al. Metformin in patients with type 2 diabetes and kidney disease. A systematic review. JAMA 2014;312:2668–75.

52. Sharif A. Should metformin be our antiglycemic agent of choice post-transplantation? Am J Transplant 2011;11:1376–81.

53. Kurian B, Joshi R, Helmuth A. Effectiveness and long-term safety of thiazolidinediones and metformin in renal transplant recipients. Endocr Pract 2008;14(8):979–84.

54. Soliman AR, Fathy A, Khashab S, et al. Sitagliptin might be a favorable antiobesity drug for new onset diabetes after a renal transplant. Exp Clin Transplant 2013;11(6):494–8.

55. Jonsson A, Rydberg T, Sterner G, et al. Pharmacokinetics of glibenclamide and its metabolites in diabetic patients with impaired renal function. Eur J Clin Pharmacol 1998;53(6):429–35.

56. Rosenkranz B, Profozic V, Metelko Z, et al. Pharmacokinetics and safety of glimepiride at clinically effective doses in diabetic patients with renal impairment. Diabetologia 1996;39(12):1617–24.

57. Asplund K, Wiholm BE, Lundman B. Severe hypoglycaemia during treatment with glipizide. Diabet Med 1991;8(8):726–31.

58. Holstein A, Beil W. Oral antidiabetic drug metabolism: pharmacogenomics and drug interactions. Expert Opin Drug Metab Toxicol 2009;5(3):225–41.

59. Holstein A, Plaschke A, Hammer C, et al. Hormonal counterregulation and consecutive glimepiride serum concentrations during severe hypoglycaemia associated with glimepiride therapy. Eur J Clin Pharmacol 2003;59(10):747–54.

60. Balant L, Zahnd G, Gorgia A, et al. Pharmacokinetics of glipizide in man: influence of renal insufficiency. Diabetologia 1973;9(Suppl):331–8.

61. Arjona Ferreira JC, Marre M, Barzilai N, et al. Efficacy and safety of sitagliptin versus glipizide in patients with type 2 diabetes and moderate-to-severe chronic renal insufficiency. Diabetes Care 2013;36(5):1067–73.

62. Islam SI, Masuda QN, Bolaji OO, et al. Possible interaction between cyclosporine and glibenclamide in posttransplant diabetic patients. Ther Drug Monit 1996;18(5):624–6.

63. Räkel A, Karelis AD. New-onset diabetes after transplantation: risk factors and clinical impact. Diabetes Metab 2011;37:1–14.

64. Sagedal S, Asberg A, Hartmann A, et al. Glipizide treatment of post-transplant diabetes does not interfere with cyclosporine pharmacokinetics in renal allograft recipients. Clin Transplant 1998;12(6):553–6.

65. Tan A, Holmes HM, Kuo Y-F, et al. Coadministration of co-trimoxazole with sulfo-nylureas: hypoglycemia events and pattern of use. J Gerontol A Biol Sci Med Sci 2015;70(2):247–54.

66. Inoue T, Shibahara N, Miyagawa K, et al. Pharmacokinetics of nateglinide and its metabolites in subjects with type 2 diabetes mellitus and renal failure. Clin Nephrol 2003;60(2):90–5.

67. Hasslacher C. Safety and efficacy of repaglinide in type 2 diabetic patients with and without impaired renal function. Diabetes Care 2003;26(3):886–91.

68. Türk T, Peitruck F, Dolff S, et al. Repaglinide in the management of new-onset diabetes mellitus after renal transplantation. Am J Transplant 2006;6:842–6.

69. Kajosaari LI, Niemi M, Neuvonen M, et al. Cyclosporine markedly raises the plasma concentrations of repaglinide. Clin Pharmacol Ther 2005;78:388–99.

70. Home P. Safety of PPAR agonists. Diabetes Care 2011;34(Suppl 2):S215–9.

71. Zhu ZN, Jiang YF, Ding T. Risk of fracture with thiazolidinediones: an updated meta-analysis of randomized clinical trials. Bone 2014;68:115–23.

72. Budde K, Neumayer HH, Frische L, et al. The pharmacokinetics of pioglitazone in patients with impaired renal function. Br J Clin Pharmacol 2003;55(5):368–74.

73. Baldwin D, Duffin KE. Rosiglitazone treatment of diabetes mellitus after solid or-gan transplantation. Transplantation 2004;77(7):1009–14.

74. Luther P, Baldwin D Jr. Pioglitazone in the management of diabetes mellitus after transplantation. Am J Transplant 2004;4:2136–8.

75. Voytovich MH, Simonsen C, Henssen T, et al. Short-term treatment with rosigli-tazone improves glucose tolerance, insulin sensitivity and endothelial function in renal transplant recipients. Nephrol Dial Transplant 2005;20:413–8.

76. Lovshin JA, Drucker DJ. Incretin-based therapies for type 2 diabetes mellitus. Nat Rev Endocrinol 2009;5(5):262–9.

77. Scheen AJ. Pharmacokinetics of dipeptidylpeptidase-4 inhibitors. Diabetes Obes Metab 2010;12:648–58.

78. Giorda CB, Nada E, Tartaglino B. Pharmacokinetics, safety, and efficacy of DPP-4 inhibitors and GLP-1 receptor agonists in patients with type 2 diabetes mellitus and renal or hepatic impairment. A systematic review of the literature. Endocrine 2014;46:406–19.

79. Su H, Boulton DW, Barros A Jr, et al. Characterization of the in vitro and in vivo metabolism and disposition and cytochrome P450 inhibition/induction profile of saxagliptin in humans. Drug Metab Dispos 2012;40:1345–56.

80. Lane JT, Odegaard DE, Haire CE, et al. Sitagliptin therapy in kidney transplant recipients with new-onset diabetes after transplantation. Transplantation 2011; 92(10):e56–7.

81. Boerner RP, Miles CD, Shivaswamy V. Efficacy and safety of sitagliptin for the treatment of new-onset diabetes after renal transplantation. Int J Endocrinol 2014;2014:617638.

82. Halden TAS, Åsberg A, Vik K, et al. Short-term efficacy and safety of sitagliptin treatment in long-term stable renal recipients with new-onset diabetes after transplantation. Nephrol Dial Transplant 2014;29:926–33.

83. Sanyal D, Gupta S, Das P. A retrospective study evaluating efficacy and safety of linagliptin in treatment of NODAT (in renal transplant recipients) in a real world setting. Indian J Endocrinol Metab 2013;17(Suppl 1):s203–5.

84. Monami M, Dicembrini I, Mannucci E. Dipeptidyl peptidase-4 inhibitors and pancreatitis risk: a meta-analysis of randomized clinical trials. Diabetes Obes Metab 2014;16:48–56.

85. Clifton P. Do dipeptidyl IV (DPP-IV) inhibitors cause heart failure? Clin Ther 2014; 36(12):2072–9.

86. Udell JA, Bhatt DL, Braunwald E, et al, for the SAVOR-TIMI 53 Steering Committee and Investigators. Saxagliptin and cardiovascular outcomes in patients with type 2 diabetes and moderate or severe renal impairment: observations from the SAVOR-TIMI 53 trial. Diabetes Care 2015;38:696–705.

87. Linnebjerg H, Kothare PA, Park S, et al. Effect of renal impairment on the pharmacokinetics of exenatide. Br J Clin Pharmacol 2007;64(3):317–27.

88. Johansen OE, Whitfield R. Exenatide may aggravate moderate diabetic renal impairment: a case report. Br J Clin Pharmacol 2008;66(4):568–9.

89. Jacobsen LV, Hindsberger C, Robson R, et al. Effect of renal impairment on the pharmacokinetics of the GLP-1 analogue liraglutide. Br J Clin Pharmacol 2009; 68(6):898–905.

90. Thomsen RW, Pedersen L, Møller N, et al. Incretin-based therapy and risk of acute pancreatitis: a nationwide population-based case-control study. Diabetes Care 2015;38:1089–98.

91. Pinelli NR, Patel A, Salinitri FD. Coadministration of liraglutide with tacrolimus in kidney transplant recipients: a case series. Diabetes Care 2013;36:e171–2.

92. Ghofaili KA, Fung M, Ao Z, et al. Effect of exenatide on beta cell function after islet transplantation in type 1 diabetes. Transplantation 2007;83(1):24–8.

93. Froud T, Faradji RN, Pileggi A, et al. The use of exenatide in islet transplant recipients with chronic allograft dysfunction: safety, efficacy, and metabolic effects. Transplantation 2008;86(1):36–45.

94. Cariou B, Bernard C, Cantarovich D. Liraglutide in whole-pancreas transplant patients with impaired glucose homoeostasis: a case series. Diabetes Metab 2014;41(3):252–7.

95. Yamout H, Perkovic V, Davies M, et al. Efficacy and safety of canagliflozin in patients with type 2 diabetes and stage 3 nephropathy. Am J Nephrol 2014;40: 64–74.

96. Peters AL, Buschur EO, Buse JB, et al. Euglycemic diabetic ketoacidosis: a potential complication of treatment with sodium-glucose cotransporter 2 inhibition. Diabetes Care 2015;38(9):1687–93.

97. Devineni D, Vaccaro N, Murphy J, et al. Effects of rifampin, cyclosporine A, and probenecid on the pharmacokinetic profile of canagliflozin, a sodium glucose co-transporter 2 inhibitor, in health participants. Int J Clin Pharmacol Ther 2015;53(2):115–28.

98. Muhlhauser I, Toth G, Sawicki PT, et al. Severe hypoglycemia in type I diabetic patients with impaired kidney function. Diabetes Care 1991;14(4):344–6.

99. Hasslacher C, Wittmann W. Severe hypoglycemia in diabetics with impaired renal function. Dtsch Med Wochenschr 2003;128(6):253–6.

100. Baldwin D, Zander J, Munoz C, et al. A randomized trial of two weight-based doses of insulin glargine and glulisine in hospitalized subjects with type 2 diabetes and renal insufficiency. Diabetes Care 2012;35(10):1970–4.

101. Keddis T, el Ters M, Rodrigo E, et al. Enhanced posttransplant management of patients with diabetes improves patient outcomes. Kidney Int 2014;86:610–8.

De Novo Malignancies After Transplantation
Risk and Surveillance Strategies

Iliana Doycheva, MD[a], Syed Amer, MBBS[b], Kymberly D. Watt, MD[c],*

KEYWORDS

- Incidence • Mortality • Skin cancer • Posttransplant lymphoproliferative disorder
- Solid organ tumors • Risk factors • Surveillance

KEY POINTS

- De novo malignancies are one of the most common late complications in transplant recipients with functioning graft with 2 to 4 times higher incidence than that in the general population.
- Immunosuppression plays a central role in pathogenesis in addition to other transplant-related and traditional risk factors.
- Nonmelanoma skin cancer is the most common malignancy, followed by posttransplant lymphoproliferative disorder and solid organ tumors.
- De novo malignancies in transplant recipients are more aggressive with increased cancer-specific mortality compared with the general population.
- Surveillance strategies are largely based on general population data but should be individualized based on risk factors of each recipient.

INTRODUCTION

De novo malignancies represent one of the leading causes of mortality in both liver and renal transplant recipients (LTRs, RTRs).[1–3] In large transplant registry studies, cancer was found to be the most common cause of death in the second decade after liver transplantation (LT)[1] and after 20 years in RTRs with functioning grafts.[2] Morbidity and quality of life are also affected in posttransplant cancer survivors. The late occurrence of de novo malignancies is mainly attributed to intensity and cumulative

Disclosure: All authors report no conflict of interest.
[a] Division of Gastroenterology and Hepatology, Medical University-Sofia, 1 G. Sofiisky Boulevard, Sofia 1431, Bulgaria; [b] Division of Internal Medicine, Mayo Clinic, 5777 East Mayo Boulevard, Phoenix, AZ 85054, USA; [c] Division of Gastroenterology and Hepatology, Mayo Clinic and Foundation, CH-10, 200 First Street Southwest, Rochester, MN 55905, USA
* Corresponding author.
E-mail address: watt.kymberly@mayo.edu

Med Clin N Am 100 (2016) 551–567
http://dx.doi.org/10.1016/j.mcna.2016.01.006
0025-7125/16/$ – see front matter © 2016 Elsevier Inc. All rights reserved.

exposure to immunosuppression. Multiple risk factors have been established in general population studies and are likely applicable to the transplant recipient, but the data available are mixed affecting the elaboration of surveillance strategies and preventive measures.

The aim of this review is to summarize current knowledge on the frequency and risk factors of de novo malignancy in LTRs and RTRs. In addition, the authors analyze outcomes of the most frequently encountered de novo malignancies in RTRs and LTRs to outline optimal screening programs to improve long-term outcomes for these patients.

INCIDENCE AND MORTALITY

When compared with the general population, the overall incidence of de novo malignancies is 2- to 4-fold greater in all solid organ transplantation (SOT) recipients.[4–9] Standardized incidence ratio (SIR) for any cancer ranges between 2.4 and 6.5 for RTRs and 1.9 and 3.4 for LTRs (**Table 1**).[4–8,10–12] The reported 5-, 10-, and 15-year cumulative incidence of any de novo malignancy in LTRs is 6.0% to 11.9%, 20.0% to 21.7%, and 55.0%[3,13] and for nonskin cancers 6.7% to 9.0%, 13.6% to 18.0%, and 25.0%, respectively.[3,14] Similarly, by 20 years after kidney transplant, almost 50% of RTRs have 1 or more skin cancers[15] and 10% to 27% have nonskin cancer.[15,16]

De novo malignancies in SOT recipients have a worse prognosis. Large transplant registry data analysis showed significantly lower stage-specific survival in transplant recipients compared with the general population.[17] Mortality rates associated with

Table 1
Cancer incidence and mortality in RTRs and LTRs

Cancer Site	Incidence in RTRs (Expressed as SIR)	Incidence in LTRs (Expressed as SIR)
All sites	2.4–6.5	1.9–3.4
NMSC	16.6–57.7	6.6–38.5
Lip	46.0–65.6	19.0–21.3
PTLD/NHL	3.8–12.5	7.8–20.8
Solid organ tumors		
Oropharyngeal	4.2–5.2	4.4–14.8
Lung	1.5–2.1	1.4–2.0
Liver	1.1–2.7	14.0–43.8[a]
Kidney	5.2–7.9	1.8–4.2
Colorectal	1.4–2.4	1.4–2.6
Genitourinary: cervix	1.6–2.4	2.5–2.6
Vulva (and vagina)	5.5–14.0	6.9–23.8
Cancer Site	Mortality in RTRs (Expressed as SMR)	Mortality in LTRs (Expressed as SMR)
SMR for all sites	1.0–2.3	1.96–2.93

The presented SIRs are based on the following references: Collett et al,[4] 2010; Engels et al,[5] 2011; Villeneuve et al,[8] 2007; Jiang et al,[10] 2008; Schrem et al,[6] 2013; Krynitz et al,[11] 2013; Adami et al,[7] 2003; and Aberg et al,[12] 2008. SMRs in kidney recipients are based on Kiberd et al,[21] 2009 and Cheung et al,[22] 2012; SMRs in liver recipients are based on Na et al,[18] 2013 and Herrero et al,[19] 2005.

Abbreviations: NHL, non-Hodgkin lymphoma; NMSC, nonmelanoma skin cancer; PTLD, posttransplant lymphoproliferative disorder; SMR, standardized mortality ratio.

[a] The elevated SIR for liver cancer in LTRs likely reflects recurrent but not de novo cancer.

Data from Refs.[4–8,10–12,18,19,21,22]

nonskin malignancy were 40% and 55% at 1 and 5 years after cancer diagnosis compared with 21% and 36% in the general population, in one study of LTRs,[3] and 2- to 3-fold greater risk of cancer-related death in 2 other studies.[18,19] The most common cancers causing death were lung cancer, colon cancer, and posttransplant lymphoproliferative disorder (PTLD).[20] Standardized mortality ratio (SMR) for all cancers ranges between 1.0 and 2.3 in RTRs.[21,22] SMR for nonskin cancers was 1.5 in a large multicenter cohort study of RTRs with 5- and 10-year survival of 86% and 71%, respectively.[23] Significant difference in mortality rate between recipients less than 50 years of age (SMR 4.3) and those greater than 50 years of age (SMR 1.2) was also noted in this study. The highest cancer mortality in RTRs was observed in recipients with non-Hodgkin lymphoma (NHL) (SMR 14.1) and carcinoma of the native kidneys (SMR 9.6).

RISK FACTORS FOR ALL MALIGNANCIES

The pivotal role of immunosuppression for development of de novo malignancies has been demonstrated in a study comparing cancer incidence in the same cohort before and after kidney transplantation.[24] Immunosuppression may facilitate carcinogenesis by lowering immunosurveillance mechanisms and directly damaging host DNA.[25] Another mechanism is the potentiation of the effect of pro-oncogenic viruses, such as human herpes virus type 8 (HHV-8) for Kaposi sarcoma, Epstein-Barr virus (EBV) for PTLD, and human papillomavirus (HPV) for oropharyngeal and anogenital carcinomas. Additional transplant-related risk factors include type of immunosuppression, with protective effects of mammalian target of rapamycin (mTOR) inhibitors (albeit controversial),[9] underlying disease before grafting,[3] type of transplant (living vs deceased donor),[26,27] history of malignancy before transplant,[27] as well as established risk factors, such as age,[5,7,13,27] sex,[5,7,12] ethnicity,[28] geographic location,[29] and smoking.[3,30,31]

SPECIFIC MALIGNANCIES
Skin Cancer

Nonmelanoma skin cancer (NMSC) is the most common and usually the first detected de novo malignancy in both LTRs and RTRs.[4,11,32] NMSC is more common in RTRs (SIR 16.6–57.7 for kidney and 6.6–38.5 for liver recipients),[4] which may relate to the higher immunosuppression needs of RTRs compared with LTRs. In addition, an observed baseline higher risk has been noted patients with kidney failure when compared with patients with other chronic diseases awaiting SOT.[32] Squamous cell carcinoma (SCC) incidence in RTRs is 60 to 250 times greater than in the general population, but only a 10-fold increase in basal cell carcinoma (BCC) incidence is noted.[33] However, this ratio was not confirmed in a subsequent study.[34] An initial increased BCC prevalence has been noted in LTRs with ratio of BCC to SCC close to that in the general population (4:1), but reversal of the ratio occurs with time.[35] Mean time to skin cancer detection ranges between 3 and 5 years.[35–37]

Once diagnosed with SCC, increased cumulative incidence of subsequent SCC was noted[11,38,39] with a 5-year risk more than 80% in RTRs[11] and 46% in LTRs.[39] Moreover, a study of RTRs demonstrated that prior SCC confers a 3-fold higher adjusted risk of developing other internal malignancy,[40] although no such association was noted in LTRs.[35] An increased incidence of lip cancer was found in all SOT recipients[5] but significantly higher in RTRs than in LTRs (SIR for RTRs 46.0–65.6 vs SIR for LTRs 19.0–20.0).[4,11]

The main risk factors for NMSC in LTRs are older age at transplantation, skin type, and sun exposure burden (**Table 2**).[35,39,41,42] No clear association with underlying liver

Table 2
Risk factors for de novo malignancies in LTRs and RTRs

Cancer	Liver Transplant	Kidney Transplant
NMSC	Older age[35,37,39,44]; skin type[37,41,44]; sun burden[35,41]; PSC[3,37]; ALD[42,43]; smoking[43]; cyclosporine use[37,44]; nonskin cancer or HCC before transplant[39,42]; duration of IS[35]; male sex[3]	Older age[34,38]; duration of IS[45,46,121]; skin type[34]; sun exposure[34]; male sex[38]
Head & neck cancer	Oropharyngeal cancer: ALD[84,86] and smoking[30,85]	Thyroid cancer: unclear risk factors
Lung cancer	ALD[3,74]; smoking[30,85]	Smoking[31,89]
Renal cell carcinoma	Smoking[30]	ACKD and dialysis duration before transplant[91]
Hepatocellular carcinoma	Hepatitis C (cirrhosis)[99,100]; type 2 diabetes[99,100]; older age[99]; male sex[99]	Hepatitis C; hepatitis B; type 2 diabetes[100]
Colorectal cancer	PSC + IBD[102,103]	Older age[109]
Anogenital cancers	High-risk HPV infection[112]	High-risk HPV infection[112] Cervical cancer and genital dysplasia: smoking[31]; young age at transplant[116]; retransplant[116]
PTLD	Early PTLD: EBV mismatch[68,69,78]; receipt of T-cell depleting Ab[69]; CMV (−) status[68] Late: older age, time since transplant, current use of CNI[69] For liver recipients: hepatitis C[74,75]	

Abbreviations: Ab, antibody; ACKD, acquired cystic kidney disease; ALD, alcoholic liver disease; CMV, cytomegalovirus; CNI, calcineurin inhibitor; HCC, hepatocellular carcinoma; IBD, inflammatory bowel disease; IS, immunosuppression; NMSC, nonmelanoma skin cancer; PSC, primary sclerosing cholangitis.

disease before transplant was noted, although a few studies suggested alcoholic cirrhosis,[42,43] primary sclerosing cholangitis (PSC),[37] and hepatocellular carcinoma (HCC) or other nonskin cancer[39,42] before transplant. Similarly, no definite association has been seen with immunosuppression type in LTRs,[42] although reports of cyclosporine as a risk factor exist.[37,44] Duration of immunosuppression was implicated to play role in RTRs.[45,46] Two randomized, multicenter trials assessed the benefit of preventing skin cancer by switching RTRs to mammalian target of rapamycin (mTOR) inhibitor, sirolimus-based regimen versus calcineurin inhibitor (CNI) continuation.[47,48] Sirolimus was effective for both primary and secondary prevention with lower rates of NMSC[48] and decreased risk of recurrent/additional SCC.[47] Notably, sirolimus was noted to be beneficial in preventing skin cancer even when combined with cyclosporine.[49]

Systematic reviews and meta-analysis have shown a greater than 2-fold risk of melanoma in SOT recipients[50,51] with a higher risk and shorter median time to detection in liver than in kidney recipients (2.0 years for LTRs[35] vs 8.5 years for RTRs[52]). Data are controversial regarding melanoma stage at the time of diagnosis, although a large cohort study reported more advanced disease at diagnosis and poor survival.[53] Risk factors are similar to those of NMSC.

Current clinical practice guidelines for care of RTRs recommend providing patients at high risk with oral and written information on the risk of skin and lip cancer, advising on minimum sun exposure and regular use of sun-protecting agents, monthly self-examination, and annual skin and lip examination by an experienced physician or dermatologist.[54,55] Although the American Association for the Study of Liver Disease's (AASLD) guidelines recommend annual dermatology examination after 5 or more years after transplant,[56] a strong argument should be made for annual screening before 5 years for all kidney and liver transplant recipients.

Kaposi sarcoma (KS), rarely seen in the immunocompetent population, occurs up to 1000 times more often in SOT recipients and commonly presents with skin involvement but frequently has visceral manifestations.[57] The highest KS incidence is detected in the first 2 years after transplant.[58] Reports have shown higher incidence in RTRs.[4,59] HHV-8 plays an important role in the etiopathogenesis of KS.[60] Increased KS prevalence in certain ethnic groups parallels geographic areas with high HHV-8 seroprevalence (Central and South Africa, Mediterranean, Caribbean, and Middle East).[57] Screening RTRs and LTRs that originate from these areas might be considered before transplant in order to identify patients at risk and adjust immunosuppression accordingly.

Posttransplant Lymphoproliferative Disorder

PTLD is the second most common de novo malignancy after transplantation. Based on the 2008 World Health Organization's classification, PTLD encompasses 4 categories: early lesions, polymorphic PTLD, monomorphic PTLD (B-cell and T-cell lymphomas), and classic Hodgkin lymphoma–type PTLD.[61] Most common is diffuse large B-cell lymphoma, which belongs to monomorphic B-cell PTLD.

EBV plays a key role in the pathogenesis of PTLD, although increasing numbers of EBV (−) PTLD have been reported.[62,63] Primary EBV infection (or reactivation) triggers a vigorous immune response.[64] Cytotoxic T cells are needed to control viral proliferation. After achieving control of the primary infection, EBV persists for life in infected B cells and can be transmitted to EBV (−) recipients through B cells in the graft or can reactivate in EBV (+) recipients in the setting of intense immunosuppression after transplant. The progression of infection is secondary to the inability of specific cytotoxic T cells to mount an adequate immune response. Primary EBV infection in EBV (−) recipients usually occurs in the first 3 to 6 months after transplant. The pathogenesis of EBV (−) PTLD is not yet clearly understood.

The most important risk factors for PTLD are age, immunosuppression, EBV serostatus of donor and recipient, and type of allograft.[65] PTLD occurs more frequently in children, as they are more likely to be EBV (−) before transplant.[5] PTLD has greater SIR and cumulative incidence in LTRs than in RTRs.[4,5,7,11,66] It usually presents in a bimodal pattern with the highest incidence in the first year and another peak after the fifth year.[5,67,68] In RTRs, early onset PTLD has been associated with EBV (−) recipient status,[67–69] cytomegalovirus seronegativity,[68] extranodal disease with higher involvement of the graft,[68] and after T-cell depleting antibodies administration.[69] The identified risk factors for late-onset PTLD are older age, longer time since transplant, and current use of CNI[69] while maintenance steroid therapy was noted to have a protective role in one study.[68] Donor (+)/recipient (−) adult RTRs are 2 to 3 times more likely to develop PTLD when compared with donor (−)/recipient (−) recipients, whereas in EBV (−) pediatric recipients, the risk is up to 17 times greater.[70] In addition, deceased donor recipients have a significantly higher rate of PTLD than living donors possibly reflecting a role of HLA mismatch.[70] Data regarding immunosuppression regimens and PTLD are controversial. One large retrospective cohort study showed no role in antibody induction and antirejection therapies.[68] Another study demonstrated immunosuppression type did not influence the PTLD rate in EBV (+) RTRs, but EBV

(−) recipients with both mTOR inhibitor and tacrolimus had the highest risk compared with other regimens.[71] Previously, an association between belatacept and PTLD (particularly central nervous system involvement) was reported[72]; but a recent systematic review suggested belatacept confers no additional risk.[73] The black box warning for its use in EBV (−) individuals exists, so screening and counseling for central nervous symptoms is still recommended before using this agent.

Similar risk factors apply to LTRs. In addition, small studies suggested that PTLD occurs more often in hepatitis C positive recipients[74,75]; but the exact pathogenic mechanism has not been elucidated, and more data are needed.

Single-center analysis of more than 30 years experience on PTLD in SOT recipients identified 3 poor prognostic factors: graft organ involvement, monomorphic disease, and poor performance status.[76] Overall survival after PTLD diagnosis in RTRs ranges broadly between studies: 51% to 67% at 1 year and 39% to 60% at 5 years.[62,67,77] Poor 5-year survival was noted in LTRs as well (38.7% vs 45%–69% of the NHL in the general population).[6] Additional predictors of poor survival in RTRs include acute kidney injury at diagnosis, impaired kidney function, early onset, T-cell disease, and history of antithymocyte globulin therapy.[78]

EBV serostatus is tested in both donor and recipient before transplant. The utility of routine EBV surveillance by using quantitative polymerase chain reaction (PCR) in high-risk EBV (−) recipients to predict PTLD development has been studied in pediatric LTRs whereby frequent EBV monitoring and reduction of immunosuppression if a high viral load was detected led to a decreased incidence of PTLD.[79] The European Renal Best Practice Advisory Board's (ERBPAB) guidelines recommend monitoring EBV-PCR in EBV (−) RTRs during the first year after transplant and reducing immunosuppression if increasing viral load is detected (**Table 3**).[80] In addition, preemptive therapy with anti-CD20 monoclonal antibody rituximab was used in EBV donor (+)/recipient (−) adult RTRs who became viremic and symptomatic during the first year after transplant with good effect.[81] However, because of insufficient evidence on EBV progression after transplant, low specificity of EBV for prediction of PTLD development, and lack of standardized test for EBV measurement, surveillance remains controversial.

Solid Organ Tumors

Head and neck cancer

LTRs have a higher risk for head and neck cancer when compared with other SOT recipients.[82] Meta-analysis of 10 studies including more than 56,000 LTRs showed SIR of 3.8 and detection time as early as 34 months after transplant.[83] Alcoholic liver disease (ALD) as an indication for transplant has an even higher SIR of 11.8.[84] Among those patients, cancer of the tongue was noted to be 23 times more frequent. Additional risk factors are smoking[30,85] and HPV infection.[86] Advanced stage at diagnosis,[6] poor outcome after treatment, and low overall and disease-free survival after transplant[82] imposes the need for regular surveillance of the oropharynx, particularly in smokers with a history of ALD.

Thyroid cancer is also a high-risk de novo malignancy, especially in RTRs. Meta-analysis of 9 studies including more than 50,000 kidney recipients found a 7-fold increased risk of papillary thyroid cancer with a mean time to diagnosis of 72 months.[87]

Lung cancer

Lung cancer is the most common solid organ tumor in both RTRs (SIR 1.4–1.9) and LTRs (SIR 1.4–2.1) (see **Table 1**).[59] The mean time to diagnosis starts increasing 6

Table 3
Summary of suggested surveillance strategies for LTRs and RTRs

Cancer	LTRs	RTRs
NMSC	Sun protective measures, annual skin examination	Education of high-risk patients, use of sun-protecting agents, monthly skin self-examination, annual total body skin examination
Head & neck cancer	Annual otolaryngology examination in smokers and if history of ALD	Annual thyroid ultrasound 6 y after transplant
Lung cancer	Annual low-dose CT for adults, aged 55–80 y with ≥30-pack smoking history and smoking cessation <15 y Smoking cessation Annual chest radiograph in other recipients	
Renal cell carcinoma	No guidelines	Imaging or urine cytology not recommended by AST and ERBPAB; consider screening ultrasound in cystic kidneys every 2 y (no data)
Hepatocellular carcinoma	Abdominal imaging every 6 mo if allograft cirrhosis	Abdominal ultrasound every 6 mo if liver cirrhosis or hepatitis B carrier
Colorectal cancer	Annual colonoscopy in PSC and IBD; general population guideline for all other recipients	Per general population guidelines
Anogenital cancers	Annual Papanicolaou test and pelvic examination, inspection of anal, vaginal, and vulvar regions Potential benefit: HPV vaccine before transplant	
Prostate cancer	Per general population guidelines	
Breast cancer	Per general population guidelines	
PTLD	No specific recommendations for EBV monitoring of adult liver recipients from AASLD	Monitor EBV-PCR in high-risk (EBV [+]/EBV [−]) recipients: once in the first wk after transplant, then at least monthly for the first 3–6 mo, then every 3 mo for the first yr, and after treatment of acute rejection

Abbreviations: ALD, alcoholic liver disease; AST, American Society of Transplantation; CT, computed tomography; IBD, inflammatory bowel disease.

to 12 months after transplant and peaks after the fifth year after transplant.[5] A recent study of almost 600 transplant recipients with non–small cell lung cancer found SCC more than adenocarcinoma (P = .02) and earlier stages (P = .02) of disease.[88] In contrast, another study observed more than 70% of lung cancer cases in LTRs were in advanced stage.[6] Similar to the general population, the most important risk factor is smoking.[89] Underlying disease may contribute to risk, as the highest risk for lung cancer occurred in LTRs with ALD compared with other causes and 5- and 10-year cumulative risk of 2.0% and 4.8% compared with 0.15% and 1.3%, respectively.[3] No change in lung cancer–specific survival was noted in nonlung transplant recipients.[88]

In December 2013, the United States Preventive Services Task Force (USPSTF) changed the general population guidelines for lung cancer screening, recommending annual low-dose computed tomography for adults, aged 55 to 80 years who have a 30-pack or greater smoking history and currently smoke or have quit within the past 15 years.[90] Because lung cancer is the most common solid organ malignancy in both LTRs and RTRs and more frequent than the general population, following these recommendations is likely to be beneficial for transplant recipients. This topic requires study in the transplant population. Annual screening with a chest radiograph has been recommended for all other (nonsmoker) RTRs and LTRs. Additionally, current smokers should be extensively counseled on smoking cessation.

Renal cell carcinoma, bladder, and prostate cancer

The SIR for renal cell carcinoma (RCC) in kidney recipients ranges between 5.2 and 7.9, whereas the risk of this cancer in LTRs is only slightly increased at 1.8 to 1.9[4,5,11] with 4.1 reported only in one study.[12] In RTRs, RCC mainly occurs in native kidneys and has been associated with acquired cystic kidney disease (ACKD).[91] It is estimated that 7% to 20% of patients with chronic kidney disease have ACKD but 60% to 80% after 4 years of dialysis. RTRs with preexisting cysts and longer dialysis duration before transplant were the strongest risk factors.[91] A bimodal distribution occurs with up to 10 times increased risk in the first year, likely reflecting undetected cancer in the cysts before transplant and a second peak 4 to 15 years after transplant.[5] A very high risk of RCC was noted in RTRs before 30 years of age (SIR 40) in one study,[8] although other large studies demonstrated the risk peaked in the 60-years-and-older age group.[4] Overall cumulative incidence seems to increase steeply after 35 years of age.[92]

The reason for RCC in LTRs (in one study) is not completely clear, although continuous smoking after transplant plays role for both RCC and other urinary tract malignancies.[30] One study noted that most LTRs with RCC were diagnosed at an earlier stage because of regular ultrasound imaging of liver recipients.[6]

Comparable 2-fold increased risk of bladder cancer was found in both RTRs and LTRs.[11,59] Most cases have histology of transitional cell carcinoma.[7] Two studies found recipients of expanded criteria deceased donor kidneys had almost 2-fold increased risk of genitourinary cancer (adjusted hazard ratio [HR] 1.79, $P = .038$),[93] whereas longer duration of dialysis before transplant augmented the risk of this cancer 2.5 times (adjusted HR 2.57, $P = .005$).[94]

Current clinical guidelines of the American Society of Transplantation (AST) and ERBPAB do not recommend screening for RCC in kidney recipients because of the lack of sufficient evidence for benefit[54,95]; however, recent guidelines of the European Association of Urology recommends annual ultrasonography of native kidneys and graft.[55] Another suggested strategy is starting in the first month after transplant and then every 2 years for those with cysts and every 5 years for recipients without cysts.[91] As there is no clear consensus, the best screening strategy for different populations warrants further study.

All studies based on large transplant databases showed no increased risk of prostate cancer in RTRs and LTRs and rates similar to those in the general population.[4,5,11] This lack of increased risk may reflect the strict cancer screening before or after transplant.

In 2010, the American Cancer Society (ACS) recommended the decision for prostate cancer screening to be made after discussion with patients of the risks and potential benefit and to start at 50 years of age (or 45 years for African American patients).[96] Interval follow-up is to be based on initial prostate-specific antigen (PSA) values. Later in 2012, the USPSTF recommended against PSA-based screening for prostate cancer in the general population.[97] Because no increased risk of prostate cancer was noted in RTRs, current guidelines from the ERBPAB do not recommend for or against screening.[54] The authors suggest following the ACS' guidelines and screen both LTRs and RTRs with PSA after explaining risks and benefits to patients. However, it is important to note that PSA depends on renal function; one study found it decreased significantly in RTRs on sirolimus when compared with those on tacrolimus.[98]

Hepatocellular carcinoma

Most cases of HCC after LT are recurrent disease; thus, the authors only review in RTRs. HCC risk is not increased in RTRs,[5] although those who are hepatitis B surface antigen (HBsAg) or hepatitis C virus antibody positive show higher incidence (SIR 6.5 and SIR 3.4, respectively).[99] Diabetes mellitus was noted to be an independent risk factor as well.[99,100]

All LTRs with allograft cirrhosis should be screened with abdominal ultrasound every 6 months.[56] RTRs who have cirrhosis or are HBsAg carriers at high risk should be also followed per guidelines.[101]

Colorectal cancer

Large studies have shown slightly elevated colorectal cancer (CRC) risk in RTRs (SIR 1.4–2.4) and up to 3-fold increased incidence in LTRs (SIR 2.3–2.9) (see **Table 1**). Most CRCs in LTRs occur in PSC liver recipients with concomitant inflammatory bowel disease (IBD) because of the known increased risk of CRC in this population.[102,103] LTRs with PSC and associated IBD with intact colon are at increased risk of gastrointestinal malignancy (HR 3.51, $P = .005$).[3] Three significant risk factors for CRC in these patients were identified: colonic dysplasia after transplant, duration of ulcerative colitis greater than 10 years, and pancolitis.[102]

A single-center study stratified by patients with PSC and non-PSC patients noted no increased CRC risk in the non-PSC cohort compared with age-adjusted general population (SIR 1.26, $P = .314$).[104] The same investigators also performed a meta-analysis on 29 studies and found persistently elevated CRC incidence rate even when excluding patients with PSC but concluded these data are insufficient to recommend more intensive screening because of several limitations of the analyzed studies.[105] Currently, most transplant centers require colonoscopy before LT, which should put LTRs at lower risk than the general population. No other transplant-related factors for CRC were identified in another meta-analysis.[106]

Results regarding CRC survival are controversial. Poor 5-year survival (30.7% in LTRs vs 63.5% in the general population) was found in a single-center US study,[107] but the opposite result was noted in a European center study (76.2% in LTRs vs 53%–63% in the general population).[6]

One prospective study evaluated CRC incidence in RTRs and noted kidney recipients had 12 times greater risk of CRC than age- and sex-matched controls.[108] CRC frequency increased with age and duration of immunosuppression. The study also assessed EBV in cancer tissue and noted that 31% were positive suggesting a possible role of EBV in the pathogenesis of CRC, although there are no further reports of this finding. A recent retrospective study also reported a higher risk of developing advanced colonic neoplasms in RTRs and especially in those older than 50 years.[109]

The AASLD's current guidelines for LTRs with concomitant PSC and IBD recommend annual colonoscopy with surveillance biopsies.[56] LTRs with PSC without IBD should also be followed closely with colonoscopies every 1 to 2 years. There are no convincing data to support more intensive colonoscopy surveillance in non-PSC LTRs than that in the general population. Despite the noted increased risk of CRC in RTRs, current guidelines recommend starting screening with colonoscopies at 50 years of age in recipients with good graft function and life expectancy and continue per general population guidelines.[110] Another suggested surveillance strategy is starting at 40 years of age or 5 years after transplant,[111] but this approach has not been tested.

Anogenital malignancies

Anogenital malignancies include cervical, vulvar, vaginal, penile, and anal cancer. All these cancers have been associated with high-risk HPV infection[112] with possible augmentation of its effect in the setting of immunosuppression. It is estimated that these patients have a 14-fold higher risk of cervical cancer, up to 50-fold greater risk of vulvar cancer, and up to 100-fold risk of anal cancer.[113] A large population of SOT recipients included in the US Transplant Cancer Match Study showed the most common HPV-related cancer was vulvar (SIR 20.3), followed by penile (SIR 18.6), anal (SIR 11.6), and vaginal (SIR 10.6).[86] Transplant recipients had significantly higher incidence for all in situ and invasive cancers except invasive cervical carcinoma (likely reflecting screening). Median time to diagnosis for both in situ and invasive cancers was 2.6 to 5.7 years. Women were noted to have higher anal cancer incidence. Meeuwis and colleagues[114] assessed the incidence of anogenital malignancies in more than 1000 female RTRs and found high-risk HPV in 92% of the detected vulvar, cervical, and anal lesions. More importantly, 75% of the patients with malignancies never had a cervical smear before transplant. Interestingly, 16% of pre-LT women had high-risk HPV with almost half of them having atypical cytology on a Papanicolaou test, suggesting the necessity for pre-LT screening.[115] Other identified risk factors for cervical cancer in RTRs are continuous smoking after transplant,[31] young age at the time of transplant, and retransplantation.[116]

The risk for vulvar cancer in LTRs was also noted to be very high in one study (SIR 23.8), although most of the lesions were at an early stage at the time of diagnosis; no change in survival was found.[6] No increased risk of uterine and ovarian cancer was seen in both liver and kidney recipients.[4,5]

In 2012 the ACS and USPSTF released new cervical cancer screening guidelines advising against annual screening and recommending, for low-risk individuals, a Papanicolaou test every 3 years between 21 and 65 years of age or cotesting (cytology/HPV) every 5 years between 30 and 65 years of age.[117] However, these guidelines are not applicable to transplant recipients because of their high risk of cervical cancer; thus, following the recommendations of the AST and ERBPAB for annual Papanicolaou test and pelvic examination with careful inspection of anal, vaginal, and vulvar regions should be followed.[54,95] Data are scarce as to whether regular additional testing of HPV would be beneficial in this population.

The effect of quadrivalent HPV vaccine was assessed in a cohort of young adult SOT recipients, but the conferred immunogenicity was suboptimal suggesting that pretransplant vaccination might be more beneficial.[118] There are no established guidelines for HPV vaccination in SOT recipients.

Breast cancer

Similar to prostate cancer, the incidence of breast cancer in RTRs is the same as that of the general population[4] and even lower in some studies with LTRs.[6,10] This finding likely again reflects the pretransplant and posttransplant cancer screening that already exists.

The last breast cancer screening guidelines of the USPSTF were issued in 2009.[119] They recommend starting biennial mammography at 50 years of age and continue until 75 years of age. There are controversies regarding screening between 40 and 50 years of age. Because of the equal risk of breast cancer in RTRs and LTRs, following the general population guidelines are recommended.

SURVEILLANCE STRATEGIES

Based on the guidelines from the AST and ERBPAB,[54,95] the AASLD's practice guideline,[56] the present data, and the recommendations from the general population guidelines, **Table 3** summarizes the recommendations for cancer screening.

Two European, retrospective, single-center studies including LTRs have assessed the efficacy of more intensive screening protocols.[85,120] More cancers were detected at earlier stages, and the cancer detection rate increased significantly from 4.9% to 13.0%.[85] Both studies found improved overall survival in the intensive screening group,[85,120] and one of them also noted significant improvement in median nonskin cancer–related mortality.[85] However, these findings have not been validated in prospective studies and their cost-effectiveness has not been tested yet.

SUMMARY

Significant progress in surgical techniques, better management strategies, and advances in immunosuppression led to improved overall survival of both LTRs and RTRs. Despite these advances, de novo malignancies remain one of the leading causes of late mortality. Immunosuppression plays a central role for cancer development, although many other transplant-related and traditional risk factors are also involved. More study is needed for optimal immunosuppression regimens that can reduce the risk of malignancy in these patients. Future prospective multicenter studies should evaluate feasibility and cost-effectiveness of more intensive screening strategies and compare them with current practices in order to elaborate the best approach for care of these complicated patients.

REFERENCES

1. Schoening WN, Buescher N, Rademacher S, et al. Twenty-year longitudinal follow-up after orthotopic liver transplantation: a single-center experience of 313 consecutive cases. Am J Transplant 2013;13:2384–94.
2. McCaughan JA, Courtney AE. The clinical course of kidney transplant recipients after 20 years of graft function. Am J Transplant 2015;15:734–40.
3. Watt KD, Pedersen RA, Kremers WK, et al. Long-term probability of and mortality from de novo malignancy after liver transplantation. Gastroenterology 2009; 137:2010–7.
4. Collett D, Mumford L, Banner NR, et al. Comparison of the incidence of malignancy in recipients of different types of organ: a UK registry audit. Am J Transplant 2010;10:1889–96.
5. Engels EA, Pfeiffer RM, Fraumeni JF Jr, et al. Spectrum of cancer risk among US solid organ transplant recipients. JAMA 2011;306:1891–901.
6. Schrem H, Kurok M, Kaltenborn A, et al. Incidence and long-term risk of de novo malignancies after liver transplantation with implications for prevention and detection. Liver Transpl 2013;19:1252–61.
7. Adami J, Gabel H, Lindelof B, et al. Cancer risk following organ transplantation: a nationwide cohort study in Sweden. Br J Cancer 2003;89:1221–7.
8. Villeneuve PJ, Schaubel DE, Fenton SS, et al. Cancer incidence among Canadian kidney transplant recipients. Am J Transplant 2007;7:941–8.
9. Piselli P, Serraino D, Segoloni GP, et al. Risk of de novo cancers after transplantation: results from a cohort of 7217 kidney transplant recipients, Italy 1997-2009. Eur J Cancer 2013;49:336–44.
10. Jiang Y, Villeneuve PJ, Fenton SS, et al. Liver transplantation and subsequent risk of cancer: findings from a Canadian cohort study. Liver Transpl 2008;14:1588–97.
11. Krynitz B, Edgren G, Lindelof B, et al. Risk of skin cancer and other malignancies in kidney, liver, heart and lung transplant recipients 1970 to 2008–a Swedish population-based study. Int J Cancer 2013;132:1429–38.

12. Aberg F, Pukkala E, Hockerstedt K, et al. Risk of malignant neoplasms after liver transplantation: a population-based study. Liver Transpl 2008;14:1428–36.

13. Haagsma EB, Hagens VE, Schaapveld M, et al. Increased cancer risk after liver transplantation: a population-based study. J Hepatol 2001;34:84–91.

14. Marques Medina E, Jimenez Romero C, Gomez de la Camara A, et al. Malignancy after liver transplantation: cumulative risk for development. Transplant Proc 2009;41:2447–9.

15. Matas AJ, Gillingham KJ, Humar A, et al. 2202 kidney transplant recipients with 10 years of graft function: what happens next? Am J Transplant 2008;8:2410–9.

16. Gallagher MP, Kelly PJ, Jardine M, et al. Long-term cancer risk of immunosuppressive regimens after kidney transplantation. J Am Soc Nephrol 2010;21: 852–8.

17. Miao Y, Everly JJ, Gross TG, et al. De novo cancers arising in organ transplant recipients are associated with adverse outcomes compared with the general population. Transplantation 2009;87:1347–59.

18. Na R, Grulich AE, Meagher NS, et al. De novo cancer-related death in Australian liver and cardiothoracic transplant recipients. Am J Transplant 2013;13: 1296–304.

19. Herrero JI, Lorenzo M, Quiroga J, et al. De Novo neoplasia after liver transplantation: an analysis of risk factors and influence on survival. Liver Transpl 2005; 11:89–97.

20. Watt KD, Pedersen RA, Kremers WK, et al. Evolution of causes and risk factors for mortality post-liver transplant: results of the NIDDK long-term follow-up study. Am J Transplant 2010;10:1420–7.

21. Kiberd BA, Rose C, Gill JS. Cancer mortality in kidney transplantation. Am J Transplant 2009;9:1868–75.

22. Cheung CY, Lam MF, Chu KH, et al. Malignancies after kidney transplantation: Hong Kong renal registry. Am J Transplant 2012;12:3039–46.

23. Tessari G, Naldi L, Boschiero L, et al. Incidence of primary and second cancers in renal transplant recipients: a multicenter cohort study. Am J Transplant 2013; 13:214–21.

24. Vajdic CM, McDonald SP, McCredie MR, et al. Cancer incidence before and after kidney transplantation. JAMA 2006;296:2823–31.

25. Buell JF, Brock GN. Risk of cancer in liver transplant recipients: a look into the mirror. Liver Transpl 2008;14:1561–3.

26. Shin M, Moon HH, Kim JM, et al. Comparison of the incidence of de novo malignancy in liver or kidney transplant recipients: analysis of 2673 consecutive cases in a single center. Transplant Proc 2013;45:3019–23.

27. Farrugia D, Mahboob S, Cheshire J, et al. Malignancy-related mortality following kidney transplantation is common. Kidney Int 2014;85:1395–403.

28. Hall EC, Segev DL, Engels EA. Racial/ethnic differences in cancer risk after kidney transplantation. Am J Transplant 2013;13:714–20.

29. Chapman JR, Webster AC, Wong G. Cancer in the transplant recipient. Cold Spring Harb Perspect Med 2013;3:1–15.

30. Herrero JI, Pardo F, D'Avola D, et al. Risk factors of lung, head and neck, esophageal, and kidney and urinary tract carcinomas after liver transplantation: the effect of smoking withdrawal. Liver Transpl 2011;17:402–8.

31. Opelz G, Dohler B. Influence of current and previous smoking on cancer and mortality after kidney transplantation. Transplantation 2016;100(1):227–32.

32. Jensen AO, Svaerke C, Farkas D, et al. Skin cancer risk among solid organ recipients: a nationwide cohort study in Denmark. Acta Derm Venereol 2010;90: 474–9.

33. de Fijter JW. Use of proliferation signal inhibitors in non-melanoma skin cancer following renal transplantation. Nephrol Dial Transplant 2007;22(Suppl 1):i23–6.

34. Bernat Garcia J, Morales Suarez-Varela M, Vilata JJ, et al. Risk factors for non-melanoma skin cancer in kidney transplant patients in a Spanish population in the Mediterranean region. Acta Derm Venereol 2013;93:422–7.

35. Ducroux E, Boillot O, Ocampo MA, et al. Skin cancers after liver transplantation: retrospective single-center study on 371 recipients. Transplantation 2014;98: 335–40.

36. Baccarani U, Adani GL, Montanaro D, et al. De novo malignancies after kidney and liver transplantations: experience on 582 consecutive cases. Transplant Proc 2006;38:1135–7.

37. Mithoefer AB, Supran S, Freeman RB. Risk factors associated with the development of skin cancer after liver transplantation. Liver Transpl 2002;8:939–44.

38. Mackenzie KA, Wells JE, Lynn KL, et al. First and subsequent nonmelanoma skin cancers: incidence and predictors in a population of New Zealand renal transplant recipients. Nephrol Dial Transplant 2010;25:300–6.

39. Herrero JI, Espana A, D'Avola D, et al. Subsequent nonmelanoma skin cancer after liver transplantation. Transplant Proc 2012;44:1568–70.

40. Wisgerhof HC, Wolterbeek R, de Fijter JW, et al. Kidney transplant recipients with cutaneous squamous cell carcinoma have an increased risk of internal malignancy. J Invest Dermatol 2012;132:2176–83.

41. Herrero JI, Espana A, Quiroga J, et al. Nonmelanoma skin cancer after liver transplantation. Study of risk factors. Liver Transpl 2005;11:1100–6.

42. Modaresi Esfeh J, Hanouneh IA, Dalal D, et al. The incidence and risk factors of de novo skin cancer in the liver transplant recipients. Int J Organ Transplant Med 2012;3:157–63.

43. Jimenez-Romero C, Manrique Municio A, Marques Medina E, et al. Incidence of de novo nonmelanoma skin tumors after liver transplantation for alcoholic and nonalcoholic liver diseases. Transplant Proc 2006;38:2505–7.

44. Belloni-Fortina A, Piaserico S, Bordignon M, et al. Skin cancer and other cutaneous disorders in liver transplant recipients. Acta Derm Venereol 2012;92: 411–5.

45. Ramsay HM, Fryer AA, Hawley CM, et al. Non-melanoma skin cancer risk in the Queensland renal transplant population. Br J Dermatol 2002;147:950–6.

46. Moloney FJ, Comber H, O'Lorcain P, et al. A population-based study of skin cancer incidence and prevalence in renal transplant recipients. Br J Dermatol 2006; 154:498–504.

47. Euvrard S, Morelon E, Rostaing L, et al. Sirolimus and secondary skin-cancer prevention in kidney transplantation. N Engl J Med 2012;367:329–39.

48. Alberu J, Pascoe MD, Campistol JM, et al. Lower malignancy rates in renal allograft recipients converted to sirolimus-based, calcineurin inhibitor-free immunotherapy: 24-month results from the CONVERT trial. Transplantation 2011;92: 303–10.

49. Mathew T, Kreis H, Friend P. Two-year incidence of malignancy in sirolimus-treated renal transplant recipients: results from five multicenter studies. Clin Transplant 2004;18:446–9.

50. Dahlke E, Murray CA, Kitchen J, et al. Systematic review of melanoma incidence and prognosis in solid organ transplant recipients. Transplant Res 2014;3:10.

51. Green AC, Olsen CM. Increased risk of melanoma in organ transplant recipients: systematic review and meta-analysis of cohort studies. Acta Derm Venereol 2015;95(8):923–7.

52. Le Mire L, Hollowood K, Gray D, et al. Melanomas in renal transplant recipients. Br J Dermatol 2006;154:472–7.

53. Krynitz B, Rozell BL, Lyth J, et al. Cutaneous malignant melanoma in the Swedish organ transplantation cohort: a study of clinicopathological characteristics and mortality. J Am Acad Dermatol 2015;73:106–13.e2.

54. Kidney Disease: Improving Global Outcomes Transplant Work Group. KDIGO clinical practice guideline for the care of kidney transplant recipients. Am J Transplant 2009;9(Suppl 3):S1–155.

55. Urology EAo. Guidelines on renal transplantation. 2014. Available at: http://uroweb.org/wp-content/uploads/27-Renal-Transplant_LRV2-May-13th-2014.pdf. Accessed August 1, 2015.

56. Lucey MR, Terrault N, Ojo L, et al. Long-term management of the successful adult liver transplant: 2012 practice guideline by the American association for the study of liver diseases and the American Society of Transplantation. Liver Transpl 2013;19:3–26.

57. Penn I. Kaposi's sarcoma in transplant recipients. Transplantation 1997;64:669–73.

58. Mbulaiteye SM, Engels EA. Kaposi's sarcoma risk among transplant recipients in the United States (1993-2003). Int J Cancer 2006;119:2685–91.

59. Sampaio MS, Cho YW, Qazi Y, et al. Posttransplant malignancies in solid organ adult recipients: an analysis of the U.S. national transplant database. Transplantation 2012;94:990–8.

60. Frances C, Marcelin AG, Legendre C, et al. The impact of preexisting or acquired Kaposi sarcoma herpesvirus infection in kidney transplant recipients on morbidity and survival. Am J Transplant 2009;9:2580–6.

61. Swerdlow S, Campo E, Harris N, et al. WHO classification of tumours of haematopoietic and lymphoid tissues. Lyon (France): IARC Press; 2008.

62. Caillard S, Lamy FX, Quelen C, et al. Epidemiology of posttransplant lymphoproliferative disorders in adult kidney and kidney pancreas recipients: report of the French registry and analysis of subgroups of lymphomas. Am J Transplant 2012;12:682–93.

63. Koch DG, Christiansen L, Lazarchick J, et al. Posttransplantation lymphoproliferative disorder–the great mimic in liver transplantation: appraisal of the clinicopathologic spectrum and the role of Epstein-Barr virus. Liver Transpl 2007;13:904–12.

64. Hislop AD, Taylor GS, Sauce D, et al. Cellular responses to viral infection in humans: lessons from Epstein-Barr virus. Annu Rev Immunol 2007;25:587–617.

65. Aucejo F, Rofaiel G, Miller C. Who is at risk for post-transplant lymphoproliferative disorders (PTLD) after liver transplantation? J Hepatol 2006;44:19–23.

66. Green M, Michaels MG. Epstein-Barr virus infection and posttransplant lymphoproliferative disorder. Am J Transplant 2013;13(Suppl 3):41–54 [quiz: 54].

67. Morton M, Coupes B, Roberts SA, et al. Epidemiology of posttransplantation lymphoproliferative disorder in adult renal transplant recipients. Transplantation 2013;95:470–8.

68. Quinlan SC, Pfeiffer RM, Morton LM, et al. Risk factors for early-onset and late-onset post-transplant lymphoproliferative disorder in kidney recipients in the United States. Am J Hematol 2011;86:206–9.

69. van Leeuwen MT, Grulich AE, Webster AC, et al. Immunosuppression and other risk factors for early and late non-Hodgkin lymphoma after kidney transplantation. Blood 2009;114:630–7.

70. Sampaio MS, Cho YW, Shah T, et al. Impact of Epstein-Barr virus donor and recipient serostatus on the incidence of post-transplant lymphoproliferative disorder in kidney transplant recipients. Nephrol Dial Transplant 2012;27:2971–9.

71. Sampaio MS, Cho YW, Shah T, et al. Association of immunosuppressive maintenance regimens with posttransplant lymphoproliferative disorder in kidney transplant recipients. Transplantation 2012;93:73–81.

72. Grinyo J, Charpentier B, Pestana JM, et al. An integrated safety profile analysis of belatacept in kidney transplant recipients. Transplantation 2010;90:1521–7.

73. Masson P, Henderson L, Chapman JR, et al. Belatacept for kidney transplant recipients. Cochrane Database Syst Rev 2014;(11):CD010699.

74. Benlloch S, Berenguer M, Prieto M, et al. De novo internal neoplasms after liver transplantation: increased risk and aggressive behavior in recent years? Am J Transplant 2004;4:596–604.

75. Kim RD, Fujikawa T, Mizuno S, et al. Adult post-transplant lymphoproliferative disease in the liver graft in patients with recurrent hepatitis C. Eur J Gastroenterol Hepatol 2011;23:559–65.

76. Ghobrial IM, Habermann TM, Maurer MJ, et al. Prognostic analysis for survival in adult solid organ transplant recipients with post-transplantation lymphoproliferative disorders. J Clin Oncol 2005;23:7574–82.

77. Faull RJ, Hollett P, McDonald SP. Lymphoproliferative disease after renal transplantation in Australia and New Zealand. Transplantation 2005;80:193–7.

78. Morton M, Coupes B, Ritchie J, et al. Post-transplant lymphoproliferative disorder in adult renal transplant recipients: survival and prognosis. Leuk Lymphoma 2015;1–23 [Epub ahead of print].

79. Lee TC, Savoldo B, Rooney CM, et al. Quantitative EBV viral loads and immunosuppression alterations can decrease PTLD incidence in pediatric liver transplant recipients. Am J Transplant 2005;5:2222–8.

80. Heemann U, Abramowicz D, Spasovski G, et al. Endorsement of the Kidney Disease Improving Global Outcomes (KDIGO) guidelines on kidney transplantation: a European Renal Best Practice (ERBP) position statement. Nephrol Dial Transplant 2011;26:2099–106.

81. Martin SI, Dodson B, Wheeler C, et al. Monitoring infection with Epstein-Barr virus among seromismatch adult renal transplant recipients. Am J Transplant 2011;11:1058–63.

82. Nelissen C, Lambrecht M, Nevens F, et al. Noncutaneous head and neck cancer in solid organ transplant patients: single center experience. Oral Oncol 2014;50: 263–8.

83. Liu Q, Yan L, Xu C, et al. Increased incidence of head and neck cancer in liver transplant recipients: a meta-analysis. BMC Cancer 2014;14:776.

84. Piselli P, Burra P, Lauro A, et al. Head and neck and esophageal cancers after liver transplant: results from a multicenter cohort study. Italy, 1997-2010. Transpl Int 2015;28:841–8.

85. Finkenstedt A, Graziadei IW, Oberaigner W, et al. Extensive surveillance promotes early diagnosis and improved survival of de novo malignancies in liver transplant recipients. Am J Transplant 2009;9:2355–61.

86. Madeleine MM, Finch JL, Lynch CF, et al. HPV-related cancers after solid organ transplantation in the United States. Am J Transplant 2013;13:3202–9.

87. Karamchandani D, Arias-Amaya R, Donaldson N, et al. Thyroid cancer and renal transplantation: a meta-analysis. Endocr Relat Cancer 2010;17:159–67.
88. Sigel K, Veluswamy R, Krauskopf K, et al. Lung cancer prognosis in elderly solid organ transplant recipients. Transplantation 2015;99(10):2181–9.
89. Genebes C, Brouchet L, Kamar N, et al. Characteristics of thoracic malignancies that occur after solid-organ transplantation. J Thorac Oncol 2010;5: 1789–95.
90. Moyer VA, US Preventive Services Task Force. Screening for lung cancer: U.S. preventive services task force recommendation statement. Ann Intern Med 2014;160:330–8.
91. Goh A, Vathsala A. Native renal cysts and dialysis duration are risk factors for renal cell carcinoma in renal transplant recipients. Am J Transplant 2011;11: 86–92.
92. Hall EC, Pfeiffer RM, Segev DL, et al. Cumulative incidence of cancer after solid organ transplantation. Cancer 2013;119:2300–8.
93. Ma MK, Lim WH, Turner RM, et al. The risk of cancer in recipients of living-donor, standard and expanded criteria deceased donor kidney transplants: a registry analysis. Transplantation 2014;98:1286–93.
94. Wong G, Turner RM, Chapman JR, et al. Time on dialysis and cancer risk after kidney transplantation. Transplantation 2013;95:114–21.
95. Kasiske BL, Vazquez MA, Harmon WE, et al. Recommendations for the outpatient surveillance of renal transplant recipients. American Society of Transplantation. J Am Soc Nephrol 2000;11(Suppl 15):S1–86.
96. Wolf AM, Wender RC, Etzioni RB, et al. American Cancer Society guideline for the early detection of prostate cancer: update 2010. CA Cancer J Clin 2010; 60:70–98.
97. Moyer VA, U.S. Preventive Services Task Force. Screening for prostate cancer: U.S. Preventive Services Task Force recommendation statement. Ann Intern Med 2012;157:120–34.
98. Chamie K, Ghosh PM, Koppie TM, et al. The effect of sirolimus on prostate-specific antigen (PSA) levels in male renal transplant recipients without prostate cancer. Am J Transplant 2008;8:2668–73.
99. Hoffmann CJ, Subramanian AK, Cameron AM, et al. Incidence and risk factors for hepatocellular carcinoma after solid organ transplantation. Transplantation 2008;86:784–90.
100. Koshiol J, Pawlish K, Goodman MT, et al. Risk of hepatobiliary cancer after solid organ transplant in the United States. Clin Gastroenterol Hepatol 2014;12: 1541–9.e3.
101. Bruix J, Sherman M. AASLD Practice guideline. Management of hepatocellular carcinoma: an update. Hepatology 2011;53(3):1020–2.
102. Vera A, Gunson BK, Ussatoff V, et al. Colorectal cancer in patients with inflammatory bowel disease after liver transplantation for primary sclerosing cholangitis. Transplantation 2003;75:1983–8.
103. Loftus EV Jr, Aguilar HI, Sandborn WJ, et al. Risk of colorectal neoplasia in patients with primary sclerosing cholangitis and ulcerative colitis following orthotopic liver transplantation. Hepatology 1998;27:685–90.
104. Sint Nicolaas J, Tjon AS, Metselaar HJ, et al. Colorectal cancer in post-liver transplant recipients. Dis Colon Rectum 2010;53:817–21.
105. Sint Nicolaas J, de Jonge V, Steyerberg EW, et al. Risk of colorectal carcinoma in post-liver transplant patients: a systematic review and meta-analysis. Am J Transplant 2010;10:868–76.

106. Singh S, Edakkanambeth Varayil J, Loftus EV Jr, et al. Incidence of colorectal cancer after liver transplantation for primary sclerosing cholangitis: a systematic review and meta-analysis. Liver Transpl 2013;19:1361–9.

107. Johnson EE, Leverson GE, Pirsch JD, et al. A 30-year analysis of colorectal adenocarcinoma in transplant recipients and proposal for altered screening. J Gastrointest Surg 2007;11:272–9.

108. Park JM, Choi MG, Kim SW, et al. Increased incidence of colorectal malignancies in renal transplant recipients: a case control study. Am J Transplant 2010;10:2043–50.

109. Kwon JH, Koh SJ, Kim JY, et al. Prevalence of advanced colorectal neoplasm after kidney transplantation: surveillance based on the results of screening colonoscopy. Dig Dis Sci 2015;60:1761–9.

110. Lieberman DA, Rex DK, Winawer SJ, et al. Guidelines for colonoscopy surveillance after screening and polypectomy: a consensus update by the US Multi-Society Task Force on Colorectal Cancer. Gastroenterology 2012;143:844–57.

111. Asch WS, Bia MJ. Oncologic issues and kidney transplantation: a review of frequency, mortality, and screening. Adv Chronic Kidney Dis 2014;21:106–13.

112. Watson M, Saraiya M, Ahmed F, et al. Using population-based cancer registry data to assess the burden of human papillomavirus-associated cancers in the United States: overview of methods. Cancer 2008;113:2841–54.

113. Hinten F, Meeuwis KA, van Rossum MM, et al. HPV-related (pre)malignancies of the female anogenital tract in renal transplant recipients. Crit Rev Oncol Hematol 2012;84:161–80.

114. Meeuwis KA, Melchers WJ, Bouten H, et al. Anogenital malignances in women after renal transplantation over 40 years in a single center. Transplantation 2012; 93:914–22.

115. Tarallo PA, Smolowitz J, Carriero D, et al. Prevalence of high-risk human papilloma virus among women with hepatitis C virus before liver transplantation. Transpl Infect Dis 2013;15:400–4.

116. Marschalek J, Helmy S, Schmidt A, et al. Prevalence of genital dysplasia after kidney transplantation - a retrospective, non-interventional study from two centers. Acta Obstet Gynecol Scand 2015;94:891–7.

117. Moyer VA, US Preventive Services Task Force. Screening for cervical cancer: U.S. Preventive Services Task Force recommendation statement. Ann Intern Med 2012;156:880–91. W312.

118. Kumar D, Unger ER, Panicker G, et al. Immunogenicity of quadrivalent human papillomavirus vaccine in organ transplant recipients. Am J Transplant 2013; 13:2411–7.

119. US Preventive Services Task Force. Screening for breast cancer: U.S. Preventive Services Task Force recommendation statement. Ann Intern Med 2009; 151:716–26. W-236.

120. Herrero JI, Alegre F, Quiroga J, et al. Usefulness of a program of neoplasia surveillance in liver transplantation. A preliminary report. Clin Transplant 2009;23: 532–6.

121. Carroll RP, Ramsay HM, Fryer AA, et al. Incidence and prediction of nonmelanoma skin cancer post-renal transplantation: a prospective study in Queensland, Australia. Am J Kidney Dis 2003;41:676–83.

Metabolic Bone Disease in the Post-transplant Population

Preventative and Therapeutic Measures

Johan Daniël Nel, MBChB, MMed (Int Med), Cert Neph (CMSA)[a,*],
Sol Epstein, MD, FRCP[b,c,1]

KEYWORDS

- Transplantation • Bone loss • Immunosuppressive agents • Fractures
- Investigations • Treatment

KEY POINTS

- Post-transplant bone disease contributes substantially to morbidity and mortality after fractures and leads to significant loss of quality of life.
- The mechanisms inducing bone loss are multifactorial and include preexisting bone disease before transplantation, glucocorticoids (GCs), and other immunosuppressive medications, among others.
- Monitoring via biochemistry and imaging is essential in decision making regarding treatment. A bone biopsy remains vital in excluding low-turnover bone disease where there is any doubt.
- The use of bisphosphonates, combined with vitamin D and calcium supplementation, remains the backbone of treatment.

INTRODUCTION

Transplantation is recognized as the treatment of choice in end-stage kidney disease (ESKD) and is well established in chronic liver failure. Due to refinements in surgical technique and, more importantly, advances in immunosuppressive medication, both patient and graft survival have improved. This has led to more frequent observation of the long-term complications of transplantation and the need for improvement in its management.

Disclosure Statement: The Authors have nothing to disclose.
[a] Division of Nephrology, Department of Medicine, Tygerberg Hospital and University of Stellenbosch, PO Box 241, Cape Town, Western Cape 8000, South Africa; [b] Mt Sinai School of Medicine, New York, NY, USA; [c] University of Pennsylvania School of Medicine, Philadelphia, PA, USA
[1] Present address: 231 Jeffrey Lane, Newtown Square, PA 19073.
* Corresponding author.
E-mail address: johannel@sun.ac.za

Med Clin N Am 100 (2016) 569–586
http://dx.doi.org/10.1016/j.mcna.2016.01.007
0025-7125/16/$ – see front matter © 2016 Elsevier Inc. All rights reserved.

Post-transplant bone disease and bone loss commonly cause significant morbidity and mortality and induce significant loss in patients' quality of life due to fractures, pain, and subsequent loss of mobility and independence. This article reviews some of the multiple pathogenic mechanisms at play and discusses the investigations, monitoring, and treatment needed for the management of both preexisting and post-transplantation bone disease related to kidney and liver organ transplantation.

EPIDEMIOLOGY: BONE MINERAL DENSITY AND FRACTURE RISK

Low bone mass and fractures commonly antedate renal transplantation. Patients with ESKD on dialysis are 4-fold more likely to have hip fractures than the general population, with a 21% increase in vertebral fracture.[1] The most significant subsequent bone loss takes place within the first 6 to 12 months after transplantation and is predominantly due to large doses of GCs. Reported rates of decrease in bone mineral density (BMD) in the first year vary between 3% and 9%.[2–4] Not only do kidney recipients have an increased fracture risk compared with the general population but also they have a 30% increase in hip fractures compared with dialysis patients awaiting transplantation.[5]

By 18 months, bone loss has been shown to be 9% from baseline, and 60% of patients have BMD less than the fracture threshold.[2,3,6] The initial rate of loss declines steeply but persists at 1% to 2% per year. This may be due to calcineurin inhibitor (CNI) effects. At 5 years after transplant, 22% of patients have been reported to have had fractures. This rises to as high as 57% at 10 years, and the cumulative incidence at 15 years is considered 3 times greater than expected.[7,8]

In liver transplant recipients, the incidence of new fractures mirrors the timing of the most rapid bone loss within the first year.[9–11] Prospective studies have shown that bone loss at the lumbar spine occurred during the first 4 to 6 months with gradual improvement thereafter, with BMD nearing or even exceeding baseline by the second post-transplant year. BMD at the femur neck also improved after 3 to 5 years but was still below baseline,[10–12] likely due to the differences between trabecular and cortical bone pathophysiology.

In kidney recipients, fractures tend to occur more commonly in cortical bone with lower limb fractures, accounting for 35% of all fractures, followed by fractures in the ribs, upper extremities, and vertebrae.[8] In contrast, liver transplant patients have a predilection for fractures of the spine, hips, and ribs. Vertebral fractures have been reported in 21% of patients in the first 2 years.[13]

The rate of post-transplant fractures may be declining due to awareness of GC side effects, introduction of GC-sparing regimens and immunosuppressive agents, and treatment of bone disease before and after transplantation.

CAUSES OF POST-TRANSPLANT BONE DISEASE

Although this review focuses on bone disease after transplantation, the impact of pretransplantation bone density and disease on subsequent bone disease is substantial. The pathogenesis of bone disease before and after transplantation is multifactorial and complex. Some but not all of the risk factors are discussed.

Pretransplantation

Risks also seen in the general population
Advanced age, smoking, excessive alcohol use, and vitamin D deficiency undoubtedly contribute to low BMD in patients with kidney failure and liver failure as well as a history of previous fractures, immobility, and being either white or female. Low muscle

mass/body weight along with poor nutrition, postmenopausal status, and hypogonadism are also important.[5,7,14,15] Falls may be a significant contributor to hip fractures in this population.

Risks contributed by underlying diseases to bone abnormalities

Diabetes mellitus Both type 1 diabetes mellitus (DM) and type 2 DM are associated with increased fracture risk in the general population[16] as well as those with solid organ transplants.[17] In type 1 DM, this stems from decreased BMD and failure to achieve peak bone mass. The decrease of insulin and amylin may also lead to impaired bone formation.[18] Patients with type 2 DM may have normal or even elevated BMD, but poor bone quality is the cardinal issue.[19] Numerous factors contribute, including advanced glycation end products, drugs, vitamin D deficiency, and increased marrow adiposity, which are linked to the development of osteoporosis and increased fragility.[20]

Systemic lupus erythematosus Systemic lupus erythematosus (SLE) is a common cause of ESKD. Low BMD is well described in these patients, with sun avoidance (leading to vitamin D deficiency) as well as corticosteroids and premature menopause after the use of cyclophosphamide contributing; however, a recent study showed similar deleterious changes in porosity and bone strength in patients without steroid exposure, thus implicating the disease itself.[21]

Human immunodeficiency virus disease Low BMD is common in patients with human immunodeficiency virus, stemming from multiple population-related factors but with both the infection as well as highly effective antiretroviral therapy contributing significantly.[16]

Medications associated with osteoporosis

A multitude of drugs used in patients with chronic kidney disease (CKD), dialysis patients, and those with liver failure have been implicated as contributing to the development of osteoporosis. These include the thiazolidinediones, proton pump inhibitors, heparin, loop diuretics, and angiotensin-converting enzyme inhibitors.[16,22] Although the effects of these drugs have been studied in healthy and osteoporotic patients as independent risk factors for decreased BMD, studies are needed to clarify their contribution to bone disease in transplantation.

Chronic kidney disease–mineral and bone disorder

CKD initiates a cascade of events leading to renal osteodystrophy. A full discussion of the complete pathophysiology of CKD–mineral and bone disorder (MBD), which increases fracture risk both before and after transplant, is beyond the scope of this review. The interplay between kidney, gut, bone, and parathyroid is complex, with phosphate retention playing a major role. This is followed by secondary hyperparathyroidism and elevation in fibroblast growth factor 23 levels. Subsequent decreased calcitriol synthesis, with hypocalcemia and the accumulation of β_2-microglobulin and aluminum, all contribute. The disease starts early and worsens with duration on dialysis. Tertiary hyperparathyroidism may occur due to polyclonal parathyroid cell proliferation, causing diffuse hyperplasia, or monoclonal expansion of adenomatous cells that do not respond to their normal suppressors. Hyperparathyroidism frequently persists after transplantation.[7,23]

Based on histologic features, CKD-MBD is classified into 4 subtypes, with various mechanisms contributing to each type. The incidence of adynamic bone disease has been on the increase,[23] especially in diabetics. In patients receiving hemodialysis, it now occurs with equal frequency as osteitis fibrosa cystica[24] and it predominates in patients on peritoneal dialysis. Patients may present with more than one defined disorder or mixed disorders.[25]

There is no clear relationship between BMD measurement and the different subtypes of CKD-MBD. The measurement of BMD and World Health Organization criteria cannot be applied to diagnose osteoporosis in patients with ESKD due to the inability to distinguish between osteoporosis and the various histologic subtypes of CKD-MBD.[15,26] Bone biopsy remains the gold standard but it is invasive and expensive and suffers from a lack of sufficient expert histomorphometrists. Newer noninvasive technologies, such as microindentation and high-resolution peripheral quantitative CT, may assist in assessing bone quality but currently these are still mostly research tools (discussed later).

Hepatic osteodystrophy

Osteoporosis is prevalent in 11% to 52% of patients awaiting liver transplantation, with common associations including smoking, immobilization, alcohol abuse, hypogonadism, and vitamin D deficiency.[11,27] Cholestatic diseases, such as primary biliary cirrhosis, induce the retention of toxins that inhibit normal osteoblast function, causing low-turnover bone disease. Unconjugated bilirubin has been shown to significantly decrease plasma mitogenic activity, thus impairing osteoblast proliferation.[28] The exact role of vitamin D deficiency is contentious due to the variance in vitamin D assays in reported studies as well as a lack of response after repletion in a small series. Vitamin D metabolism may still play a pivotal role. Due to insufficient 25-hydroxylation of cholecalciferol by the hepatocyte in end-stage liver disease, patients frequently have low serum levels of 25-hydroxyvitamin D (25[OH] vitamin D). This is worsened by fat malabsorption, increased vitamin D catabolism, and reduced levels of vitamin D–binding protein. The serum level of 25(OH) vitamin D may be misleading because vitamin D–binding proteins may be low and, therefore, free 25(OH) vitamin D levels may be increased. Some studies report improved BMD scores with supplementation pretransplantation.[11] Bone turnover converts to high turnover status after transplantation as demonstrated by significant increases in osteoprotegerin and receptor activator of nuclear factor κB ligand (RANKL) levels in the first 2 weeks after surgery. Histomorphometric studies indicate that in contrast to kidney recipients, bone loss stops at 6 months and subsequent gains follow mainly at cancellous bone in the next 18 months.[12] The gains in BMD are significantly higher in premenopausal than postmenopausal women, demonstrating the protective effects of estrogen to the skeleton.[29] It is clear from studies monitoring longer-term changes in bone mass, however, that although spinal BMD may recover fully, this is not the case in BMD measurements of the femoral neck. Frequently there is delayed and incomplete recovery of femoral neck BMD at 36 months post-transplant,[12] which may remain consistently below pretransplant values.[10]

Post-transplantation

In general, the initial severe loss of BMD after both kidney and liver transplantation is due to the use of large doses of GCs. In contrast to liver recipients, who may see ongoing gain in BMD from 6 months after transplantation onward, kidney recipients experience ongoing loss, albeit at a much slower rate than in the first year. Many aspects contributing to CKD-MBD may improve significantly after kidney transplantation, but the degree of recovery is frequently incomplete. Hyperparathyroidism may persist in 30% to 50%, partly due to delayed involution of the glands.[30] Refractory hyperparathyroidism occurs in up to 25% of recipients at 1 year after transplantation,[31] often as a result of monoclonal hyperplasia. Phenotypically, diffuse hyperplasia classically regresses whereas remaining nodular hyperplasia does not.[32] Hyperparathyroidism is associated with both increased mortality and graft loss in otherwise stable kidney recipients.[33] Unfortunately, there is limited clarity in the management of hyperparathyroidism after transplantation, and further study is much needed for the development of evidence-based guidelines.

Hypophosphatemia occurs due to increased phosphate excretion with both ongoing hyperparathyroidism and persistently elevated levels of fibroblast growth factor 23 contributing to ongoing phosphate losses. In addition, both GCs and CNIs cause decreased proximal tubular reabsorption. Hypophosphatemia induces decreased osteoblast activity and osteomalacia and muscle weakness (also related to vitamin D deficiency) anemia as well as increased mortality risks.[34]

It is worthwhile remembering that significantly new CKD-MBD may also occur in varying degrees depending on the level of function of the renal allograft.

Simultaneous pancreas-kidney transplantation

Previous studies demonstrated a significantly higher fracture risk in patients after simultaneous pancreas-kidney (SPK) transplantation compared with patients receiving kidney transplant alone.[35] More recently, a retrospective study compared hospitalization rates for fractures between adults with type 1 DM undergoing kidney-alone transplantation versus SPK transplantation. The incidence of fractures was based on billing by Medicare and data from the US Renal Data System. Fractures occurred in significantly fewer (4.7%) of SPK transplants compared with the kidney-alone transplant cohort (5.9%), showing a 31% risk reduction, particularly in men undergoing SPK transplantation.[36] Many but certainly not all fracture covariates were ascertained and compared between the 2 groups, with the similar unadjusted prevalence of prior fractures reported supporting the validity of the findings.[37] The exact reason why no benefit was found in women is unclear and needs further confirmatory study. Possibilities include an under-reported detection rate due to nonhospitalization and a higher likelihood that women may have undergone screening and subsequent treatment with medication aimed at fracture reduction. Regardless, the restoration of endogenous insulin production and euglycemia may account for the observed benefit in the study and prompt decision making in future transplants for patients with type 1 DM.

Immunosuppressive drugs

Glucocorticoids GCs are undoubtedly the major contributor to bone loss after transplantation, with most substantial BMD losses (5.5%–19.5%) occurring during the first 6 months in kidney recipients after the use of large doses in the direct post-transplant period.[34] Continued bone loss is seen with continued therapy even at doses as low as 2.5 mg daily, with annual loss at a rate of 1% to 2% seen in the subsequent years.[38] Osteoblast function may recover once GC doses are tapered to below 5 mg per day, slowing down the rate of bone loss and even leading to some recovery, but this is mainly in cancellous bone.[26,39] Minimizing steroid use has been shown to be beneficial both in kidney transplant recipients, where absence of bone loss at the lumbar spine and proximal femur was reported,[40] as well as in liver transplant recipients, where steroid withdrawal accelerated recovery of lumbar spine density.[41]

GCs predominantly reduce bone formation but also significantly increase reabsorption, both directly and indirectly. Directly, production of osteoblast precursors are decreased through inhibition of Wnt signaling via enhanced expression of Dickkopf-1 and sclerostin,[42] and both osteoblast proliferation and function are decreased by inhibiting the gene expression of osteocalcin and insulinlike growth factor 1. Enhanced apoptosis of osteocytes, which contribute to the ability to withstand compressive forces, take place through increased expression of 11β-hydroxysteroid dehydrogenase type 1, which increases active metabolites of adrenal hormone.[43] Both lifespan and activity of osteoclasts are increased via increased production of RANKL and suppression of osteoprotegrin (which acts as natural decoy receptor for RANKL). An independent prosurvival effect is also conferred.[16] Indirectly, GCs contribute to increased bone resorption through several mechanisms. Along with low levels of 1,25-*dihydroxyvitamin* vitamin D, GCs cause decreased intestinal calcium reabsorption and increased renal calcium wasting, further encouraging secondary hyperparathyroidism. In addition, GCs promote hypogonadism through the decreased production of testosterone and estrogen. Corticosteroids also increase the potential for fractures by increasing fall risk: they can induce a profound myopathy, impair mobility and balance, and decrease weight-bearing activity.[15,26]

GCs are viewed as the major contributor to the development of debilitating osteonecrosis/avascular necrosis through compromise of the vascular supply to bone via microfractures, fat embolism, adipocyte hyperplasia, increased intramarrow pressure, and bone necrosis. GC-free maintenance regimes demonstrated low rates of avascular necrosis at 3-year follow-up.[44]

Calcineurin inhibitors The use of CNIs has benefitted transplant patients significantly by reducing the number of episodes of acute rejection and allowing for decrease or even discontinuation of GCs. The impact of CNIs on bone loss may seem confusing and contradictory in the literature. In vitro studies showed that they inhibit bone resorption, but in vivo studies with cyclosporine in rat models demonstrated severe accelerated high-turnover bone disease and extensive bone resorption.[45] An explanation for this apparent contradiction lies in the issues that in vitro studies could not mimic: the mediation of T lymphocytes in vivo and their subsequent production of osteoclast-stimulatory cytokines, which overwhelms the effect of CNIs on calcineurin in bone.[46]

It remains difficult to evaluate the true impact of CNIs on bone loss due to concomitant contributions by preexisting factors as well as the masking effect from GCs. Some investigators report no BMD loss over the 18 months after transplant with the use of a steroid-free regimen, resulting in significantly fewer bone complications after 4 years.[47] The impact of cyclosporine is significantly more prominent in long-term follow-up: a study analyzing bone mass loss via BMD and histology found no difference between kidney recipients on cyclosporine monotherapy versus either patients on azathioprine combined with GCs or patients on triple therapy.[48] A more recent study evaluated the impact of CNIs while correcting for as many modifiable and non-modifiable factors as possible, enrolling only patients with good renal function (estimated glomerular filtration rate [eGFR] >60 mL/min) and with intact parathyroid hormone (PTH) levels less than 100 pg/mL. Although slight bone formation was demonstrated, it was overwhelmed by potent and clinically relevant bone resorption in patients on cyclosporine and tacrolimus.[49]

Several differences conferring benefit to tacrolimus over cyclosporine have been highlighted in liver transplantation but should be carefully interpreted because they often represent different eras in transplantation with several variables that have changed over these 2 major periods of time. In studies claiming fewer fractures and faster bone architecture recovery with tacrolimus, the use of GCs in patients given cyclosporine was significantly higher.[50,51] Tacrolimus is as deleterious as cyclosporine in murine models[52] and may be beneficial mainly by allowing the use of significantly fewer corticosteroids.

Other immunosuppressive agents Both azathioprine and mycophenolic acid/mycophenylate mofetil are bone neutral. Of the mechanistic target of rapamycin (mTOR) inhibitors, sirolimus caused resistance to insulinlike growth factor 1 and subsequent impaired longitudinal bone growth in rats[53] but seems to offer lower bone resorption in humans.[54] Everolimus may be bone sparing or even protective, but clinical studies are lacking.[55] In addition, a review of available studies has indicated that the mTOR inhibitors can impair gonadal function, but the impact of this effect is unknown.[56] The use of interleukin-2 receptor monoclonal antibodies and T-cell depleting agents have no direct impact on BMD but using drugs, such as basiliximab or thymoglobulin, in induction therapy may allow for significantly less GC use during the first months without an increase in the rate of acute rejection. Potentially this will be beneficial to bone health, but this hypothesis has not yet been validated.

New-onset diabetes after transplantation
New-onset diabetes after transplantation (NODAT) is well known as a clinical entity in transplant patients. It is a common complication after transplantation, occurring at a rate of 20% to 50% in kidney recipients and 9% to 21% in liver recipients at 12 months after transplant, respectively.[57] Patients who develop NODAT have individual susceptibility factors that are exacerbated by mainly the immunosuppressive agents used but also by cytomegalovirus infection and acute rejection. NODAT leads to higher rejection rates and poorer graft survival along with an increase in cardiovascular morbidity and mortality as well as more frequent infections.[57] The effects of NODAT on bone disease after transplantation are as yet unknown, but considering the impact of diabetes on bone health in general and on fracture risk after solid organ transplantation, it warrants further study.

MONITORING AND INVESTIGATING POST-TRANSPLANT BONE DISEASE
Biochemistry

Kidney
In kidney transplantation, regular monitoring of calcium, phosphate, vitamin D, PTH, and bone-specific alkaline phosphatase is used in an attempt to identify and monitor post-transplant CKD-MBD as well as its treatment. Recommendations based on Kidney Disease: Improving Global Outcomes (KDIGO) and Kidney Disease Outcomes Quality Initiative (KDOQI) guidelines are well summarized elsewhere.[58] Correction of abnormalities have to be individually tailored based on targets governed by degree of kidney impairment in the absence of studies specific to transplant patients. Calcium and phosphate levels should be monitored frequently until stable due to the severe changes in this period. The optimal level for PTH after transplant remains an enigma and should be assessed in conjunction with serum calcium and phosphate levels as well as eGFR after transplantation. Bone turnover correlates poorly with PTH levels after transplantation. Still, assessment of PTH contributes significantly to identifying patients at risk: recently persistent intact PTH levels exceeding 130 ng/L 3 months after transplantation were identified as a major determinant of fractures in the first 5 years of follow-up.[59,60] The management of persistent hyperparathyroidism is extremely complex and the decision to observe treat medically or perform surgery, as well as the choice of operation, is not in the realm of this review but readers can refer to Messa and colleagues'[60] article. Likewise, ectopic or heterotopic calcification are not discussed.

Liver
The majority of bone loss in liver transplantation takes place rapidly and in the first 6 months, during which bone disease frequently converts from a low-turnover state

to a high-turnover state. It is prudent to assess and monitor biochemical parameters in this period but no clear guidelines exist as to frequency. Frequency of monitoring depends on the abnormality prior to transplantation as well as post-transplantation, taking into consideration the treatment offered as well as concurrent kidney function. Evaluation of vitamin D, calcium, and PTH is cardinal. In addition, monitoring of kidney function is required both before and after the administration of specific antiosteoporosis medications.

Bone Biomarkers

Biomarkers for both bone formation (bone-specific alkaline phosphatase, osteocalcin, and procollagen type 1 N-terminal propeptide) and resorption (tartrate-resistant acid phosphatase 5b and C-terminal telopeptide of type 1 collagen [CTX]) have been studied but found wanting in CKD. Many bone turnover markers are cleared by the kidney and retained with worsening glomerular filtration rate, which complicates their interpretation. These markers have yet not been shown to predict fracture risk in kidney recipients.[58] Bone-specific alkaline phosphatase has been advocated to help recognize low-turnover bone disease.

In liver recipients, raised levels of CTX at the time of transplant as well as a rise in bone-specific alkaline phosphatase 6 months hence have been shown to predict, respectively, bone loss and fracture risk in the first post-transplant year.[61]

Imaging

Conventional radiographs have little role in post-transplant bone disease apart from identifying fractures. Screening for asymptomatic spinal fractures may contribute to identifying patients at higher risk for the development of fractures after transplantation. Bone densitometry measured via dual energy x-ray absorptiometry (DEXA) is the clinical tool for determining fracture risk in a general population, but its use in CKD and kidney transplantation has been controversial. Bone strength is dependent both on bone density and bone material quality and includes aspects, such as microarchitecture, bone turnover, and mineralization. Bone quality cannot be assessed by DEXA. In addition, DEXA cannot identify the underlying cause of CKD-MBD. Notwithstanding, newer studies in both the CKD population[62] and in kidney transplant recipients[63] have demonstrated that low-areal BMD measured by DEXA at the hip and femur neck does predict fracture risk in multiple CKD populations, prompting KDIGO to re-examine current guidelines regarding the routine performance of DEXA.[64] Practically, this means DEXA should be obtained as soon as possible within the first 3 months after transplantation and at yearly intervals for the first 2 years after transplant. Sequential measurements may be of benefit in monitoring antiresorptive therapy,[58] although its exact role is still to be determined. Less controversy exists in liver transplantation, where it is recommended that patients (especially those with primary biliary cirrhosis and other risk factors for bone disease) undergo routine assessment while awaiting transplant, again at 3 months post-transplant and then after 1 year. Low BMD along with preexisting fractures remain the major risk determinants for fractures in liver transplant recipients.[50] No clear consensus exists regarding subsequent follow-up measures and further DEXA evaluation should be individualized depending on circumstances, T-score, and continuation of GC and immunosuppressant therapy.

Significant new research is being done on the role of high-resolution quantitative CT as well as micro-MRI in the assessment of bone microarchitecture. In addition, finite element analysis to quantify bone strength can be applied to CT to measure strength of either whole-bone or individual cortical/trabecular components.[65] Of particular interest is microindentation. A recent study has shown reference point indentation to confirm increases in bone material strength index in patients with GC-induced osteoporosis treated with selected bisphosphonates, whereas no DEXA-measured bone densitometry changes were found.[66] Currently, all these are mostly costly tools used for research and not readily available. These utilities need significant validation both in patients with CKD and after transplantation before being applied widely, but the possibility exists that, in combination with DEXA, bone turnover markers, or both, bone status will be able to be assessed through a virtual biopsy in the near future.

Bone Biopsy

Tetracyclin double-labeled transiliac crest bone biopsy with histomorphometry is the gold standard for assessing bone disease and renal dystrophy in particular. Yet bone biopsy is invasive and expensive and needs skilled histomorphometrists for accurate analysis. As a result, it has been performed with significantly less frequency in the past decade and may not be readily available for clinicians. KDIGO still acknowledges several factors that would prompt the performance of bone biopsies, the foremost being prior to bisphosphonate therapy in patients with possible adynamic bone disease,[65] although with the advent of alternative therapies, such as denosumab and teriparatide, this is being reconsidered.

TREATMENT
General

The treatment of post-transplant bone disease and subsequent reduction of fractures starts well before transplantation. All patients must be examined thoroughly and potential risks identified (**Box 1**). Regardless of pretransplant BDM measurements, all patients should follow the same recommendations to prevent osteoporosis in the general population. Smoking and alcohol use must be avoided, poor nutritional status addressed, and calcium intake supplemented where indicated. The use of prolonged courses of GCs before transplantation should be considered carefully. Where possible, any medication that could contribute to osteoporosis should be replaced by safer alternatives. In patients with previous fractures or T-score below −2.5 on DEXA, other secondary causes for osteoporosis (such as hypogonadism) should be searched for and treated. Measures for fall prevention should be taught, especially in patients with poor balance or gait deficits. Structured weight-bearing exercise has shown benefits in other solid organ transplants and may be beneficial in both pre-transplant and post-transplant periods. A planned physical rehabilitation program can be prescribed to prevent prolonged immobilization after surgery.

Pretransplantation

The disorders associated with CKD-MBD need to be investigated and treatment tailored accordingly. Several guidelines from KDIGO regarding fracture risk assessment and treatment in CKD-MBD are being revisited.[64] Post hoc analyses of agents approved for treating postmenopausal osteoporosis have been shown to be tolerated well and with few adverse events in patients with stage 3 or stage 4 CKD.[67] Significant further studies are required but these agents may be potentially efficacious with respect to fracture risk reduction. The presence of adynamic bone disease must be ruled out because bisphosphonates may significantly worsen it. In addition, no bisphosphonate is approved for treatment in ESKD.

Patients awaiting liver transplantation should all receive supplementation of calcium and vitamin D, the latter in substantial doses if 25(OH) vitamin D levels are less than

---

Box 1
Factors contributing to bone disease after transplantation

Pretransplant

General
- Age greater than 45
- Caucasian
- Hypogonadism
- Excessive alcohol use
- Smoking
- Vitamin D deficiency
- Immobility
- Body mass index below 23/malnutrition
- Neuropathy or balance deficits predisposing to falls
- Previous fractures or fragility fractures

Comorbid diseases
- For example, diabetes mellitus, SLE

Medications
- Prolonged corticosteroid use, loop diuretics, others (see text)

Kidney transplant patients
- CKD-MBD, duration of dialysis, high or low PTH levels (>700 pg/mL or <100 pg/mL, respectively), previous parathyroidectomy

Liver transplant patients
- Cholestatic liver diseases (eg primary sclerosing cholangitis)

Post-transplant
- Immunosuppression: GCs as main contributor but also CNIs
- Hyperparathyroidism
- Hypercalcemia
- Hypophosphatemia

---

50 nmol/L.[15,26] Supplementation is underutilized, with some studies indicating supplementation in as few as 7.5% of patients.[68] Although no consensus exists, the use of bisphosphonates pretransplant may be beneficial if indicated, provided the patient does not have low-turnover bone disease. Liver disease patients do not have adynamic bone disease, according to the definition, but low turnover where bisphosphonates may be ineffectual or renal insufficiency with eGFR less than 35 mL/min.

Post-transplantation

There is consensus regarding both kidney transplantation and liver transplantation that ongoing supplementation with calcium and vitamin D, where patients are insufficient, is indicated in the immediate post-transplant period, provided that it is carefully monitored. These agents may not prevent clinically significant bone loss but have been used concomitantly in most trials evaluating antiresorptive therapy and enhance bisphosphonate effects.[69] Hypercalcemia may limit the use of vitamin D and calcium in kidney transplant patients but if due to excess parathyroid hormone, vitamin D or analogs may aid through PTH suppression and improve bone loss. Hypophosphatemia in kidney recipients may need replenishment, but, considering the risks of hypocalcemia and nephrocalcinosis, it should only be given in patients with serum levels below mg/dL 1 to 1.5 mg/dL or those who are symptomatic.[70]

Steroid withdrawal and avoidance

The rationale for minimizing GC use relates to its established risks of severely accelerated bone loss in the initial post-transplant period as well as the established risks of osteoporosis and avascular necrosis observed in other populations requiring steroids. Some studies have linked withdrawal at various time points to improved BMD values, specifically a reduced fracture risk in patients discharged without steroids after transplantation,[71] although this is not confirmed in all studies.[72] The dose of GCs in the studies as well as the timing of withdrawal may explain the discrepancy. Observational data in an article by NinKovic and colleagues[73] support the benefits of reduction in both dose and duration of GCs: vertebral fractures decreased from 27% to 5% between 2 studies in liver patients where the use of cyclosporine and tacrolimus barely changed but fewer GCs were used in the second group.[73] Care needs to be taken in kidney transplantation because of a higher risk of rejection. Significant advances has been made with newer and more potent agents both for induction and maintenance immunosuppression therapy, creating the hope that omission of GCs may become a distinct possibility, but prospective trials are needed.

Hormone replacement therapy

Hypogonadism is common in solid organ transplant patients due to chronic illness and compounded by GC therapy. Low testosterone and dehydroepiandrosterone levels predict mortality in men, independent of other confounders.[74] Although replacement therapy is known to increase BMD in hypogonadal women and men with osteoporosis, published data for the transplant population is limited and studies have small numbers. Transdermal estradiol improved BMD similar to healthy postmenopausal women in a study on 33 female liver recipients.[75] It makes sense to use gonadal hormone therapy in the short term to slow bone loss, but growing concerns are expressed about potential side effects in a population already prone to ischemic heart disease and malignancy after transplantation. General opinion is to start with caution, 1 to 3 months after transplantation, so that the engrafted organ has fully settled and GC doses are weaned. Patients need to be screened carefully for contraindications and the associated risks should be well explained. In addition, patients should be retested after withdrawal or minimization of GCs to assess gonadal status because the hormonal levels may have returned to normal levels and replacement is not required.

Pharmaceutical intervention

Current treatment of bone disease in transplant patients is significantly hampered by the lack of randomized control studies evaluating the effect of treatment in terms of hard outcomes, such as fracture rates, hospitalizations, and mortality. Many studies involve small numbers or no randomization or control groups and often do not take into consideration the multiple comorbid factors contributing to bone disease or severity of bone disease equally in their groups. In addition, many studies are underpowered to provide the answers requested. Patients are often treated with different immunosuppressive agents or GCs in varying doses or with concomitant drugs that potentially affect bone health. In many studies, an increase in BMD has been accepted as substitute for reduction in facture risk. That said, 2 meta-analyses offer significant insight. A Cochrane review by Palmer and colleagues[76] of 24 trials in kidney transplantation showed that no single therapy prevented fractures in randomized control studies, but meta-analysis of all available such trials combined shows that any intervention (bisphosphonate, vitamin D sterol, or calcitonin) for bone disease does reduce the risk of fracture in this population.[76] Only 11 of the studies in this review reported on fracture incidence. Stein and colleagues'[77] meta-analysis, which included randomized trials in solid organ transplantation only if fracture data were reported, concluded that treatment with either bisphosphonates or vitamin D receptor analogs in the first year after transplantation was associated with a reduction in fractures.

Bisphosphonates are currently deemed the most effective treatment of post-transplant bone disease. The use of bisphosphonates is recommended in guidelines by KDIGO after kidney transplantation[78] and by the American Society for Transplantation in liver recipients.[79] The multitude of studies with bisphosphonates are well summarized elsewhere and are not repeated here.[15,23,26,58,80] In kidney transplantation, bisphosphonates should be used with caution in patients with reduced kidney function and avoided where the eGFR is less than 30 mL/min. Bisphosphonates accumulate and have a prolonged duration of action, which can induce or worsen adynamic bone disease. Given the rapidity of bone loss in the first months, it is advisable to start therapy early after transplant in appropriate candidates with preexisting fractures or low BMD. If adynamic bone disease is suspected, a bone biopsy is imperative to rule it out, because bisphosphonates perpetuate adynamic bone disease and potentially increase fracture risk in this group. Some investigators argue that it may be prudent to offer bisphosphonates for all except patients with potential adynamic bone disease because fractures occur in patients with an initially normal BMD as well—more so in liver transplantation where fracture rates are excessively high and active pretransplant therapy may be beneficial. Other investigators are significantly more cautious and wish to reserve bisphosphonate use for patients with a particularly high fracture risk.[81] An individualized approach to treatment is indicated[34] and possible: Mainra and Elder[82] argue for the use of bisphosphonates in patients who have BMD levels in the osteoporotic or osteopenic range or those with multiple fracture risk factors, while treating those with near-normal BMD and potential low bone turnover with calcitriol. Data are lacking for both kidney and liver transplants to support the use of one bisphosphonate over another, and choice may be left to individual doctor and patient preference, depending on local availability, compliance, and ease of administration. Intravenous ibandronate has an excellent renal safety profile[83] and adherence to therapy has been shown better in patients with primary biliary cirrhosis and osteoporosis, likely due to dosing with extended (3-month) intervals.[84] Further studies are needed to determine the appropriate duration of therapy but current consensus is that 12 to 18 months may be sufficient considering the initial impact of GCs.

The vitamin D receptor analogs, calcidiol and calcitriol, are beneficial in prevention of bone loss and the latter in reduction of fracture risk,[77,85] but the evidence for this is less strong than the benefits for using bisphosphonates. Care needs to be taken in regular monitoring for hypercalcemia as well as regarding the risk of oversuppression of the parathyroid gland. As described previously, it is the safest treatment option in kidney recipients with adynamic bone disease confirmed by biopsy or suggested by bone markers.[58,82]

Cinacalcet, a calcimimetic, is effective in the treatment of persistent post-transplant hyperparathyroidism and hypercalcemia in kidney recipients. It has been shown to improve BMD in small studies[86] but the effect on fracture risk has not been established.

Teriparatide is a recombinant PTH that has been shown to increase BMD and lower vertebral fractures in GC-induced osteoporosis through its anabolic effects.[87] Its benefit in kidney recipients remains to be confirmed. A small prospective study involving 62 patients did not show benefit,[88] and further studies are needed.

Denosumab is a fully humanized monoclonal antibody to RANKL that decreases the function and survival of osteoclasts. It increases BMD and decreases fractures in postmenopausal women and is Food and Drug Administration approved for the treatment of postmenopausal osteoporosis. It does not depend on kidney clearance for metabolism or excretion, and secondary data analysis among postmenopausal women with varying degrees of renal impairment has shown that it is effective at reducing fracture risk without an increase in adverse events.[89] No clinical trials have been performed, however, to validate benefit after transplantation, and case reports regarding profound hypocalcemia as well as dramatic unexplained increase in PTH need clarification.

OSTEONECROSIS/AVASCULAR NECROSIS

Osteonecrosis, in essence the death of all cellular elements of bone, is the most debilitating of bone diseases after transplantation. The femoral head is most commonly affected but also other joints such as the proximal humerus, knee, and ankle. The incidence varies between 3% and 41% in kidney recipients, with significant decrease to 4% seen since the standard use of CNIs.[90] The Mayo Clinic reported an incidence of 9% between 1985 and 2001 in their liver recipients.[50] GC use (described previously) is the major contributor to its development. Ischemia may occur as early as 2 weeks after transplant, but patients may present with symptoms only later. A majority of cases are diagnosed within the first 2 years after transplantation. Both intravenous methylprednisolone pulse therapy for the treatment of acute rejection and cumulative doses of greater than 2 g for greater than 3 months significantly increase the risk. A new classification of osteonecrosis has been developed by the Association Research Circulation Osseous and summarized along with recommendations for stage-related therapy by Drescher and colleagues.[90] Early detection remains crucial, and MRI is the best imaging modality commonly available for early detection because radiographs may appear normal in the initial stage.[91] Although bisphosphonates have been used in the treatment of osteonecrosis, there are insufficient data to justify their use for this indication[92] and they are not currently recommended.[90]

SUMMARY

In summary, understanding of post-transplant bone disease has grown significantly alongside the advances in transplantation over the past 3 decades. Advances in immunosuppression may well mean that a significant decrease in fracture rates may be seen with use of fewer GCs, whereas advances in imaging and the investigation of bone quality and strength may assist in further individualization of treatment. Newer anabolic therapy with antisclerostin antibodies, PTHrP, PTH patches, or weekly administration also seem promising and would be welcome additions to the bone treatment arsenal.

REFERENCES

1. Alem AM, Sherrard DJ, Gillen DL, et al. Increased risk of hip fracture among patients with end-stage renal disease. Kidney Int 2000;58:396–9.
2. Julian BA, Laskow DA, Dubovsky J, et al. Rapid loss of vertebral mineral density after renal transplantation. N Engl J Med 1991;325(8):544–50.
3. Mikuls TR, Julian BA, Bartolucci A, et al. Bone mineral density changes within six months of renal transplantation. Transplantation 2003;75(1):49–54.
4. Almond MK, Kwan JT, Evans K, et al. Loss of regional bone mineral density in the first 12 months following renal transplantation. Nephron 1994;66(1):52–7.

5. Ball AM, Gillen DL, Sherrard D, et al. Risk of hip fractures among dialysis and renal transplant recipients. JAMA 2002;288(23):3014–8.

6. Casez JP, Lippuner K, Horber FF, et al. Changes in bone mineral density over 18 months following kidney transplantation: the respective roles of prednisone and parathyroid hormone. Nephrol Dial Transplant 2002;17(7):1318–26.

7. Nikkel LE, Hollenbeak CS, Fox EJ, et al. Risk of fractures after renal transplantation in the United States. Transplantation 2009;87(12):1846–51.

8. Vautour LM, Melton LJ 3rd, Clarke BL, et al. Long-term fracture risk following renal transplantation: a population-based study. Osteoporos Int 2004;15(2):160–7.

9. Eastell R, Dickson ER, Hodgson SF, et al. Rates of vertebral bone loss before and after liver transplantation in women with primary biliary cirrhosis. Hepatology 1991;14(2):296–300.

10. Krol CG, Dekkers OM, Kroon HM, et al. Longitudinal changes in BMD and fracture risk in orthotopic liver transplant recipients not using bone-modifying treatment. J Bone Miner Res 2014;29(8):1763–9.

11. Guichelaar MM, Kendall R, Malinchoc M, et al. Bone mineral density before and after OLT: long-term follow-up and predictive factors. Liver Transpl 2006;12:1390.

12. Monegal A, Navasa M, Guañabens N, et al. Bone disease after liver transplantation: a long-term prospective study of bone mass changes, hormonal status and histomorphometric characteristics. Osteoporos Int 2001;12:484.

13. Leidig-Bruckner G, Hosch S, Dodidou P, et al. Frequency and predictors of osteoporotic fractures after cardiac or liver transplantation: a follow-up study. Lancet 2001;357:342.

14. Black DM, Steinbuch M, Palermo L, et al. An assessment tool for predicting fracture risk in postmenopausal women. Osteoporos Int 2001;12(7):519–28.

15. Maalouf NM, Shane E. Osteoporosis after solid organ transplantation. J Clin Endocrinol Metab 2005;90(4):2456–65.

16. Emkey GR, Epstein S. Secondary osteoporosis: pathophysiology & diagnosis. Best Pract Res Clin Endocrinol Metab 2014;28:911–35.

17. Rakel A, Sheehy O, Rahme E, et al. Does diabetes increase the risk for fractures after solid organ transplantation? A nested case-control study. J Bone Miner Res 2007;22:1878.

18. Fowlkes JL, Bunn RC, Thrailkill KM. Contributions of the insulin/insulin-like growth factor-1 axis to diabetic osteopathy. J Diabetes Metab 2011;1. S1–003.

19. Burghardt AJ, Issever AS, Schwartz AV, et al. High resolution peripheral quantitative computed tomographic imaging of cortical and trabecular bone microarchitecture in patients with type-2 diabetes mellitus. J Clin Endocrinol Metab 2010;95:5045–55.

20. Rosen CJ, Bouxsein ML. Mechanisms of disease: is osteoporosis the obesity of bone? Nat Clin Pract Rheumatol 2006;2:35–43.

21. Tang XL, Griffith JF, Qin L, et al. SLE disease contributes to deterioration in bone mineral density, microstructure, and bone strength. Lupus 2013;22:1162–8.

22. Bislev LS, Sikjaer T, Rolighed L, et al. Relationship between aldosterone and parathyroid hormone, and the effect of angiotensin and aldosterone inhibition on bone health. Clin Rev Bone Miner Metab 2015;13:194–205.

23. Weisinger JR, Carlini RG, Rojas E, et al. Bone disease after transplantation. Clin J Am Soc Nephrol 2006;1:1300–13.

24. Malluche HH, Mawad H, Monier-Faugere MC. The importance of bone health in end-stage renal disease: out of the frying pan, into the fire? Nephrol Dial Transplant 2004;19(Suppl 1):i9–13.

25. Hruska KA, Teitelbaum SL. Renal osteodystrophy. N Engl J Med 1995;333(3): 166–74.
26. Hawkins FG, Guadalix S, Sanchez R, et al. Post-transplant bone disease. In: Dionyssiotis Y, editor. Osteoporosis. InTech; 2012. ISBN: 978-953-51-0026-3. Available at: http://www.intechopen.com/books/osteoporosis/post-transplantation-bone-disease.
27. Compston JE. Osteoporosis after liver transplantation. Liver Transpl 2003;9(4): 321–30.
28. Janes CH, Rolland Dickson E, Okazaki R, et al. Role of hyperbilirubinemia in the impairment of osteoblast proliferation associated with cholestatic jaundice. J Clin Invest 1995;95:2581–6.
29. Baccaro LF, Boin IF, Pedro AO, et al. Decrease in bone mass in women after liver transplantation: associated factors. Transplant Proc 2011;43(4):1351–6.
30. Heaf J, Tvedegaard E, Kanstrup IL, et al. Hyperparathyroidism and long-term bone loss after renal transplantation. Clin Transplant 2003;17:268.
31. Evenepoel P, Claes K, Kuypers D, et al. Natural history of parathyroid function and calcium metabolism after kidney transplantation: a single-centre study. Nephrol Dial Transplant 2004;19(5):1281–7.
32. Taniguchi M, Tokumodu M, Matsua D, et al. Persistent hyperparathyroidism in renal allograft recipients: Vitamin D receptor, calcium-sensing receptor, and apoptosis. Kidney Int 2006;70:363–70.
33. Pihlstrom H, Dahle DO, Mjoen G, et al. Increased risk of all-cause mortality and renal graft loss in stable renal transplant patients with hyperparathyroidism. Transplantation 2015;99(2):351–9.
34. Kalantar-Zadeh K, Molnar MZ, Kovesdy CP, et al. Management of mineral and bone disorders after kidney transplantation. Curr Opin Nephrol Hypertens 2012;21(4):389–403.
35. Chiu MY, Sprague SM, Bruce DS, et al. Analysis of fracture prevalence in kidney-pancreas allograft recipients. J Am Soc Nephrol 1998;9(4):677–83.
36. Nikkel LE, Iyer SP, Mohan S, et al. Pancreas-kidney transplantation is associated with reduced fracture risk compared with kidney-alone transplantation in men with type-1 diabetes. Kidney Int 2013;83:471–8.
37. Scialla JJ. Choices in kidney transplantation in type 1 diabetes: are there skeletal benefits of the endocrine pancreas? Kidney Int 2013;83:356–8.
38. LoCascio V, Bonucci E, Imbimbo B, et al. Bone loss in response to long-term glucocorticoid therapy. Bone Miner 1990;8:39–51.
39. Kulak CAM, Shane E. Transplantation osteoporosis: biochemical correlates of pathogenesis and treatment. In: Seibel MJ, Robbins SP, Bilezikian JP, editors. Dynamics of bone and cartilage metabolism. 2nd edition. San Diego (CA): Academic Press; 2006. p. 515–26.
40. Goffin E, Devogelaer JP, Depresseux G, et al. Osteoporosis after transplantation. Lancet 2001;357(9268):1623.
41. Martinez Diaz-Guerra G, Gomez R, Jodar E, et al. Long-term follow up of bone mass after orthotopic liver transplantation: effect of steroid withdrawal from the immunosuppressive regimen. Osteoporos Int 2002;13(2):147–50.
42. Gifre L, Ruis-Gaspa S, Monegal A, et al. Effect of glucocorticoid treatment on Wnt signalling antagoniss (sclerostin and Dkk-1) and their relationship with bone turn-over. Bone 2013;57:272–6.
43. Weinstein RS, Wan C, Liu Q, et al. Endogenous glucocorticoids decrease skeletal angiogenesis, vascularity, hydration and strength in aged mice. Aging Cell 2010; 9:147–61.

44. Khwaja K, Asolati M, Harmon J, et al. Outcome at 3 years with prednisone-free maintenance regimen: a single centre experience with 349 kidney transplant recipients. Am J Transplant 2002;4:980–7.

45. Movsowitz C, Epstein S, Ismail F, et al. Cyclosporin A in the oophorectomized rat: unexpected severe bone resorption. J Bone Miner Res 2004;22:554–60.

46. Epstein S, Inzerillo AM, Caminis J, et al. Disorders associated with acute rapid and severe bone loss. J Bone Miner Res 2003;18:2083–94.

47. Ponticelli C, Aroldi A. Osteoporosis after transplantation. Lancet 2001;357:1623.

48. Cueto-Manzano A, Konel S, Hutchison AJ, et al. Bone loss in long-term renal transplantation: histopathology and densitometry analysis. Kidney Int 1999;55: 2021–9.

49. Bozkaya G, Nart A, Uslu T, et al. Impact of calcineurin inhibitors on bone metabolism in primary kindey transplant patients. Transplant Proc 2008;40:151–5.

50. Guichelaar MM, Schmoll J, Malinchoc M, et al. Fractures and avascular necrosis before and after orthotopic liver transplantation: long-term follow-up and predictive factors. Hepatology 2007;46(4):1198–207.

51. Monegal A, Navasa M, Guanabens N, et al. Bone mass and mineral metabolism in liver transplant patietns treated with FK506 or cyclosporine A. Calcif Tissue Int 2001;68(2):83–6.

52. Epstein S. Post-transplantation bone disease: the role of immunosuppressive agents and the skeleton. J Bone Miner Res 1996;11(1):1–7.

53. Alvares-Garcia O, Garcia-Lopes E, Lored V. rapamycin induces growth retardation by disrupting angiogenesis in the growth plate. Kidney Int 2010;78:561–8.

54. Campistol JM, Holt DW, Epstein S. Bone metabolism in renal transplant patients treated with cyclosporine or sirolimus. Transpl Int 2005;18(9):1028–35.

55. Blaslov K, Katalinic L, Kes P, et al. What is the impact of immunosuppressive treatment on the post-transplant renal osteodystrophy? Int Urol Nephrol 2014; 46:1019–24.

56. Huyghe E, Zairi A, Nohra J, et al. Gonadal impact of target of rapamycin inhibitors (sirolimus and everolimus) in male patients: an overview. Transpl Int 2007;20(4): 305–11.

57. Lane JT, Dagogo-Jack S. Approach to the patient with new-onset diabetes after transplant (NODAT). J Clin Endocrinol Metab 2011;96(11):3289–97.

58. Alshayeb HM, Sprague SM, Josephson MA. Management of Transplantational renal bone disease: interplay of bone mineral density and decisions regarding bisphosphonate use. In: Weir MR, Lerma EV, editors. Kidney transplantation: practical guide to management. Springer Science +Business Media; 2014.

59. Perrin P, Caillard S, Javier RM, et al. Persistent hyperparathyroidism is a major risk factor for fractures in the five years after kidney transplantation. Am J Transplant 2013;13:2653–63.

60. Messa P, Regalia A, Alfieri CM, et al. Current indications to parathyroidectomy in CKD patients before and after renal transplantation. J Nephrol 2013;26(6): 1025–32.

61. Krol C, Meiland D, Dekkers O, et al. Pitfalls in the interpretation of bone turnover markers in liver transplantation. Poster Presented at the 17th European Congress of Endocrinology. Dublin, May 16–20, 2015. Available from: Endocrine Abstracts (2015). p. 37.EP226.

62. Imori S, Mori Y, Akita W, et al. Diagnostic usefulness of bone mineral density and biochemical markers of bone turnover in predicting fracture in CKD stage 5D patients – a single-center cohort study. Nephrol Dial Transplant 2012;27:345–51.

63. Akaberi S, Simonsen O, Lindergard B, et al. Can DXA predict fractures in renal transplant patients? Am J Transplant 2008;8:2647–51.
64. Ketteler M, Elder GJ, Evenepoel P, et al. Revisiting KDIGO clinical practice guideline on chronic kidney disease-mineral and bone disorder: a commentary from a kidney disease: improving global outcomes controversies conference. Kidney Int 2015;87(3):502–28.
65. Babyev R, Nickolas TL. Can one evaluate bone disease in chronic kidney disease without a biopsy? Curr Opin Nephrol Hypertens 2014;23(4):431–7.
66. Mellibovsky L, Prieto-Alhambra D, Mellibovsky F, et al. Bone tissue properties measurement by reference point indentation in glucocorticoid-induced osteoporosis. J Bone Miner Res 2015;30(9):1651–6.
67. Goldenstein P, Jamal S, Moyses RMA. Fractures in chronic kidney disease: pursuing the best screening and management. Curr Opin Nephrol Hypertens 2015; 24(4):317–23.
68. Monegal A, navasa M, Pilar P, et al. Bone disease in patients awaiting liver transplantation. Has the situation improved in the last two decades? Calcif Tissue Int 2013;93:571–6.
69. Adamai S, Gianini G, Bianchi L, et al. Vitamin D status and response to treatment in post-menopausal osteoporosis. Osteoporos Int 2009;20:239–44.
70. Evenepoel P, Lerut E, Naesens M, et al. Localisation, etiology and impact of calcium phosphate deposits in renal allografts. Am J Transplant 2009;9(11):2470–8.
71. Nikkel LE, Mohan S, Zhang A, et al. Reduced fracture risk with early corticosteroid withdrawal after kidney transplant. Am J Transplant 2012;12:649–59.
72. Edwards BJ, Desai A, Tsai J, et al. Elevated incidence of fractures in solid-organ transplant recipients on glucocorticoid-sparing immunosuppressive regimens. J Osteoporos 2011;2011:591793. Article ID 591793.
73. NinKovic M, Love S, Tom BD, et al. lack of effect of intravenous pamidronate on fracture incidence and bone mineral density after orthotopic liver transplantation. J Hepatol 2002;37(1):93–100.
74. Grossmann M, Hoerman R, Ng Tang Fui M, et al. Sex steroid levels in chronic kidney disease and kidney transplant recipients: associations with disease severity and predictions of mortality. Clin Endocrinol 2015;82:767–75.
75. Isoniemi H, Appelberg J, Nilsson CG, et al. Transdermal oestrogen therapy protects postmenopausal liver transplant women from osteoporosis. A 2-year follow-up study. J Hepatol 2001;34:299–305.
76. Palmer SC, McGregor DO, Strippoli GF. Interventions for preventing bone disease in kidney transplant recipients. Cochrane Database Syst Rev 2007;(3):CD005015.
77. Stein EM, Ortiz D, Jin Z, et al. Prevention of fractures after solid organ transplantation: a meta-analysis. J Clin Endocrinol Metab 2011;96(11):3457–65.
78. Kidney Disease: Improving Global Outcomes (KDIGO) CKD-MBD Work Group. KDIGO clinical practice guideline for the diagnosis, evaluation, prevention and treatment of CKD-MBD. Kidney Int 2009;76:S1–130.
79. Lucey MR, Terrault N, Oju L, et al. Long-term management of the successful adult liver transplant: 2012 practice guidelines by the American association for the study of liver diseases and the American transplant society. Liver Transpl 2013; 19:3–26.
80. Molnar M, Naser MS, Rhee CM, et al. Boen and mineral disorders after kidney transplantation: therapeutic strategies. Transplant Rev 2014;28:56–62.
81. Brandenburg VM, Floege J. Transplantation: an end to bone disease after renal transplantation? Nat Rev Nephrol 2013;9:5–6.

82. Mainra R, Elder GJ. Individualized therapy to prevent bone mineral density loss after kidney and kidney-pancreas transplantation. Clin J Am Soc Nephrol 2010; 5:117–24.

83. Smerud KT, Dolgos S, Olsen IC, et al. a 1-year randomized, double-blind, placebo-controlled study of intravenous ibandronate on bone loss following renal transplantation. Am J Transplant 2012;12:3316–25.

84. Guanabens N, Monegal A, Cerda D, et al. Randomized trial comparing gmonthly ibandronate and weekly alendronate for osteoporosis in patients with primary biliary cirrhosis. Hepatology 2013;58(6):2070–8.

85. Josephson MA, Schumm LP, Chiu MY, et al. Calcium and calcitriol prophylaxis attenuates posttransplant bone disease. Transplantation 2004;78:1233–6.

86. Bergua C, Torregrosa JV, Fuster D, et al. Effect of cinacalcet on hypercalcemia and bone mineral density in renal transplanted patients with secondary hyperparathyroidism. Transplantation 2008;86:413–7.

87. Saag KG, Shane E, Boonen S, et al. Teriparatide or alendronate in glucocorticoid-induced osteoporosis. N Engl J Med 2007;357(20):2028–39.

88. Cejka D, benesh T, Krestan C, et al. Effect of teriparatide on early bone loss after kidney transplantation. Am J Transplant 2008;8(9):1864–70.

89. Jamal S, Ljunggren O, Stehman-Breen C, et al. Efects of denosumab on fracture and bone mineral density by level of kidney function. J Bone Miner Res 2001; 26(8):1829–35.

90. Drescher W, Schlieper G, Floege J, et al. Steroid-related osteonecrosis- an update. Nephrol Dial Transplant 2011;26:2728–31.

91. Hiralal AK, Udiya AT, Jha MK, et al. Avascular necrosis of the hip (AVN) in post renal transplant recipient: case report & review of literature. Indian J Transplant 2014;8(1):32–5.

92. Cardozo JB, Andrade DM, Santiago MB. The use of bisphosphontates in the treatment of avascular necrosis: a systematic review. Clin Rheumatol 2008;27: 685–8.

Infectious Complications and Vaccinations in the Posttransplant Population

 CrossMark

William G. Greendyke, MD, Marcus R. Pereira, MD, MPH*

KEYWORDS

- Kidney transplant • Liver transplant • Vaccination • Infections • Prophylaxis
- Complications

KEY POINTS

- Because of immunosuppression, solid organ transplant recipients are vulnerable to a wider variety of common and opportunistic infections and may not demonstrate classic signs and symptoms of infection, so a heightened knowledge and awareness of these risks are required for accurate diagnosis and proper care.
- The first month after transplant is characterized by hospital-acquired and postsurgical infections as well as donor-derived infections.
- From 1 to 6 months, liver and kidney transplant recipients are susceptible to a variety of opportunistic infections, including cytomegalovirus, herpes simplex virus, varicella zoster virus, *Aspergillus*, and tuberculosis.
- After 6 months, transplant recipients are usually infected with more common infections, such as *Pneumococcus*, *Legionella*, and respiratory viruses, although the risk of opportunistic infections is never eliminated.
- Although most vaccines are safe to give transplant recipients and their close contacts, live-attenuated vaccines are contraindicated for the recipients and may require some caution in close household contacts.

INTRODUCTION

For many patients with end-stage liver or kidney disease, solid organ transplant is the therapy of choice because it improves quality of life and overall survival. The Organ Procurement and Transplantation Network reports that in 2014 there were more than 17,000 kidney and more than 6700 liver transplantations in the United States. Because of a combination of improved surgical techniques, more multidisciplinary

Disclosure Statement: The authors have nothing to disclose.
Division of Infectious Diseases, Columbia University College of Physicians and Surgeons, 622 West 168th Street, Box 82, New York, NY 10032, USA
* Corresponding author.
E-mail address: Mp2323@cumc.columbia.edu

http://dx.doi.org/10.1016/j.mcna.2016.01.008
0025-7125/16/$ – see front matter © 2016 Elsevier Inc. All rights reserved.
medical.theclinics.com

care, and more effective immunosuppressant agents, survival rates for solid organ transplant recipients have increased over the last decades. The 5-year survival rate with a functioning allograft for kidney transplant recipients is now approximately 75%, and for liver transplant recipients is around 70%. With better access and this improvement in long-term patient survival, the number of transplant recipients has also increased several-fold. In 2012, it was reported that there were nearly 57,000 and more than 180,000 adults in the United States living with a transplanted liver or kidney, respectively.[1]

In this growing population of immunocompromised patients, infections with both common and opportunistic pathogens remain a major cause of morbidity and mortality. Although transplant specialists in tertiary centers manage most of these infections, an increasing number are cared for, diagnosed, and treated by non-transplant-specialized physicians. Therefore, it is increasingly important for the internist to be familiar with the differential diagnosis and management of infections in individuals that have received a solid organ transplant and are maintained on immunosuppressive medications.

GENERAL PRINCIPLES OF INFECTIONS AFTER LIVER OR KIDNEY TRANSPLANTATION

Although it is well recognized that liver and kidney transplant recipients are at an increased risk of infection, there are several important elements that are unique to these patients when compared with the general population.[2]

It Is More Difficult to Recognize an Infection in Transplant Recipients

Many of the classic clinical markers of infection are related to the body's immune responses to infection rather than the infection itself. When patients are being treated with immunosuppressive agents, the classic inflammatory signs and symptoms associated with infection are muted, so, for example, fever or leukocytosis is not always present; a wound infection is not necessarily erythematous or warm, lesions may not be discolored, and patients may not be febrile. Altered anatomy and organ denervation affect the presentation of infection, such that the location and intensity of pain are not always reliable markers. Because infections in these patients can go unrecognized for longer periods of time, a diagnosis is often only made at an advanced stage, thus increasing risk of morbidity and mortality. Therefore, a high index of suspicion for infection should always be maintained in these patients, especially during periods of increased immunosuppression.

There Are a Wide Variety of Infections That a Transplant Recipient Is at Risk for, Both Common and Uncommon

These infections include common pathogens, such as *Klebsiella pneumoniae*, *Streptococcus pneumoniae*, and community-acquired respiratory viruses, as well as opportunistic infection caused by cytomegalovirus (CMV), *Pneumocystis jiroveci* pneumonia (PJP), *Nocardia*, and *Aspergillus*. Among common bacterial pathogens, multidrug resistance (MDR) is of increasing concern.[3] Generating a broad and appropriate differential is essential for a prompt diagnosis and good outcomes.

There Are Important Limitations in Diagnostic Tools Among Transplant Recipients

Although helpful in determining past infections and exposures, serologic testing is generally not useful in the diagnosis of acute disease after transplant. Bacterial and fungal cultures often have lower yields when compared with the general population. Radiographs are often insufficient for diagnosing infections such as PJP or aspergillosis. Instead, the diagnostic workup is often reliant on molecular methods such as polymerase chain reaction (PCR) or direct antigen testing. In addition, use of computed tomography or MRI is often necessary to evaluate subtle findings. Often, when the above methods are not illustrative, a biopsy is necessary to establish the diagnosis.

The Treatment of Many Infections After Liver and Kidney Transplant May Be Toxic and Complex and May Require Invasive Procedures

Treatment of CMV infection requires antiviral agents that either cause pronounced bone marrow suppression (ganciclovir) or significant nephrotoxicity (foscarnet, cidofovir). MDR gram-negative infections such as carbapenem-resistant *Enterobacteriaceae* (CRE) are currently treated with polymyxin or aminoglycosides, which can also be nephrotoxic. Drug-drug interactions between common antimicrobials (such as azole antifungals) and calcineurin inhibitors must be considered. It is imperative that the transplant team is aware of decisions to initiate or discontinue these medications so that proper adjustments can be made to the immunosuppressive regimen. Intra-abdominal abscesses require prompt drainage, whether surgical or via interventional radiology, for diagnosis and source control. Anatomic problems that can lead to infections, such as anastomotic breakdown or obstruction in the biliary tree or ureters, require prompt surgical correction.

For all of these reasons, disease prevention is critical and includes both prophylactic medications and vaccination against the most common pathogens.

RISK FACTORS FOR INFECTIONS AFTER KIDNEY AND LIVER TRANSPLANT

There are many factors that impact the risk of infection in kidney and liver transplant recipients. Although some of these factors are present in the donor or recipient before transplant, others are derived from events occurring either during or after transplant (**Box 1**). A careful assessment of these factors is essential.

Latent and Active Infections in the Recipient

Like most adults, liver and kidney transplant recipients carry many latent infections that can reactivate in the setting of immunosuppression. These latent infections commonly include herpesviruses, such as CMV, herpes simplex virus (HSV), Epstein-Barr virus (EBV), and varicella zoster virus (VZV), as well as hepatitis B (HBV) and C (HCV). All are important pathogens that can predictably cause major morbidity and mortality in the posttransplant period. Serologic testing for these pathogens is routinely done during pretransplant evaluation, and preventative protocols are in place in most transplant centers.[4] Many centers are now transplanting patients

---

Box 1
Risk factors for infection posttransplant

Latent and active infections in the organ recipient

Recipient comorbidities (eg, diabetes, chronic obstructive pulmonary disease)

Active and latent infections in the organ donor

Operative factors and complications

Health care exposures before and after transplant

Immunosuppressive therapy

with well-controlled human immunodeficiency virus infection (ie, a sustained CD4 count >200 cells/mm^3 along with an undetectable viral load). However, these patients require careful pretransplant assessment of their immune status and the potential for prior opportunistic infection (eg, *Cryptococcus* and *Mycobacterium avium intracellulare*) to recur posttransplant.[5,6] In an era of increasingly mobile populations, an expanded assessment is conducted for geographically important organisms, such as tuberculosis, *Trypanosoma cruzi*, *Brucella*, and *Strongyloides*.[7]

In addition to latent infections, recipients can also harbor active infections that are unrecognized and therefore untreated at the time of transplant. In the particular case of liver transplant recipients, for example, these infections can be in the biliary tree or the peritoneum and cause major postoperative mortality.

Latent and Active Infections in the Donor

Donor-derived infections play a major role in posttransplant infections. Careful assessment of potential organ donors is imperative. Like recipients, donors are routinely screened for common latent infections outlined above. Consideration for these pathogens will be made in devising the posttransplant prophylaxis regimen. In addition, geographically important pathogens, such as tuberculosis (in the case of living donors), *T cruzi*, *Brucella*, and *Strongyloides*, are also evaluated.[7] Deceased organ donors are also carefully evaluated when the clinical presentation is suggestive of an infection. Some infections such as West Nile virus are contraindications to proceeding with donation, others, such as *S pneumoniae* bacteremia or meningitis, can be safely managed in the recipient.[8]

Operative Complications and Organ Quality

Intraoperative events, such as prolonged warm and cold ischemia time, excessive bleeding, or organ injury, greatly impact the risk of infection posttransplant. Even if successful, the procedure itself can impact the risk of infection. Among liver transplant recipients, for example, the choice of biliary anastomosis impacts the rate of postoperative biliary complications.[9] The complex anatomic issues around liver transplants from living donors increase risk for biliary leaks and subsequent infections.[10] The quality of the organ is also an important determinant of the risk of posttransplant complications. For example, deceased donor kidney allografts are generally more prone to postoperative dysfunction, leading to higher rates of urinary tract infection (UTI), and use of extended criteria donor liver allografts is associated with an increased risk of infection.[9]

Immunosuppressive Therapies

Both induction and maintenance immunosuppression critically impact the risk of posttransplant infections. Agents that cause lympholysis such as antithymocyte globulin or alemtuzumab can be used for either induction or treatment of rejection, have a profound effect on the immune system, and result in prolonged (>1 year) immunosuppression.[11] At any time after transplant, treatment of rejection resets this increased risk of infection and restarts the transplant clock, prompting reinitiation of prophylaxis and monitoring.[8]

TIMELINE OF INFECTIONS AFTER LIVER AND KIDNEY TRANSPLANT

Although infections after transplant are affected by the risk factors discussed above, they largely follow somewhat predictable patterns in relation to time after transplant as it correlates with hospital discharge, healing, decreased immunosuppression, decreased numbers of procedures, and increased community exposures. In addition, reactivation of latent infections usually occurs in the first 180 days after transplant.[2] Therefore, this timeline helps not only with generating a differential diagnosis after transplant but also with developing measures for the prevention and mitigation of infections after transplant (**Table 1**).

Within the first month of transplant, the patient is at highest risk of infectious complications related to surgical anatomy, other nosocomial infections, and donor-derived infections from the allograft. Once the immediate postoperative window has passed, the most common infections that occur within the first 1 to 6 months are due to opportunistic pathogens. After 6 months, the transplant recipient is at highest risk for community-acquired pathogens.[2]

INFECTIONS IN THE FIRST MONTH POSTTRANSPLANT

Most infections in the first month following liver and kidney transplant are hospital acquired and are usually due to complications from the surgical procedure or from untreated/unrecognized infections in the donor or the recipient.[12] Bacterial and fungal pathogens are most common and acquisition of MDR bacteria is a major concern.

Among liver transplant recipients, postoperative infections are usually a function of the complex hepatobiliary anatomy and can be initially difficult to detect. Superficial wound infections can often indicate a more serious, deeper process and should prompt further investigation. Deep surgical site infections include peritonitis and intra-abdominal abscesses. Biliary leaks, usually at the anastomosis, can often lead to infected bilomas. The use of a Roux-en-Y anastomosis (rather than duct-to-duct) is associated with increased rates of biliary obstruction and subsequent infections.[9] These infections are often polymicrobial with enteric pathogens, such as *Enterococcus*, *Enterobacteriaceae*, or *Candida* spp. Most are endogenous to the recipient. The increase of MDR gram-negative infections in this setting is an area of major concern because it leads to poor outcomes.[13] Sepsis frequently occurs in this setting; 12% of liver recipients in one cohort developed bloodstream infection (BSI) within 30 days of transplant.[14] Treatment is usually complex and requires a combination of prolonged antimicrobial therapy and drainage (often by interventional radiology or

Table 1 Timeline of infections from date of transplantation		
Transplant to 1 mo Posttransplant	**1–6 mo Posttransplant**	**6+ mo Posttransplant**
Donor-derived infection	Chronic infections from	Community-acquired
Surgical site infection	time of transplant	pathogens
Intra-abdominal infection	Reactivation of latent/	*S pneumoniae*
Central line–associated BSI	transmitted infections:	Legionella
UTI	CMV	Listeria
Hospital-acquired	Herpes viruses: HSV, VZV,	Aspergillus
pneumonia	HHV6	EBV/PTLD
C difficile	HBV and HCV	
	Tuberculosis	
	Strongyloides	
	T cruzi	
	Syphilis	
	Opportunistic infections:	
	PJP	
	Cryptococcus	

endoscopy). Surgical repair of the disrupted anatomy is frequently required.[9] A key point is that achievement of source control is essential for successful resolution of these deep infections.

Compared with liver transplant recipients, kidney transplant patients have higher rates of UTI in the postoperative period. Kidney transplants are heterotopic and are most commonly placed in the pelvis with a short ureter, no nerves, and no ureteral valve. Uncomplicated cystitis is most routinely seen; however, pyelonephritis is also quite common. Symptoms of UTI can be minimal; urinalysis findings may be nonspecific and are not considered sensitive, and it is often difficult to distinguish colonization or contamination from true infection. Treatment according to culture and susceptibilities is sufficient for resolution, but recurrence rates are high. It is also common for patients to develop *Candida* colonization of the urinary tract while on broad spectrum antibiotics for other infections.[15] In general, it is not necessary to treat candiduria unless the patient is symptomatic. Ureteral obstructions can lead to the formation of strictures, or leakage of urine can lead to the formation of urinomas. These complications provide opportunities for secondary infection.[16]

When operative complications occur, intensive care unit and overall length of stays are prolonged and frequently lead to hospital-acquired infections such as ventilator-associated pneumonias, central line–associated BSI, or catheter-associated UTIs. Because of extensive antibiotic exposures, the prevalence of *Clostridium difficile* infection among liver and kidney recipients is 9% and 4%, respectively.[17]

Finally, donor-derived infections are a major concern in this period as well. Many active bacterial infections in the donor can be safely managed, allowing for the transplant to proceed. An exception to this situation may be MDR organisms, which are associated with increased morbidity and mortality.[18] Viral infections, however, particularly those with no established treatment, lead to major morbidity and mortality and are contraindications for donation. When transmission occurs via the allograft, signs and symptoms in the recipient can be difficult to recognize, often leading to a delayed diagnosis.[19]

INFECTIONS BETWEEN 1 AND 6 MONTHS POSTTRANSPLANT

Although postoperative and hospital-acquired problems may persist after the first month, opportunistic infections pose the greatest challenge to the transplant recipient during this period.[8] Immunosuppression is greatest at this time, triggering the reactivation of latent pathogens. These problems, however, can often be prevented with antimicrobial prophylaxis.

In the absence of antiviral prophylaxis, CMV is a major pathogen in this period. Like all herpes viruses, it establishes latency after primary infection and reactivates in the setting of immunosuppression.[20] The risk of CMV reactivation is highest in seronegative recipients who receive a seropositive organ.[21,22] CMV disease can manifest in a myriad of signs and symptoms ranging from asymptomatic viremia, to a nonspecific viral syndrome to tissue invasive disease, such as hepatitis, pneumonitis, or colitis. Given this diverse array, CMV should be considered in most individuals when infection is suspected, in particular in recipients at high risk. CMV is detected and monitored through the use of a serum CMV PCR assay, although biopsy is sometimes required for diagnosis of gastrointestinal disease. Ganciclovir is the treatment of choice; however, toxicities (bone marrow suppression) are common, and resistance can be a major problem. In addition to direct effects of infection, CMV is also associated with allograft rejection and can precipitate coinfections with other viral, bacterial, or fungal pathogens.[23]

Other viral infections commonly causing problems during this period include HSV and VZV, both of which can reactivate in localized (mucocutaneous and dermatomal, respectively) or more rarely in disseminated (hepatic, pulmonary, and gastrointestinal disease) fashion. Human herpesvirus-6 (HHV6) can occasionally cause severe encephalitis. Treatment of both HSV and VZV infection is with acyclovir, whereas treatment of HHV6 requires therapy with ganciclovir.

The management of recurrent HCV in liver transplant recipients has changed dramatically in the past few years with the development of direct-acting agents, and treatment protocol for both before and after transplant is changing rapidly.[24] Further details on management of post-transplant HCV infection are provided elsewhere in this issue (see Fenkel JM, Halegoua-DeMarzio DL: Management of the Liver Transplant Recipient: Approach to Allograft Dysfunction, in this issue).

Infection with BK virus (a polyoma virus genetically similar to JC virus) is a particular problem among kidney transplant recipients. In immunocompetent individuals, BK virus infection does not cause clinical disease; however, in individuals who have received a kidney transplant, it may cause a characteristic nephropathy and frequently leads to allograft failure. Treatment beyond reduction of immunosuppression has not been optimized.[25]

Aspergillosis occurs more frequently in liver transplant recipients, with an incidence estimated at up to 6%, but remains a major problem in kidney transplant recipients as well.[26] Although in the past it occurred most frequently in the first month after transplant, the epidemiology has changed to later infections. Invasive infections most commonly affect the lungs, but rhinosinusitis and brain abscesses are also common. Treatment with voriconazole has greatly improved outcomes.[27]

Rarely, anatomic problems persist despite interventions. For example, liver transplant recipients with unresolved biliary obstruction are likely to experience recurrent episodes of cholangitis. Kidney transplant recipients with ureteral reflux are likely to experience recurrent UTIs. In both situations, recurrent infections are likely to eventually produce MDR organisms that require complex and toxic antimicrobial regimens, rehospitalizations, and even need for repeat transplantation.[3]

INFECTIONS AFTER 6 MONTHS POSTTRANSPLANT

In the absence of major complications or rejection, patients 6 months beyond liver or kidney transplant generally experience reduced immunosuppression. In addition, anastomoses and wounds have largely healed, and hospital readmissions are less frequent. The potential for MDR bacterial and *Candida* infections is reduced. These developments provide for patients to resume their jobs and other everyday activities. As such, patients in this period are more likely to be infected with organisms endemic to the community, such as *S pneumoniae*, *Legionella*, and respiratory viruses.[2] Other infections related to environmental exposure include *Nocardia*, *Aspergillus*, and *Cryptococcus*, all of which may have subtle presentations over many months and can unfortunately be diagnosed late. *Listeria* is a food-borne pathogen and important cause of bacterial meningitis in this group.

Despite this improved immune status, transplant recipients remain at risk for opportunistic infections during this time period. Late CMV, for example, is an important infection that causes significant morbidity and mortality in liver and kidney transplant recipients. Manifestations of late CMV may be subtle, but any fever without an obvious source should prompt an investigation for CMV, especially in patients that are at high risk.[21] Newer methods for assessing risk of late CMV reactivation are ongoing. For example, interferon release assays for CMV may be an important predictor of late CMV.[28]

Although prophylaxis against PJP is very effective, the risk of infection persists after it is discontinued, usually at 12 months.[29] The diagnosis of PJP can be challenging, due to the nonspecific nature of symptoms (dyspnea on exertion, cough) and the nonspecific chest imaging findings. The use of serum 1,3-β-D-glucan testing may assist in establishing the diagnosis, but definitive diagnosis requires bronchoscopy. Treatment of PJP is with trimethoprim-sulfamethoxazole (TMP-SMX).[30]

Last, posttransplant lymphoproliferative disorder (PTLD) is a major hematologic malignancy related to EBV infection that often occurs in this period as well. PTLD is primarily a result of heightened antirejection medications that impair the transplant recipient's immune system from controlling viral infections, in particular EBV. Presentation is often muted but includes "B symptoms," such as fevers, night sweats, and weight loss. Body imaging reveals lymphadenopathy and diagnosis are primarily histologic, although a detectable EBV serum PCR is suggestive. Chemotherapy and reduction of immunosuppression, rather than antiviral therapy, are the primary treatments.

DISEASE PREVENTION: PROPHYLAXIS AND VACCINES
Prophylaxis

Two complementary strategies are used to prevent the development of disease in the transplant recipient: prophylaxis and vaccination. Prophylaxis is critically important in the first months after transplant, while vaccination remains a priority before and after transplantation.

Nearly all patients receive some form of antiviral prophylaxis (**Table 2**). Although protocols vary by institution, most individuals (except patients that are D−/R−) receive CMV prophylaxis with oral valganciclovir. The duration of prophylaxis is usually for 3 to 12 months and usually depends on which organ is transplanted. The main toxicity associated with valganciclovir is bone marrow suppression. Prophylaxis is often reinstituted in individuals undergoing treatment for rejection.[21]

Like CMV, protocols for HSV prophylaxis vary by institution, but are recommended by the American Society of Transplantation for at least the first month posttransplant as well as during times of increased immunosuppression.[8] Prophylaxis is usually with acyclovir or valacyclovir. These agents are usually well tolerated, but can cause nephrotoxicity. Patients requiring valganciclovir for CMV prophylaxis do not require additional prophylaxis for HSV.

Table 2
Prophylaxis after kidney and liver transplant

Prophylaxis Regimen	Patient Population That Receives It	Prophylaxis Directed Toward
TMP-SMX/dapsone/ atovaquone	Everyone	PJP Nocardia with TMP-SMX as well
Nystatin	Everyone	Candida
Valganciclovir	Seropositive CMV recipients Seronegative CMV recipients that receive a CMV+ organ	CMV, HSV
Valacyclovir/acyclovir	Seronegative CMV recipients that receive a CMV− organ	HSV
Entecavir/tenofovir	Recipients with a positive HBV core Ab Recipients of an organ from an HBV core Ab donor	HBV

Prophylaxis with TMP-SMX usually lasts for 6 to 12 months from the time of transplant. TMP-SMX is generally well tolerated, but can be associated with marrow suppression and kidney dysfunction. Individuals who are unable to tolerate TMP-SMX are given atovaquone, or occasionally dapsone (provided they have a normal G-6PD function), for PJP prophylaxis.[31]

Patients that receive an organ from a donor with a history of HBV or a personal history of HBV require prophylaxis in order to prevent recurrence of disease. Prophylaxis generally consists of combination therapy with HBV immunoglobulin and/or a nucleos(t)ide analogue such as lamivudine, entecavir, or tenofovir.[32] Pharmacotherapy with lamivudine and entecavir is generally well tolerated without substantial side effects; tenofovir therapy has been associated with renal toxicity, although that is rare. Infectious Diseases Society of America guidelines also recommend vaccination with the HBV vaccine for chronic HBV-infected recipients (2–6 months after liver transplantation) in an attempt to eliminate the lifelong requirement for HBV immunoglobulin.[33] It should be recognized, though, that this is a weak recommendation based on low-quality evidence.

Vaccination in the Transplant Recipient

Vaccination is essential to reduce the incidence of preventable disease after transplant. Ideally, all age-appropriate vaccinations are given before transplant (**Table 3**). Many vaccines can be safely given after transplant as well, with the exception of live-attenuated vaccines.[34] The contraindicated vaccines include measles, mumps, and rubella virus (MMR), varicella and zoster vaccines, and live influenza. In general, vaccination is deferred until at least 2 to 6 months posttransplant to maximize the development of a lasting immune response. Concerns about the possibility that vaccination will precipitate rejection of the allograft have been disproven and should not be withheld in the posttransplant population.[35]

Travel-related vaccines are also important. Safe vaccines to give after transplant include hepatitis A, Japanese encephalitis, and intramuscular (inactivated) typhoid. It is important to consult with an infectious disease specialist or a travel clinic before giving these vaccines.

Vaccination of Close Contacts of the Transplant Recipient

Domestic partners, children, and pets of the transplant recipient should also remain up to date on vaccinations. Although live-attenuated vaccinations are less preferable for

Table 3
Vaccination after kidney and liver transplant

Vaccines Safe to Give After Transplant	Vaccines Contraindicated After Transplant
Hepatitis A	Anthrax
HBV	BCG (Bacillus Calmette–Guérin)
Human papilloma virus	Influenza (intranasal)
Inactivated polio	MMR
Influenza (inactivated)	Smallpox
Neisseria meningitidis	Varicella zoster
Pertussis (Tdap)	
Rabies	
S pneumoniae both PCV-13 (pneumococcal conjugate vaccine) and PPSV-23 (pneumococcal polysaccharide vaccine)	
Tetanus	

close contacts of transplant recipients when an inactivated alternative is available (for example, in the case of influenza vaccination), these can be safely administered with attention to careful hand hygiene in the weeks following vaccination. With the exception of oral polio vaccine (not currently available in the United States), there are no absolute contraindications to administration of live-attenuated vaccines to household contacts of transplant recipients.[35]

There is a theoretic risk of transmission of the attenuated virus found in the rotavirus vaccine from the vaccinated infant to the organ recipient; however, this theoretic risk of transmission is outweighed by the benefits to the infant and to the household. The transplant recipient should not be involved with changing diapers of a vaccinated infant and reasonable precautions with attention to handwashing should be undertaken by family members during the 1 to 2 weeks following vaccine administration.[36] There is no evidence of person-to-person transmission of the attenuated viruses found in the MMR vaccine.[37]

Varicella and zoster vaccines are also not contraindicated for close contacts to transplant recipients. However, because the vaccines are live attenuated, if the vaccine recipient develops a varicella-like rash, they should be isolated from the transplant recipient until resolved.[38]

REFERENCES

1. 2012 Annual Report of the U.S. Organ Procurement and Transplantation Network and the Scientific Registry of Transplant Recipients: Transplant Data 1994-2003. Department of Health and Human Services, Health Resources and Services Administration, Healthcare Systems Bureau, Division of Transplantation, Rockville, MD; United Network for Organ Sharing, Richmond, VA; University Renal Research and Education Association, Ann Arbor, MI.
2. Fishman JA. Infection in solid-organ transplant recipients. N Engl J Med 2007; 357(25):2601–14.
3. Santoro-Lopes G, de Gouvea EF. Multidrug-resistant bacterial infections after liver transplantation: an ever-growing challenge. World J Gastroenterol 2014; 20(20):6201–10.
4. Fischer SA, Avery RK, AST Infectious Diseases Community of Practice. Screening of donor and recipient prior to solid organ transplantation. Am J Transplant 2009;9(Suppl 4):S7–18.
5. Muller E, Barday Z, Mendelson M, et al. HIV-positive-to-HIV-positive kidney transplantation–results at 3 to 5 years. N Engl J Med 2015;372(7):613–20.
6. Roland ME, Barin B, Carlson L, et al. HIV-infected liver and kidney transplant recipients: 1- and 3-year outcomes. Am J Transplant 2008;8(2):355–65.
7. Fischer SA, Lu K, AST Infectious Diseases Community of Practice. Screening of donor and recipient in solid organ transplantation. Am J Transplant 2013; 13(Suppl 4):9–21.
8. Green M. Introduction: infections in solid organ transplantation. Am J Transplant 2013;13(Suppl 4):3–8.
9. Reid GE, Grim SA, Sankary H, et al. Early intra-abdominal infections associated with orthotopic liver transplantation. Transplantation 2009;87(11):1706–11.
10. Safdar N, Said A, Lucey MR, et al. Infected bilomas in liver transplant recipients: clinical features, optimal management, and risk factors for mortality. Clin Infect Dis 2004;39(4):517–25.
11. Koo S, Marty FM, Baden LR. Infectious complications associated with immuno-modulating biologic agents. Infect Dis Clin North Am 2010;24(2):285–306.

12. Patel G, Huprikar S. Infectious complications after orthotopic liver transplantation. Semin Respir Crit Care Med 2012;33(1):111–24.
13. Camargo LF, Marra AR, Pignatari AC, et al. Nosocomial bloodstream infections in a nationwide study: comparison between solid organ transplant patients and the general population. Transpl Infect Dis 2015;17(2):308–13.
14. Linares L, Garcia-Goez JF, Cervera C, et al. Early bacteremia after solid organ transplantation. Transplant Proc 2009;41(6):2262–4.
15. Hadley S, Samore MH, Lewis WD, et al. Major infectious complications after orthotopic liver transplantation and comparison of outcomes in patients receiving cyclosporine or FK506 as primary immunosuppression. Transplantation 1995; 59(6):851–9.
16. Alangaden GJ, Thyagarajan R, Gruber SA, et al. Infectious complications after kidney transplantation: current epidemiology and associated risk factors. Clin Transplant 2006;20(4):401–9.
17. Paudel S, Zacharioudakis IM, Zervou FN, et al. Prevalence of Clostridium difficile infection among solid organ transplant recipients: a meta-analysis of published studies. PLoS One 2015;10(4):e0124483.
18. Lubbert C, Becker-Rux D, Rodloff AC, et al. Colonization of liver transplant recipients with KPC-producing Klebsiella pneumoniae is associated with high infection rates and excess mortality: a case-control analysis. Infection 2014;42(2):309–16.
19. Basavaraju SV, Kuehnert MJ, Zaki SR, et al. Encephalitis caused by pathogens transmitted through organ transplants, United States, 2002-2013. Emerg Infect Dis 2014;20(9):1443–51.
20. Cannon MJ, Schmid DS, Hyde TB. Review of cytomegalovirus seroprevalence and demographic characteristics associated with infection. Rev Med Virol 2010;20(4):202–13.
21. Razonable RR, Humar A, AST Infectious Diseases Community of Practice. Cytomegalovirus in solid organ transplantation. Am J Transplant 2013;13(Suppl 4): 93–106.
22. Eid AJ, Razonable RR. New developments in the management of cytomegalovirus infection after solid organ transplantation. Drugs 2010;70(8):965–81.
23. Helantera I, Lautenschlager I, Koskinen P. The risk of cytomegalovirus recurrence after kidney transplantation. Transpl Int 2011;24(12):1170–8.
24. AASLD/IDSA HCV Guidance Panel. Hepatitis C guidance: AASLD-IDSA recommendations for testing, managing, and treating adults infected with hepatitis C virus. Hepatology 2015;62(3):932–54.
25. Hirsch HH, Randhawa P, AST Infectious Diseases Community of Practice. BK polyomavirus in solid organ transplantation. Am J Transplant 2013;13(Suppl 4): 179–88.
26. Singh N, Avery RK, Munoz P, et al. Trends in risk profiles for and mortality associated with invasive aspergillosis among liver transplant recipients. Clin Infect Dis 2003;36(1):46–52.
27. Barchiesi F, Mazzocato S, Mazzanti S, et al. Invasive aspergillosis in liver transplant recipients: epidemiology, clinical characteristics, treatment, and outcomes in 116 cases. Liver Transpl 2015;21(2):204–12.
28. Sood S, Haifer C, Yu L, et al. Targeted individual prophylaxis offers superior risk stratification for cytomegalovirus reactivation after liver transplantation. Liver Transpl 2015;21:1478–85.
29. Iriart X, Challan Belval T, Fillaux J, et al. Risk factors of Pneumocystis pneumonia in solid organ recipients in the era of the common use of posttransplantation prophylaxis. Am J Transplant 2015;15(1):190–9.

30. Limper AH, Knox KS, Sarosi GA, et al. An official American Thoracic Society statement: treatment of fungal infections in adult pulmonary and critical care patients. Am J Respir Crit Care Med 2011;183(1):96–128.
31. Fishman JA. Prevention of infection caused by Pneumocystis carinii in transplant recipients. Clin Infect Dis 2001;33(8):1397–405.
32. Terrault N, Roche B, Samuel D. Management of the hepatitis B virus in the liver transplantation setting: a European and an American perspective. Liver Transpl 2005;11(7):716–32.
33. Rubin LG, Levin MJ, Ljungman P, et al. 2013 IDSA clinical practice guideline for vaccination of the immunocompromised host. Clin Infect Dis 2014;58(3):309–18.
34. Centers for Disease Control and Prevention (CDC). Advisory Committee on Immunization Practices (ACIP) recommended immunization schedules for persons aged 0 through 18 years and adults aged 19 years and older–United States, 2013. MMWR Surveill Summ 2013;62(Suppl 1):1.
35. Danziger-Isakov L, Kumar D, AST Infectious Diseases Community of Practice. Vaccination in solid organ transplantation. Am J Transplant 2013;13(Suppl 4): 311–7.
36. Parashar UD, Alexander JP, Glass RI, et al. Prevention of rotavirus gastroenteritis among infants and children. Recommendations of the Advisory Committee on Immunization Practices (ACIP). MMWR Recomm Rep 2006;55(RR-12):1–13.
37. Watson JC, Hadler SC, Dykewicz CA, et al. Measles, mumps, and rubella–vaccine use and strategies for elimination of measles, rubella, and congenital rubella syndrome and control of mumps: recommendations of the Advisory Committee on Immunization Practices (ACIP). MMWR Recomm Rep 1998;47(RR-8):1–57.
38. Prevention of Varicella. Update recommendations of the Advisory Committee on Immunization Practices (ACIP). MMWR Recomm Rep 1999;48(RR-6):1–5.

Selection and Postoperative Care of the Living Donor

Dianne LaPointe Rudow, DNP[a], Karen M. Warburton, MD, FASN[b],*

KEYWORDS

• Live donor • Kidney • Liver • Evaluation • Follow-up • Outcomes

KEY POINTS

- Live organ donation is an acceptable method to address the deceased donor organ shortage and save lives of patients with advanced liver and kidney disease.
- Careful evaluation of the live donor is critical to ensure donor safety. Controversies exist regarding selection of donors with comorbid conditions, including increased age, obesity, hypertension, prediabetes, and complex anatomy.
- Short- and long-term risks exist, but their incidence remains low. Donors are at risk for immediate surgical complications, such as bleeding, wound complications, infection, and venous thromboembolism.
- Kidney donors are at increased risk for pre-eclampsia and have a slightly increased risk of end-stage kidney disease. Liver donors may experience bile duct injury, liver failure, or damage to vessels during surgery.

INTRODUCTION

Live organ donors are increasingly seen in primary care practices across the country. Whether considering live donation or presenting after surgery for follow-up and routine primary care, such patients require that their physician have a basic understanding of the live donor evaluation process, surgery, and outcomes. Solid organ transplantation is the preferred treatment modality for many patients with end-stage liver and kidney disease. Excellent outcomes have resulted in expanded indications for transplant and larger waitlists across the country. Currently, 100,938

Disclosure Statement: The authors have nothing to disclose.
[a] Recanati Miller Transplantation Institute, Mount Sinai Hospital, 1425 Madison Avenue, Box 1105, New York, NY 10029, USA; [b] Division of Renal, Electrolyte and Hypertension, Penn Transplant Institute, Perelman School of Medicine, University of Pennsylvania, 1 Founders, Renal Division, 3400 Spruce Street, Philadelphia, PA 19104, USA
* Corresponding author.
E-mail address: karen.warburton@uphs.upenn.edu

patients are listed for kidney and 15,098 patients are listed for liver transplant in the United States. However, there were only 11,570 deceased donor kidney and 6449 deceased donor liver transplants performed in the United States in 2014.[1] This inequity of supply and demand remains a primary motivation to expand the use of live donors in kidney and liver transplantation.

The first successful live donor kidney transplant was performed in identical twins in 1954 by Dr Murray.[2] When compared with deceased donor transplantation, live donor kidney transplantation has many advantages, including superior graft and patient survival rates, fewer immunologic complications, less exposure to dialysis, better quality of life, and greater cost-effectiveness.[1,3,4] Live kidney donation is considered safe in medically suitable donors with low morbidity and mortality, significant psychological benefit, and very low rates of regret.[5–8]

Live donor liver transplantation (LDLT), in comparison, is less frequently used in the care of patients with end-stage liver disease and has stricter recipient and donor criteria. LDLT is commonly performed in the setting of adults donating to children using the left lateral segment of the liver, because this carries much less risk to the live donor and has proven benefit to the child.[9] Adult-to-adult LDLT is reserved for a select group of transplant candidates and is more common in large academic centers and geographic regions of the country with less opportunity for deceased donor transplant.[10] Right lobe hepatectomy, performed routinely in adult-to-adult LDLT, may carry increased morbidity and mortality to the donor when compared with kidney donation[11] but is still thought to be an acceptable solution to the shortage of deceased donors.[1,12] In addition, liver donors report psychological benefit and satisfaction with the donation experience.[8,13]

Despite data to support the need for and success of live donor organ transplant, numbers have trended down over the last few years in all parts of the United States.[14] The reasons for this are multifactorial and include changes to organ allocation, increased scrutiny of transplant program outcomes by regulatory bodies, an aging population of donor and recipient candidates, and financial crisis in the country, creating disincentives to live donation.[15] The transplant community is currently partnering with professional societies, patient advocacy groups, and the federal government to investigate these issues and propose solutions. Recent recommendations include engaging the nephrology community and primary care physicians to engage in live donor conversations with patients and their families early in the disease process as one method to educate future potential donors.[16,17]

Many strategies have been used to expand the live donor pool, including the increased use of altruistic donors, use of medically complex donors, and participation in paired and pooled exchange programs. Traditionally, living donors were genetically related to their recipient. With improvements in immunosuppressive drugs and increased comfort with live kidney donation in general, this relationship has evolved over time.[18] At most transplant programs, family, spouses, friends, and community members may be evaluated for both kidney and liver donation. In addition, programs are evaluating more and more nonbiological/nonemotionally related donors, often referred to as nondirected donors or altruistic donors. The use of social media to solicit for live donors is becoming more prevalent, as is the existence of groups that helps recipients find potential donors in the community. In addition, kidney-paired exchange programs enable exchange of organs between incompatible donor-recipient pairs. Careful education, evaluation, and counseling of potential donors over time are essential to maintain live donor safety throughout the donation process.

PATIENT PREPARATION

The living donor evaluation process includes an assessment of both the immunologic compatibility between donor and recipient and the mental and physical health of the donor. Historically, transplant centers have relied on the consensus view of experts to guide the selection practice.[19–23] Survey data suggest that there is considerable variability in specific testing protocols among different transplant centers.[24,25] In 2013, the United Network of Organ Sharing/Organ Procurement and Transplantation Network (OPTN) implemented new policy requirements that specify a minimum set of required tests and procedures for the medical and psychosocial evaluation of potential living kidney donors in the United States. In 2015, the liver donor policies were approved. The OPTN requirements for evaluation include blood type, on 2 separate occasions; medical evaluation by an expert in the field; psychosocial evaluation; and visit with an independent donor advocate who is not involved in the care of the transplant candidate, advocates for the rights of the donor, ensures that there is no evidence of coercion or financial compensation, and ensures that the donor is educated about all aspects of informed consent.[26]

With this framework in mind, the general approach to the medical and psychosocial evaluation of the living donor outlined in **Box 1** is proposed.

INDICATIONS/CONTRAINDICATIONS

Donor selection criteria vary significantly among US transplant centers.[24,25,28,29] Given the ethical considerations involved in living organ donation, there are no randomized controlled trials to guide the selection process. Although OPTN guidelines define absolute contraindications, they recommend that transplant centers use their judgment when it comes to individual cases and avoid, in most circumstances, the use of rigid cutoffs.[26] Therefore, selection of appropriate candidates for live donation is a highly individualized process. In general, there are few absolute, but many relative, contraindications to both liver and kidney donation.[10,11,19,20,23,30,31] These contraindications are summarized in **Box 2**.

The variability in selection criteria among transplant centers can in part be explained by the limited long-term data on the use of medically complex donors. Most studies suggest that outcomes are generally excellent for live kidney donors but have comprised younger, nonobese donors.[6,32,33] The general population is increasingly older, heavier, and more hypertensive, and available outcomes data on these groups are less well characterized. In kidney transplantation, the medically complex live donors have been defined as donors with risk factors for the future development of kidney disease, such as hypertension, obesity, or reduced GFR.[29] Studies have shown that medically complex patients form a substantial proportion of the current donor pool.[29,34,35] The following is a review of some common areas of controversy and variability among centers.

Age

There is no universally agreed on upper age cutoff for live kidney donation.[36] Older donors may have more comorbidities, including cardiovascular disease and lower kidney function.[37] However, many think that it is acceptable to use medically complex donors if they are greater than 55 years old because there is a better sense of their health phenotype. Although US transplant centers have become more permissive with older ages, most are now stricter with younger patients.[24] In a registry study of patients who were placed on a kidney transplant waiting list after previously donating a kidney, the mean age at donation was 32, and the majority developed end-stage

---

Box 1
Medical and psychosocial evaluation of the living donor

- Patient history
  - General medical history, including history of hypertension, diabetes, cardiovascular disease, thromboembolic events, bleeding history
  - Psychiatric disease, including depression, anxiety, suicidality, substance abuse
  - Medication use, including over-the-counter drugs and herbal remedies
  - Functional status and activity level
  - Assessment of high-risk behaviors as defined by the US Public Health Service[27]
  - Organ-specific history
    - *Kidney*: History of kidney problems, including stones, infections, hematuria, proteinuria, obstetric history, including gestational hypertension or diabetes, pre-eclampsia
    - *Liver*: History liver problems, risk factors for and/or actual history of viral hepatitis, history of abnormal liver function tests, diabetes, fatty liver disease, jaundice, bleeding, pruritus
  - Family history, with particular focus on kidney disease, liver disease diabetes, hypertension, clotting disorders, malignancy
  - Motivation to donate, absence of coercion or monetary exchange
  - Assessment of financial and employment concerns, social support systems
  - Assessment of understanding of risks

- Physical examination
  - Blood pressure (for kidney donors, on at least 2 occasions, consider ambulatory blood pressure monitoring in some cases)
  - Body mass index (BMI)
  - Complete physical examination

- Clinical testing
  - ABO
  - Kidney donors: HLA typing; donor and recipient cross-matching
  - Complete blood count
  - Complete metabolic panel
  - Prothrombin time/partial thromboplastin time
  - Viral studies (hepatitis B [HBV], hepatitis C [HCV], human immunodeficiency virus [HIV], cytomegalovirus, Epstein-Barr virus, Rubeola)
  - Rapid plasma reagin
  - Lipid panel
  - Organ-specific testing
    Kidney donors
    - Assessment of renal function with one or more of the following tests
      - 24-hour urine collection to calculate creatinine clearance
      - Nuclear studies using radioactive isotope or iodinated tracer
    - Assessment of proteinuria with 24-hour urine collection
    - Urinalysis with microscopy
    - Assessment of diabetes risk with one or more of the following tests
      - Fasting blood glucose
      - Hemoglobin A1C
      - 2-hour oral glucose tolerance test
    Liver donors
    - Hepatic function panel
    - Ceruloplasmin in a donor with family history of Wilson disease
    - Iron, iron binding capacity, ferritin
    - α-1-Antitrypsin level: those with low α-1-antitrypsin levels must have a phenotype
    - Autoimmune disease
    - Hypercoagulable workup
    - Appropriate testing for genetic diseases must be assessed in relatives (donors) for recipients with such diseases
    - Liver biopsy as needed

- Imaging and additional testing
  - Computed tomography angiogram or MRI abdomen to assess parenchyma, arterial and venous anatomy, and biliary tree (liver donors)
  - Age-appropriate cancer screening
  - Electrocardiogram
  - Chest radiograph

kidney disease (ESKD) more than 15 years after donation.[38] There is concern about both the cumulative risk and the comprehension of those potential risks in younger patients. Almost all programs now have a lower limit cutoff for age, typically 18 to 21 years of age.[24]

Box 2
Contraindications to live organ donation

- Absolute contraindications
  - Age <18 and mentally incapable of making an informed decision
  - Diabetes mellitus
  - Active or incompletely treated malignancy
  - High suspicion of donor coercion
  - High suspicion of illegal financial exchange between donor and recipient
  - HIV
  - Evidence of acute symptomatic infection
  - Active mental illness that requires treatment, including any evidence of suicidality
  - Kidney specific
    - Uncontrolled hypertension, or hypertension with evidence of end-organ damage
  - Liver-specific contraindications:
    - HCV RNA positive
    - HBsAg positive
    - Donors with ZZ, Z-null, null-null, and S-null α-1-antitrypsin phenotypes and untypeable phenotypes
    - Donor remnant volume less than 30% of native liver volume
    - Prior living liver donor
- Relative contraindications
  - Age <21
  - History of certain prior malignancies or treatment with nephrotoxic therapy for malignancy
  - Chronic illness (cardiovascular, pulmonary, liver, neurologic, autoimmune disease)
  - Active substance abuse
  - Disorders requiring anticoagulation, bleeding disorders
  - Morbid obesity (BMI >35)
  - Prediabetes
  - Kidney specific
    - Glomerular filtration rate (GFR) <80 mL/min or <2 SD below the mean for donor age
    - Proteinuria greater than 300 mg/d
    - Persistent hematuria
    - Structural concerns involving renal collecting system or vasculature
    - Kidney stones with high likelihood of recurrence
    - Chronic, active viral infection (HBV, HCV)
  - Liver specific
    - Age greater than 60
    - Unexplained liver function test abnormalities
    - Vascular or biliary anatomy in the donor liver that makes the likelihood of successful transplantation low or increases the risk in the potential donor
    - Multiple or complex upper abdominal surgeries
    - Significant hepatic steatosis

Obesity

Obesity is an independent risk factor for ESKD in the general population,[39] in addition to being associated with an increased hypertension, diabetes, and overall cardiovascular risk. Among live kidney donors, BMI 35 kg/m^2 or higher has been associated with slightly longer operative times and more perioperative complications, most of them minor.[40] Long-term outcomes data are limited in this population of donors.[41] There has been no consensus about an upper limit for BMI in potential live kidney donors. Most US centers do not accept donors with a BMI of greater than 35,[24] and consideration of patients with a BMI between 30 and 35 must be judicious, particularly if they are young. Obese patients should always be counseled about weight loss, lifestyle changes, and exercise and need to be very carefully advised about potential short- and long-term risks following donation.

Hypertension

Transplant centers are increasingly willing to accept a select population of hypertensive donors. Nearly half of US programs will consider a donor on antihypertensive medications if blood pressure is well-controlled, and many will further loosen the criteria if the patient is older.[24] To the extent that it is possible, the goal is to predict who will develop ESKD from hypertension and exclude those patients. Thus, evidence of end-organ damage, uncontrolled blood pressure, or blood pressure requiring multiple medications are typically contraindications to donation. Centers may exclude potential donors with a first-degree relative who has ESKD secondary to hypertension, and young or non-white patients with hypertension must be considered very cautiously.

At Risk for Diabetes

Although the presence of diabetes is generally considered a contraindication to live kidney donation,[19,20,24] many potential donors have risk factors for the development of diabetes at the time of their evaluation. There is no clear consensus about exclusion of patients with prediabetes, as defined in recent guidelines from the American Diabetes Association,[42,43] and exclusion criteria vary greatly from center to center.[24] Younger patients with abnormal fasting blood glucose or evidence of glucose intolerance, particularly if they are obese, hypertensive, or have a family history of kidney disease from diabetes, may not be appropriate donors. Conversely, an older individual with mildly impaired glucose tolerance who is thin and exercises regularly may be a reasonable donor. The risk profile is strongly influenced by the patient's family history, age, race, and lifestyle.

Controversies for Potential Liver Donors

For live liver donation, the largest limiting factor for finding suitable donors is the reluctance of the patients with end-stage liver failure to consider LDLT[40]; this is multifactorial. The MELD (or model for end-stage liver disease) allocation[44] system for liver transplant prioritizes the sickest patients waiting, and this often gives false comfort that a suitable organ can be found. Data suggest that there is a survival benefit to LDLT versus waiting on the list.[45] Waiting for patients to decompensate before LDLT results in worse outcomes for the recipient. Other factors affecting LDLT recipient survival include increased donor and recipient age, presence of hepatocellular carcinoma or hepatitis C in the recipient, intensive care unit stay before transplant, hospitalization before surgery versus being at home, center experience, and cold ischemia time greater than 4.5 hours.[10] Donor issues that complicate the decision to consider available living donors include presence of steatosis and complex vascular and biliary anatomy; each of these factors may result in donors being declined at a higher rate because of increased risk of complications in the recipient.[46,47] Predonation predictors of donor complications include older age, male gender, and higher BMI; however, these risk factors are typically predictive of minor issues such as wound and hernia complications.[11]

In summary, the selection of live donors is an individualized process. Given that the increased use of medically complex donors is an important strategy to increase the pool of live donors, it is important to avoid being too rigid in the application of numeric cutoffs as one waits for more long-term outcomes data for this population. Generally speaking, centers have evolved to a more inclusive policy of acceptance in many areas, including the use of unrelated donors and older donors. The one exception to that trend is related to the use of younger kidney donors, which has appropriately gone in the other direction, with increased scrutiny and higher thresholds to accept risks that may magnify over the lifetime of the potential donor.

After Procedure Care

The specifics of short- and long-term management of live organ donors have been the subject of much discussion in terms of who should follow them, for how long, and using what measurements.[48] Some donors want to be followed very closely, and others refuse to return to the transplant center for care even immediately after donation.[49] Typically, kidney donors are hospitalized for 2 or 3 days after a laparoscopic procedure, are out of work 2 to 4 weeks, and feel back to normal shortly thereafter. A liver donor may be hospitalized for up to 7 days and will be out of work for about 6 weeks and may not feel completely recovered for 3 to 4 months. In an effort to collect short-term data on live organ donors, and to ensure access to care in the immediate period after donation, the OPTN has policies regarding donor follow-up.[26] All transplant programs that perform live donor transplants must report accurate, complete, and timely follow-up data for live kidney and liver donors, including the donor status and clinical information shown in **Box 3** at 6 months, 1 year, and 2 years after donation. The method of follow-up varies across programs. Some choose to perform the follow-up by telephone and local laboratory tests, whereas others see the donors at each follow-up interval, and still others send the donor to the primary care physician. Often the method of follow-up is a donor-driven process; therefore, a primary care physician may find a donor in his or her waiting room requesting assistance with mandated follow-up. Some centers have developed comprehensive live donor programs that provide education and follow-up with the goal of ensuring long-term health maintenance and healthy lifestyles.[50] There are few data to support any of the OPTN-mandated follow-up practices nor do there exist any data to suggest what might be the optimal practice after the initial 2 year after-donation period.

Outcomes and Evidence

The short-term risks of both kidney and liver donation are well described in the literature, and both surgeries are thought to be relatively safe with low incidence of complications. As with any medical procedure, there is both morbidity and mortality associated with the operation itself. Short-term risks to the live donor are shown in **Box 4**.

Risks Specific to Kidney Donation

When possible, live donor nephrectomies are performed laparoscopically versus an open approach. Surgical mortality is quite low at 3.1 per 10,000 donors in the first 90 days.[6]

Box 3
Elements of donor follow-up

Required for all live donors: 6 months, 1 year, and 2 years after donation

General

- Patient status; cause of death, if applicable and known
- Working for income, and if not working, reason for not working
- Loss of medical (health, life) insurance due to donation
- Readmissions since last follow-up

Kidney complications

- Maintenance dialysis
- Development of hypertension requiring medication
- Diabetes

Liver complications

- Abscess
- Bile leak
- Hepatic resection
- Incisional hernias due to donation surgery
- Liver failure
- Registered on the liver candidate waiting list

Required kidney laboratory data

- Serum creatinine
- Urine protein

Required liver laboratory data

- Alanine aminotransferase
- Alkaline phosphatase
- Platelet count
- Total bilirubin

In most studies, long-term survival and rate of major cardiovascular events in live kidney donors are similar to that of healthy matched controls in the general population,[6,32,51] even among older donors.[37]

Following nephrectomy and the loss of 50% of the kidney mass, there is compensatory hypertrophy in the remaining kidney, and the donor retains approximately two-thirds of the baseline kidney function.[52,53] ESKD following donation is so rare that it is difficult to study, although data support an elevated relative risk in donors when compared with healthy matched controls in the population.[32,33] In the current allocation system, OPTN prioritizes donors who have developed ESKD such that prior donors should have a very short waiting time before deceased-donor transplantation.

Some studies suggest that the risk of hypertension and chronic kidney disease after donation varies among subpopulations and is higher for African American donors.[33,54]

Box 4
Short-term risks to the live organ donor

All donors

- Potential medical or surgical risks
  - Aborted procedure
  - Bleeding requiring transfusion
  - Wound-related: wound infection, scar, hernia
  - Venous thromboembolism, including pulmonary embolism
  - Pneumonia, urinary tract infection
  - Nerve injury, pain, atelectasis, pneumothorax, and other consequences typical of any surgical procedure
  - Abdominal symptoms such as bloating, nausea, ileus, bowel obstruction

- Potential psychosocial risks
  - Problems with body image
  - Depression or anxiety
  - Feelings of emotional distress or grief if the transplant recipient experiences any recurrent disease, graft failure or death

- Potential financial risks
  - Unreimbursed personal expenses of travel, housing, child-care costs, and lost wages related to donation.
  - Need for life-long follow-up at the donor's expense
  - Loss of employment or income
  - Negative impact on the ability to obtain future employment
  - Negative impact on the ability to obtain, maintain, or afford health insurance, disability insurance, and life insurance
  - Future health problems experienced by living donors following donation may not be covered by the recipient's insurance

- Kidney donors
  - Death (3 per 10,000)
  - Conversion from laparoscopic surgery to open procedure
  - Decreased kidney function
  - End-stage renal disease (<1% in 10 years)

- Liver donors
  - Death (risk is 1–5 in 1000 transplants, likely relative to the amount of liver tissue removed)[58]
  - Acute liver failure with need for liver transplant
  - Transient liver dysfunction with recovery (degree of dysfunction depends on the amount of the total liver removed)
  - Biliary complications including leak or stricture (9%)
  - Vascular thrombus (including hepatic artery or portal vein, 0.9%)
  - Pleural effusion

Data from Refs.[6,11,26,33,61]

The racial disparity in outcomes may be due to genetic factors, such as polymorphisms in the *APOL1* genes.

Recent studies have demonstrated that gestational hypertension or pre-eclampsia is more common among live kidney donors than among nondonors, although most women have uncomplicated pregnancies following donation.[55,56] Recent consensus guidelines appropriately emphasize the need for full disclosure of these pregnancy-associated risks during the evaluation process.[16]

Psychological outcomes among kidney donors are generally good, and most report overall positive experiences.[57]

Risks Specific to Liver Donation

The short-term risks to the liver donor are often directly related to the segment of the liver removed. The larger the segment removed, the greater the risk. The estimated risk of death ranges from 0.4% to 0.6%[58] with 4 known right lobe donor perioperative deaths in the United States.[1] Forty percent of all liver donors have at least one complication, but most are Clavien grades 1 and 2 (less severe with no residual disability).[11,58] Blood transfusion requirement and intraoperative hypotension were associated with a 48% higher likelihood of complications in the multicenter A2ALL (Adult-to-Adult Living Donor Liver Transplantation Cohort) study of LDLT.[11] Elevated BMI was a risk factor for bile duct leaks. Those of older age, men, and those with elevated BMI were significantly more likely to get incisional hernias.[11]

Most untoward outcomes occur in the early preoperative period as the liver has the capacity to regenerate and resume normal function within months of surgery. Studies show that within 3 months significant regeneration occurs, and the percentage of reconstitution was 80%.[59] Despite regeneration, long-term complications can arise, but most are directly related to surgery and scar tissue. It is reported that 7% of liver donors may have a complications after 1 year, including hernia, bowel obstruction, and psychological complications.

Psychological outcomes in liver donors are generally good, most reporting psychological benefits and satisfaction with their donation experience.[8,13] Studies reveal that liver donors have above average physical and mental components scores on the Short Form-36 up to 11 years after donation.[13] There have been psychosocial complications and somatic complaints reported in national trials and signal center reports especially when the recipient has done poorly.[8,11,13,59,60] These complaints include anxiety, depression, posttraumatic stress disorder, abdominal pain requiring medication, gastrointestinal upset, and intolerance to fatty foods. Despite these occurrences, most donors do not regret donation.

In summary, live donors are healthy individuals plummeted into the health care system often with little or no health care literacy. Partnerships with the donor, their primary care physician, and the live donor team can effectively evaluate, manage, and monitor the live organ donor throughout the process.

REFERENCES

1. The Organ Procurement and Transplantation Network. National data report web site. Available at: http://optn.transplant.hrsa.gov/converge/latestData/step2.asp. Accessed August 12, 2015.
2. Murray JE, Merrill JP, Harrison JH. Kidney transplantation between seven pairs of identical twins. Ann Surg 1958;148:343–59.
3. US Renal Data System, USRDS. 2013 Annual data report: atlas of chronic kidney disease and end-stage renal disease in the United States. Bethesda (MD): National Institutes of Health, National Institute of Diabetes and Digestive and Kidney Diseases; 2013.
4. Purnell TS, Auguste P, Crews DC, et al. Comparison of life participation activities among adults treated by hemodialysis, peritoneal dialysis, and kidney transplantation: a systematic review. Am J Kidney Dis 2013;62:953–73.
5. Ibrahim HN, Foley R, Tan L, et al. Long-term consequences of kidney donation. N Engl J Med 2009;360(5):459–69.
6. Segev DL, Muzzaale AD, Caffo BS, et al. Perioperative mortality and long-term survival following live kidney donation. JAMA 2010;303(10):959–66.

7. Clemens KK, Thiessen-Philbrook H, Parikh CR, et al, Donor Nephrectomy Outcomes Research (DONOR) Network. Psychosocial health of living kidney donors: a systematic review. Am J Transplant 2006;6:2965–77.

8. LaPointe Rudow D, Charlton M, Sanchez C, et al. Kidney and liver living donors: a comparison of experiences. Prog Transplant 2005;15(2):185–91.

9. Emre S. Living-donor liver transplantation in children. Pediatr Transplant 2002; 6:43–6.

10. Olhtoff KM, Abecasis MM, Emond JC, et al, A2ALL Study Group. Outcomes of adult-to-adult living donor transplantation: comparison of the adult-to adult living donor liver transplantation cohort study and national experience. Liver Transpl 2011;17:789–97.

11. Abecasis MM, Fisher RA, Olthoff KM, et al, A2ALL Study Group. Complications of living donor hepatic lobectomy–a comprehensive report. Am J Transplant 2012; 12(5):1208–17.

12. Freise CE, Gillespie BW, Koffron AJ, et al, A2ALL Study Group. Recipient morbidity after living and deceased donor liver transplantation: findings from the A2ALL retrospective cohort study. Am J Transplant 2008;12(12):2569–79.

13. Ladner DP, Dew MA, Forney S, et al. Long-term quality of life after liver donation in the adult to adult living donor livers transplantation cohort study (A2ALL). J Hepatol 2015;62:346–53.

14. Matas AJ, Smith JM, Skeans MA, et al. OPTN/SRTR 2012 Annual data report: kidney. Am J Transplant 2013;14(1):11–44. Available at: http://onlinelibrary.wiley.com/doi/10.1111/ajt.12579/full#ajt12579-fig-0022.

15. Rodrigue JR, Schold JD, Mandelbrot DA. The decline in living kidney donation in the United States: random variation or cause for concern? Transplantation 2013; 96:767–73.

16. LaPointe Rudow D, Hays R, Cohen DJ, et al. Consensus conference on best practices in live kidney donation: recommendations to optimize education, access, and care. Am J Transplant 2015;15(4):914–22.

17. McGill RL, Ko TY. Transplantation and the primary care physician. Adv Chronic Kidney Dis 2011;18(6):433–8.

18. Reese PP, Boudville N, Garg AX. Living kidney donation: outcomes, ethics, and uncertainty. Lancet 2015;385(9981):2003–13.

19. Delmonico F. A report of the Amsterdam Forum on the Care of the Live Kidney Donor: data and medical guidelines. Transplantation 2005;79(Suppl 6):S53–66.

20. Abramowicz D, Cochat P, Claas FH, et al. European Renal Best Practice Guideline on kidney donor and recipient evaluation and perioperative care. Nephrol Dial Transplant 2014;30(11):1790–7.

21. Kasiske BL, Bia MJ. The evaluation and selection of living kidney donors. Am J Kidney Dis 1995;26(2):387–98.

22. Davis CL, Delmonico FL. Living-donor kidney transplantation: a review of the current practices for the live donor. J Am Soc Nephrol 2005;16(7):2098–110.

23. Barr ML, Belghiti J, Villamil FG, et al. A report of the Vancouver Forum on the care of the live organ donor: lung, liver, pancreas, and intestine data and medical guidelines. Transplantation 2006;81(10):1373–85.

24. Mandelbrot DA, Pavlakis M, Danovitch GM, et al. The medical evaluation of living kidney donors: a survey of US transplant centers. Am J Transplant 2007;7(10): 2333–43.

25. Bia MJ, Ramos EL, Danovitch GM, et al. Evaluation of living renal donors. The current practice of US transplant centers. Transplantation 1995;60(4):322–7.

26. Organ Procurement and Transplantation Network (OPTN) policies on live donation. Available at: http://optn.transplant.hrsa.gov/ContentDocuments/OPTN_Policies. pdf#nameddest=Policy_14. Accessed August 13, 2015.

27. PHS guideline for reducing human immunodeficiency virus, hepatitis B virus, and hepatitis C virus transmission through organ transplantation. Available at: http://www.publichealthreports.org/issueopen.cfm?articleID=2975. Accessed August 12, 2015.

28. Tong A, Chapman JR, Wong G, et al. Living kidney donor assessment: challenges, uncertainties and controversies among transplant nephrologists and surgeons. Am J Transplant 2013;13(11):2912–23.

29. Reese PP, Feldman HI, McBride MA, et al. Substantial variation in the acceptance of medically complex live kidney donors across US renal transplant centers. Am J Transplant 2008;8(10):2062–70.

30. Kher A, Mandelbrot DA. The living kidney donor evaluation: focus on renal issues. Clin J Am Soc Nephrol 2012;7(2):366–71.

31. Lobritto S, Kato T, Emond J. Living-donor liver transplantation: current perspective. Semin Liver Dis 2012;32(4):333–40.

32. Mjoen G, Hallan S, Hartmann A, et al. Long-term risks for kidney donors. Kidney Int 2014;86:162–7.

33. Muzaale AD, Massie AB, Wang MC, et al. Risk of end-stage renal disease following live kidney donation. JAMA 2014;311:579–86.

34. Taler SJ, Messersmith EE, Leichtman AB, et al. Demographic, metabolic, and blood pressure characteristics of living kidney donors spanning five decades. Am J Transplant 2013;13(2):390–8.

35. Davis CL, Cooper M. The state of US living kidney donors. Clin J Am Soc Nephrol 2010;5(10):1873–80.

36. Berger JC, Muzaale AD, James N, et al. Living kidney donors ages 70 and older: recipient and donor outcomes. Clin J Am Soc Nephrol 2011;6(12):2887–93.

37. Reese PP, Bloom RD, Feldman HI, et al. Mortality and cardiovascular disease among older live kidney donors. Am J Transplant 2014;14(8):1853–61.

38. Gibney EM, King AL, Maluf DG, et al. Living kidney donors requiring transplantation: focus on African Americans. Transplantation 2007;84(5):647–9.

39. Chertow GM, Hsu CY, Johansen KL. The enlarging body of evidence: obesity and chronic kidney disease. J Am Soc Nephrol 2006;17(6):1501–2.

40. Heimbach JK, Taler SJ, Prieto M, et al. Obesity in living kidney donors: clinical characteristics and outcomes in the era of laparoscopic donor nephrectomy. Am J Transplant 2005;5(5):1057–64.

41. Tavakol MM, Vincenti FG, Assadi H, et al. Long-term renal function and cardiovascular disease risk in obese kidney donors. Clin J Am Soc Nephrol 2009; 4(7):1230–8.

42. American Diabetes Association Position Statement. Diagnosis and classification of diabetes mellitus. Diabetes Care 2010;33(1):S62–9.

43. Hayashi K, Uchida H, Takaoka C, et al. Discrepancy in psychological attitudes toward living donor liver transplantation between recipients and donors. Transplantation 2015;99(12):2551–5.

44. Singal AK, Kamath PS. Model for end-stage liver disease. J Clin Exp Hepatol 2013;3(1):50–60.

45. Berg CL, Gillespie BW, Merion RM, et al. Improvement in survival associated with adult-to-adult living donor liver transplantation. Gastroenterology 2007;133(6): 1806–13.

46. Simpson MA, Verbesey JE, Khettry U, et al. Successful algorithm for selective liver biopsy in the right hepatic lobe live donor (RHLD). Am J Transplant 2008; 8(4):832–8.

47. Lee SG. A complete treatment of adult living donor liver transplantation: a review of surgical technique and current challenges to expand indication of patients. Am J Transplant 2015;15(1):17–38.

48. Living Kidney Donor Follow-Up Conference Writing Group, Leichtman A, Abecassis M, et al. Living kidney donor follow-up: state-of-the-art and future directions, conference summary and recommendations. Am J Transplant 2011;11(12): 2561–8.

49. Waterman AD, Dew MA, Davis CL, et al. Living-donor follow-up attitudes and practices in U.S. kidney and liver donor programs. Transplantation 2013;95(6): 883–8.

50. LaPointe Rudow D. Development of the Center for Living Donation: incorporating the role of the nurse practitioner as director. Prog Transplant 2011;21(4):312–6.

51. Garg AX, Meirambayeva A, Huang A, et al. Cardiovascular disease in kidney donors: matched cohort study. BMJ 2012;344:e1203.

52. Pabico RC, McKenna BA, Freeman RB. Renal function before and after unilateral nephrectomy in renal donors. Kidney Int 1975;8(3):166–75.

53. Fehrman-Ekholm I, Duner F, Brink B, et al. No evidence of accelerated loss of kidney function in living kidney donors: results from a cross-sectional follow-up. Transplantation 2001;72(3):444–9.

54. Lentine KL, Schnitzler MA, Xiao H, et al. Racial variation in medical outcomes among living kidney donors. N Engl J Med 2010;363:724.

55. Nevis IF, Garg AX, Donor Nephrectomy Outcomes Research (DONOR) Network. Maternal and fetal outcomes after living kidney donation. Am J Transplant 2009; 9(4):661–8.

56. Garg AX, Nevis IF, McArthur E, et al. Gestational hypertension and preeclampsia in living kidney donors. N Engl J Med 2015;372(2):124–33.

57. Johnson EM, Anderson JK, Jacobs C, et al. Long-term follow-up of living kidney donors: quality of life after donation. Transplantation 1999;67:717.

58. Cheah YL, Simpson MA, Pomposelli JJ, et al. Incidence of death and potentially life-threatening near-miss events in living donor hepatic lobectomy: a world-wide survey. Liver Transpl 2013;19(5):499–506.

59. Olthoff KM, Emond JC, Shearon TH, et al. Liver regeneration after living donor transplantation: adult-to-adult living donor liver transplantation cohort study. Liver Transpl 2015;21(1):79–88.

60. Kim-Schluger L, Florman SS, Schiano T, et al. Quality of life after lobectomy for adult liver transplantation. Transplantation 2002;73(10):1593–7.

61. Tan JC, Gordon EJ, Dew MA, et al. Living donor kidney transplantation: facilitating education about live kidney donation—recommendations from a consensus conference. Clin J Am Soc Nephrol 2015;10(9):1670–7.

Long-Term Functional Recovery, Quality of Life, and Pregnancy After Solid Organ Transplantation

Swati Rao, MD[a], Mythili Ghanta, MD[b], Michael J. Moritz, MD[c,d,e], Serban Constantinescu, MD, PhD[e,f,*]

KEYWORDS

- Kidney transplantation • Liver transplantation • Pregnancy • Quality of life
- Functional recovery

KEY POINTS

- Successful transplantation results in improved functional status, health-related quality of life (HR-QOL), and reproductive health in kidney and liver recipients. However, functional status and HR-QOL of recipients remain lower than in the general population.
- Functional status and HR-QOL are associated with patient and graft survival. Multiple factors, such as comorbidities, perioperative course, graft function, immunosuppressive medications, and patient demographics, impact HR-QOL.
- Fertility is restored soon after successful transplant. Appropriate birth control and pregnancy counseling is warranted. Transplant recipients should wait at least 1 to 2 years after transplantation before conceiving.
- Most pregnancies in kidney and liver recipients have successful maternal and newborn outcomes. These pregnancies are high risk, with increased incidences of hypertension, preeclampsia, and prematurity.

Continued

Disclosure Statement: The National Transplantation Pregnancy Registry is supported by grants from Astellas Pharma US, Pfizer, and Bristol-Myers Squibb Company.

[a] Section of Nephrology, Hypertension and Kidney Transplantation, Temple University School of Medicine, 3440 North Broad Street, Kresge West, Suite 100, Philadelphia, PA 19140, USA; [b] Pancreas Transplant Program, Section of Nephrology, Hypertension and Kidney Transplantation, Temple University School of Medicine, 3440 North Broad Street, Kresge West, Suite 100, Philadelphia, PA 19140, USA; [c] Transplant Services, Lehigh Valley Health Network, Allentown, PA 18103, USA; [d] Morsani College of Medicine, University of South Florida, Tampa, FL 33612, USA; [e] National Transplantation Pregnancy Registry, Gift of Life Institute, 401 North 3rd Street, Philadelphia, PA 19123, USA; [f] Kidney Transplant Program, Section of Nephrology, Hypertension and Kidney Transplantation, Temple University School of Medicine, 3440 North Broad Street, Kresge West, Suite 100, Philadelphia, PA 19140, USA
* Corresponding author. Section of Nephrology, Hypertension and Kidney Transplantation, Temple University School of Medicine, 3440 North Broad Street, Kresge West, Suite 100, Philadelphia, PA 19140.
E-mail address: serban.constantinescu@tuhs.temple.edu

Med Clin N Am 100 (2016) 613–629
http://dx.doi.org/10.1016/j.mcna.2016.01.010
0025-7125/16/$ – see front matter © 2016 Elsevier Inc. All rights reserved.

Continued

- The incidence of birth defects is similar to the general population, except for pregnancies exposed to mycophenolic acid products. These pregnancies are associated with higher incidences of miscarriages and birth defects, including a specific pattern of birth defects in the offspring.

INTRODUCTION

Improved health after transplantation enables kidney and liver recipients to resume many personal and social functions with an enhanced sense of well-being. Along with data on patient and allograft survival, analyses of functional recovery, health-related quality of life (HR-QOL), and pregnancy outcomes can better define the success of transplantation.[1,2]

Sexuality and fertility are adversely affected by chronic organ failure. Successful transplantation improves reproductive function. The first pregnancy after kidney transplantation occurred in 1958 and after liver transplantation in 1977.[3,4] Since then, thousands of successful posttransplant pregnancies have been reported.[5,6] Reproductive health and the opportunity for parenthood can have a major impact on overall QOL for recipients. It is estimated that as of June 2013, there were 200,000 recipients alive with a functioning kidney transplant and 65,000 recipients alive with a functioning liver transplant.[1,2] Approximately 25% of these recipients are women of reproductive age.[5,6]

Internists and family physicians play a key role in providing essential preventive care, management of comorbidities, and long-term care to this patient population. This article focuses on salient features of functional recovery, HR-QOL, and reproductive health after kidney or liver transplantation.

FUNCTIONAL RECOVERY

Functional recovery after transplantation includes improvements in cognition, physical function, and employment potential.

Cognitive Function

The positive impact of transplantation on cognitive function is an important measure of patient recovery. Pretransplant hepatic encephalopathy or uremia leads to cognitive impairment impacting every arena of life. Transplantation reverses the metabolic effects of end-stage liver or kidney failure. However, the immunosuppressive medications tacrolimus and cyclosporine do have neurologic side effects that may impact posttransplant cognition.

Liver transplant recipients demonstrate improved cognition and normalization of the electroencephalogram.[7] Similarly, kidney transplant recipients' cognitive function improves to a level at par with the general population.[8]

Physical Function

In a study of 279 transplant recipients (among them 88 kidney and 77 liver recipients), physical function improved significantly from pretransplant levels with sustained benefits at 4 years posttransplant. Despite this improvement, the functional status achieved was less than that of the general population.[9]

Because chronic illness negatively impacts functional status, physical therapy and rehabilitation should be considered in all transplant recipients. Long-term supervised physical activity in kidney and liver recipients demonstrates a positive effect on physical strength and psychological well-being, highlighting a potential target for intervention.[10]

Because most liver recipients are quite ill and severely deconditioned pretransplant, they benefit from inpatient rehabilitation. However, there is a significantly higher rate of hospital readmission and lesser functional gain compared with nontransplant rehabilitation patients. A close partnership between transplant hospitals and rehabilitation centers could facilitate posttransplant recovery.[11]

Employment

Gainful employment posttransplant is considered a hallmark of successful integration of transplant recipients into society. Patients who worked before transplant are more likely to be employed posttransplantation. Among kidney recipients between 18 and 64 years of age who were employed at the time of transplant, the employment rate 1 year after transplantation was 47% for privately insured and only 16% for the recipients with public insurance. Among kidney recipients unemployed at the time of transplantation, only 5% were working 1 year after transplantation.[12] For liver transplant recipients, employment decreased from 71% pretransplant to 27% posttransplant, with most recipients returning to work within 1 year after transplantation.[13] Reasons for the high unemployment rate include a prolonged absence from the profession because of illness or employer hesitancies to hire a transplant recipient. The inability to pursue their original line of work, such as manual labor, can be a major factor for unemployment.[14] Appropriate use of vocational training can increase the rate of return to the work force for transplant recipients.[15]

HEALTH-RELATED QUALITY OF LIFE

HR-QOL is defined as an individual's self-assessment of their health and encompasses physical status, mental health, and social well-being. By improving overall health, transplantation provides hope for a better and longer life. **Box 1** details factors that are known to determine QOL in transplant recipients.[16–25]

A meta-analysis of 218 studies, with more than 14,000 transplant recipients, revealed an overall improvement in all aspects of HR-QOL from pretransplant to posttransplant. For most of the recipients, transplantation resulted in significant gain in physical functional status, whereas the improvements were not as great in the mental health and social domains of QOL. The overall HR-QOL for transplant recipients was on par with chronically ill patients and remained lower than healthy individuals.[26]

Kidney transplant recipients' HR-QOL is improved compared with end-stage kidney disease patients on the wait list, but is lower than that of the general population. Among the transplanted patients, those who had complications after surgery showed a lower level of social functioning, general mental health, and physical status; these recipients were also found to have a higher level of anxiety than wait-listed patients on dialysis.[27] When QOL was analyzed by modality of kidney-replacement therapy, the highest QOL was reported with transplantation, followed by peritoneal dialysis, then hemodialysis.[28]

Improved overall HR-QOL has been reported in liver transplant recipients when compared with patients awaiting transplantation. Additionally, the liver recipients also reported improvement in feelings of hopelessness and anxiety, resulting in more fulfilling social interactions.[18]

Similar to the general population, depression in kidney transplant recipients is associated with decreased medication compliance.[22] In kidney recipients, lower physical

---

Box 1
Factors determining health-related quality of life in transplant recipients

Comorbidities

- Many recipients have comorbid conditions, such as hypertension and diabetes.
- Diabetes is a significant predictor of lower HR-QOL.[16]
- Anemia and osteoporosis contribute to the disease burden and impact QOL.[17]

Pretransplant course

- Primary disease: type, age of onset, duration, systemic manifestation, prior treatment modalities, and duration of treatment (eg, dialysis).
- Malnutrition, encephalopathy, and infections contribute to prolonged recovery phase.
- Potential irreversible effects of the chronic disease on cognitive and motor function.

Perioperative course

- Surgical complications and prolonged hospitalization impede the recovery process.[18]

Graft function

- Patients who had acute and chronic rejections had a lower QOL score.[19]
- Poor graft function leads to poorer physical capabilities and increased physiologic stress.
- Patients with failing graft should have increased surveillance to address emotional and general physical health issues.

Immunosuppressive medication

- Neurologic side effects of immunosuppressive medications, such as headache and tremors, can undermine the functional status of the recipients.
- Side effects of immunosuppressive medications inversely correlate with QOL score.[16]
- Among calcineurin inhibitors, tacrolimus was associated with fewer side effects than cyclosporine.[20]

Physical changes after transplantation

- Transplantation results in alteration of body image and other physical changes, such as weight gain and hirsutism, which have negative psychological effects.[16]

Reproductive health after transplantation

- Despite improvement in reproductive health, sexual dysfunction remains common after transplantation.
- Sexual dysfunction is one of the strongest predictors of lower QOL.[16]

Psychological factors

- There is a high prevalence of anxiety and depression in transplant recipients.[21]
- Patients with anxiety and depression have lower survival and are more likely to be noncompliant.[22]

Ethnicity and gender

- Although all recipients demonstrate improved QOL, the gain is less in African-American and female recipients.[23]

Socioeconomic factors

- Married kidney transplant recipients reported higher QOL and satisfaction than single or widowed patients.[24]
- Social support had a positive impact on the QOL in transplant recipients.[25]
- Gainful employment is a boost to a transplant recipient's self-esteem, provides financial stability and insurance coverage, and results in a higher QOL score.

QOL scores were associated with increased mortality and graft failure.[29] In liver transplant recipients, depression is a risk factor for decreased survival.[30]

PREGNANCY IN KIDNEY AND LIVER TRANSPLANT RECIPIENTS

Worldwide, there have been more than 4700 pregnancies reported in kidney transplant recipients and 450 pregnancies in liver recipients.[5,6,31] The National Transplantation Pregnancy Registry (NTPR), established in the United States in 1991, is the longest, continuous study of pregnancy outcomes in solid organ transplant recipients, including those fathered by transplant recipients. Many pregnancy outcomes data presented below are based on NTPR analyses.

Box 2 lists some of the specific considerations that should be addressed in women with transplanted organs who are contemplating pregnancy.

Female Fertility and Contraception After Transplantation

Most women with chronic kidney or liver disease have menstrual abnormalities, amenorrhea, and/or reduced fertility.[32,33] After successful transplantation, there is a rapid return of fertility. However, in a survey of transplant recipients, 44% were unaware that they could become pregnant posttransplant.[34] Because unintended pregnancy puts transplant recipients at greater risk, repeated counseling regarding contraceptive options and pregnancy planning must begin before transplant and continue throughout years of child-bearing potential. Although most methods of contraception are considered safe for use in transplant recipients, long-acting contraceptives, such as intrauterine devices and progesterone implants, are the most effective methods and remain reversible with additional noncontraceptive benefits.[35,36]

Timing of Pregnancy

An interval from transplant to conception is advisable to allow establishment of stable transplant function and reduction of immunosuppression to maintenance levels. NTPR data have shown higher incidences of pregnancy termination and postpartum rejection in pregnancies conceived within 6 months of transplant.[36] The American Society of Transplantation advises delaying conception for at least 1 year after kidney transplantation.[37] Transplant-to-conception intervals of more than 2 years were associated with improved mother and newborn outcomes in liver transplant recipients.[38]

Box 2
Important considerations in pregnancy after transplant

- *The Mother*: Potential for risks to her long-term health, survival, and ability to be a parent.

- *The Graft*: Potential for risks of dysfunction and/or loss related to the pregnancy itself and the potential for changes in drug metabolism during pregnancy that could increase the susceptibility to rejection.

- *The Fetus/Neonate*: High incidences of prematurity and low birth weight. Potential for teratogenic risks associated with immunosuppression and other medications. Some birth defects may comprise subtle developmental changes, which might not become apparent until later in life.

- *Family and Social Issues*: The ability of a parent with a transplant to cope with unexpected illnesses and/or graft dysfunction while child rearing and the impact on the child if the transplanted parent is ill or dies.

Teratogenic Risk of Immunosuppressive Drugs

Immunosuppression is essential to maintain the transplanted organ, thus establishing the safety of these medications during pregnancy is critical. Transplant-maintenance immunosuppressive medications and their pregnancy considerations are shown in **Table 1**.[39–52]

The most common maintenance immunosuppressive regimen is a calcineurin inhibitor (tacrolimus more often than cyclosporine) plus a mycophenolic acid (MPA) product with or without prednisone (see Malat G, Culkin C: The ABCs of Immunosuppression: a primer for primary care physicians, in this issue for a detailed review of immunosuppression in transplantation).

NTPR data and meta-analyses have shown that the incidence of birth defects in infants exposed to prednisone, azathioprine, cyclosporine, and/or tacrolimus in utero is approximately 3% to 5%, which is similar to the general population.[53,54] However, exposure to MPA during pregnancy (mycophenolate mofetil and mycophenolic sodium) shows higher incidences of miscarriages (52% vs 19%) and birth defects (14% vs 6%) compared with pregnancies without MPA exposure.[43] A specific pattern of birth defects, notably microtia (ear anomaly) and facial malformations, has been described in the offspring.[42] Thus, it is recommended that MPA be discontinued 6 weeks before conception. Depending on the recipient and the immunologic history, replacing MPA with azathioprine plus prednisone (or increased prednisone) may be the safest choice for mother and child.[44]

Pregnancy Outcomes in Kidney Transplant Recipients

Maternal and newborn outcomes

Pregnancy outcomes in kidney transplant recipients reporting to the NTPR are listed in **Table 2**.[55] Compared with the general population, kidney recipients are at greater risk for hypertension (54% vs 5%), preeclampsia (27% vs 3.8%), and diabetes (8% vs 3.9%) during pregnancy.[5,56] Hypertension in a kidney recipient is a risk factor for poorer pregnancy outcomes including prematurity and low birth weight. Preeclampsia is difficult to diagnose because many kidney recipients have pre-existing hypertension and proteinuria. Unlike nontransplant pregnancies, changes in urinary protein excretion, plasma urate levels, platelet count, or liver function tests are not as useful as markers for either the onset or the severity of preeclampsia.[57] The NTPR has reported up to 10% of kidney transplant recipients on calcineurin inhibitors required insulin during pregnancy. Optimal glucose control is desired especially in the first trimester given the association between gestational diabetes and birth defects.[58]

Infections (commonly urinary tract infections) are of concern because of the immunocompromised status of pregnant transplant recipient and routine urine cultures are recommended. Maternal to fetal transmission of infections, such as cytomegalovirus, can result in hearing/vision loss and mental retardation, hence maternal screening is vital.[59]

Approximately 75% of pregnancies in kidney recipients result in a live birth.[5,31,36,55] Kidney recipients, on average, deliver 1 month early, with a preterm (<37 weeks) delivery rate of 50% and mean birth weight of approximately 2500 g. Reports to the NTPR evaluating recipient and newborn variables do not reveal significant differences in the outcomes of pregnancies in living donor, deceased donor, and repeat transplantation; however, African American ethnicity is a risk factor for poorer pregnancy outcomes.[36,60,61]

Graft function

Pregnancy does not seem to cause deterioration of kidney graft function when pre-pregnancy function is stable.[62,63] Women with impaired transplant function before pregnancy (ie, serum creatinine >1.5 mg/dL, >133 μmol/L) have a greater likelihood

Table 1
Common maintenance immunosuppressive medications and pregnancy

Medication	Food and Drug Administration Category[a]	Special Comments
Prednisone	C	In utero exposure results in fetal malformation rate of 3.5%, similar to general population.[39] The reported association between steroid exposure and oral cleft has not been confirmed by later clinical reports.[40,41]
MPA: mycophenolate mofetil (CellCept), enteric-coated mycophenolate sodium (Myfortic)	D	Higher incidence of miscarriages and birth defects. Specific pattern of birth defects, notably microtia (ear anomaly) and facial malformations.[42–44] Contraception should be used while taking MPA. MPA should be discontinued 6 wk before conception. Replacing MPA with azathioprine has proven an effective alternative in many cases.[44]
Azathioprine (Imuran)	D	Azathioprine is currently considered a safe option for maintenance immunosuppression during pregnancy; usual dose range 0.5–1.5 mg/kg/d. Although listed as pregnancy category D, clinical data do not support teratogenic potential. Infants exposed to azathioprine have an increased risk of growth restriction and preterm delivery.[45]
Calcineurin inhibitors: cyclosporine (Sandimmune, Neoral, Gengraf), tacrolimus (Prograf, Advagraf, Astragraf XL, Hecoria)	C	The incidence of birth defects in kidney recipients on calcineurin inhibitors without adjunctive use of MPA products is similar to the general population, without any predominant pattern of malformations.[46–48]
Sirolimus (Rapamune)	C	Data are limited. To date, reports have not shown that exposure to sirolimus during pregnancy is associated with an increased risk or a pattern of birth defects.[49,50] Risk for infertility in men.[51]
Everolimus (Zortress)	C	Very limited data on pregnancy outcomes, but not an absolute contraindication.[52]
Belatacept (Nulojix)	C	Very limited pregnancy data available.

Former Category C: Animal reproduction studies have shown an adverse effect on the fetus and there are no adequate and well-controlled studies in humans, but potential benefits may warrant use of the drug in pregnant women despite potential risks.

Former Category D: there is positive evidence of human fetal risk based on adverse reaction data from investigational or marketing experience or studies in humans, but potential benefits may warrant use of the drug in pregnant women despite potential risks.

[a] These categories will soon be replaced with a narrative risk summary providing more detailed data to help providers in counseling female and male patients of reproductive potential.

Table 2
NTPR: pregnancy outcomes in female kidney transplant recipients

	Azathioprine and/or Prednisone[a]	Cyclosporine-based[b]	Tacrolimus-based[b]
Recipients	243	482	254
Maternal factors (n = pregnancies)	448	822	427
Mean transplant-to-conception interval, y	6.8 ± 4.9	4.7 ± 3.5	4.8 ± 3.3
Hypertension during pregnancy, %	25	60	53
Diabetes during pregnancy, %	5	9	9
Infection during pregnancy, %	16	21	20
Preeclampsia, %	22	32	35
Rejection episode during pregnancy, %[c]	1	1	2
Mean serum creatinine, mg/dL			
Before pregnancy	1.1 ± 0.4	1.4 ± 0.4	1.2 ± 0.3
During pregnancy	1.2 ± 0.5	1.4 ± 0.6	1.3 ± 0.9
After pregnancy	1.2 ± 0.6	1.5 ± 0.8	1.3 ± 0.5
Graft loss within 2 y of delivery, %	4	7	9
Outcomes, n[d]	463	852	439
Terminations, %	4	5	2.3
Miscarriages, %	12	16	24.4
Ectopic, %	1	1	0.5
Stillborn, %	2	2	1.4
Live births, %	81	76	71.5
Live births, n	374	645	314
Mean gestational age, wk	36.4 ± 3.3	35.8 ± 3.4	35.4 ± 3.6
Premature (<37 wk), %	47	52	52
Mean birthweight, g	2734 ± 718	2507 ± 749	2522 ± 821
Low birthweight (<2500 g), %	35	44	42
Cesarean section, %	51	51	58
Newborn complications, %	37	42	52
Birth defects, %	2.2	4	8
Neonatal deaths, n (%) (within 30 d of birth)	6 (1.3)	11 (1.7)[e]	5 (1.6)

Cyclosporine-based regimens (brand name or generic formulations of cyclosporine and cyclosporine, USP modified) and tacrolimus-based regimens (brand name and generic formulations of tacrolimus and brand name tacrolimus extended release); regimens may include azathioprine or MPA and/or prednisone.

[a] No calcineurin inhibitor.
[b] MPA exposure during pregnancy: cyclosporine (4%), tacrolimus (23%).
[c] Biopsy-proven acute rejection only.
[d] Includes multiple births.
[e] Includes 24-wk quadruplet pregnancy; all newborns died.

Data from National Transplantation Pregnancy Registry. 2014 annual report. Philadelphia: Gift of Life Institute; 2015.

of graft dysfunction during and after pregnancy with poor newborn outcomes.[64] An upward trend in serum creatinine during pregnancy warrants prompt investigation. Because serum creatinine normally decreases during pregnancy as a result of increased glomerular filtration rate, rejection during gestation may be signaled by only a minor increase in serum creatinine.

Immunosuppressive drug levels need to be closely monitored during pregnancy, and doses may be adjusted, because drug blood concentrations are likely to decrease from increased metabolism and volume of distribution.[36]

The acute rejection rate during pregnancy reported in the NTPR ranges from 1% to 4% and is comparable with nonpregnant transplant recipients.[5,55] Similarly, graft loss within 2 years of delivery does not seem to be precipitated by pregnancy.[36]

Pregnancy Outcomes in Liver Transplant Recipients

Maternal and newborn outcomes

Pregnancy outcomes in liver transplant recipients are listed in **Table 3**.[55] Compared with the general population, liver recipients have higher incidences of hypertension (27% vs 5%), preeclampsia (22% vs 3.8%), and diabetes (5% vs 3.9%) during pregnancy.[6,56] In contrast to kidney recipients, pregnancies in liver transplant recipients are characterized by lower incidences of hypertension during pregnancy and preeclampsia, without significant differences in gestational diabetes.[6,65]

The live birth rate in female liver recipients is 75%, similar to kidney recipients. However, the gestational age and birth weight are higher for liver recipients compared with kidney transplant recipients, with same incidence of birth defects.[6,55,65,66]

Graft function

Most pregnancies in liver recipients seem to be well tolerated with no apparent adverse effects on graft function. However, pruritus and cholestasis occur frequently during pregnancy. The HELLP syndrome (hemolysis, elevated liver enzymes, low platelets) occurs in 0.8% of all pregnancies, but was evident in 8% of liver recipients in a small study of 38 pregnancies.[67] Acute rejection needs to be considered and differentiated from other conditions. In a meta-analysis, the incidence of acute rejection during pregnancy ranged between 2% and 17%, which is significantly higher than in kidney recipients.[6] Rejection is diagnosed and managed as in nonpregnant recipients with similar success in controlling the acute process. Acute rejection during pregnancy is a risk factor for low birth weight and preterm birth.[68] An NTPR analysis of 161 liver recipients showed that acute rejection during pregnancy is the strongest risk factor for graft loss within 5 years of delivery, followed by younger age at the time of conception.[66] The outcomes for pregnancy after living donor liver transplantation are comparable with those after deceased donor liver transplantation.[69]

Labor and Delivery and Postnatal Care

A higher incidence of cesarean sections has been reported in kidney and liver transplant recipients than in the general population.[5,6,36,55] However, cesarean section should be performed for obstetric indications only. Immunosuppression must not be interrupted during labor and delivery.

Most oral maintenance immunosuppression drugs are easily absorbed and treatment can be resumed shortly after cesarean section. Practitioners should be aware of postpartum depression among transplant recipients and the risk of medication nonadherence. Also, changes in immunosuppressive drug metabolism occur during pregnancy and peripartum. Therefore, continued close monitoring of immunosuppressive levels and transplant function is warranted for several months postpartum.[36]

Table 3
NTPR: pregnancy outcomes in female liver transplant recipients

	Cyclosporine-based[a]	Tacrolimus-based[a]
Recipients	97	127
Maternal factors (n = pregnancies)	183	226
Mean transplant-to-conception interval, y	6.9 ± 6.2	6.8 ± 5.4
Hypertension during pregnancy, %	35	17
Diabetes during pregnancy, %	1	13
Infection during pregnancy, %	30	15
Preeclampsia, %	24	22
Rejection episode during pregnancy, %	6	3
Graft loss within 2 y of delivery, %	5	4
Outcomes, n[b]	186	237
Terminations, %	7	2
Miscarriages, %	14	26
Ectopic pregnancy, %	0.5	1
Stillbirths, %	1.6	1
Live births, %	76.9	70
Live births, n	143	167
Mean gestational age, wk	36.9 ± 3.3	36.2 ± 3.6
Premature (<37 wk), %	35	44
Mean birthweight, g	2735 ± 727	2729 ± 826
Low birthweight (<2500 g), %	29	31
Cesarean section, %	41	49
Newborn complications, %	29	40
Birth defects, %	4.2	4.0
Neonatal deaths (%) (within 30 d of birth)	1 (0.7)	1 (0.6)

Cyclosporine-based regimens (brand name or generic formulations of cyclosporine and cyclosporine, USP modified) and tacrolimus-based regimens (brand name and generic formulations of tacrolimus and brand name tacrolimus extended release); regimens may include azathioprine or MPA and/or prednisone.
[a] MPA exposure during pregnancy: cyclosporine (1%), tacrolimus (9%).
[b] Includes multiple births.
Data from National Transplantation Pregnancy Registry. 2014 annual report. Philadelphia: Gift of Life Institute; 2015.

Breastfeeding

Whether recipients should breastfeed while on immunosuppression remains unresolved. Recent studies reveal that not all immunosuppressive exposure translates to risk for the infant; that the exposure in utero is greater than via breast milk; and that no lingering effects from breastfeeding have been found to date in the infants who were breastfed while their mother were taking prednisone, azathioprine, cyclosporine, or tacrolimus. To allay any possible concerns, infant blood levels of immunosuppressive medications could be tested.[70]

A review of breastfeeding practices among NTPR participants shows an increasing trend in the number of recipients choosing to breastfed their infants while on immunosuppression (10% in 1990s to 50% in 2014).[55] For such drugs as MPA, sirolimus, everolimus, and belatacept, there are insufficient data from which to assess safety of breastfeeding.[70]

Management Options

An analysis of NTPR data along with a literature review assisted the NTPR investigators in creating management guidelines for pregnant transplant recipients (**Box 3**). The guidelines, derived primarily from studies of the kidney transplant recipient pregnancies, are in large part applicable to other organ recipient groups.

Box 3
Pregnancy after transplantation: management options

Prepregnancy

Patients should defer conception for at least 1 year after transplantation, with adequate contraception

Assessment of graft function (organ specific)
- Maintenance immunosuppression options
- Recent biopsy
- Proteinuria
- Hepatitis B and C status; consider treatment before conception
- Cytomegalovirus, toxoplasmosis, herpes simplex status

The effect of comorbid conditions (ie, diabetes, hypertension) should be considered and their management optimized; nonkidney recipients should have their baseline kidney function and proteinuria assessed

Vaccinations should be given if needed (ie, rubella vaccine before transplantation)

Explore cause of original disease; discuss genetic issues if relevant

Discuss the effect of pregnancy on graft function

Discuss the risks of intrauterine growth restriction, prematurity, low birthweight

Prenatal

Accurate early diagnosis and dating of pregnancy

Clinical and laboratory monitoring of functional status of transplanted organ and immunosuppressive drug levels every 4 weeks until 32 weeks, then every 2 weeks until 36 weeks, and then weekly until delivery

Monthly urine culture

Graft dysfunction may require biopsy

Surveillance for bacterial or viral presence (eg, cytomegalovirus, toxoplasmosis, hepatitis)

Fetal surveillance

Monitor for hypertension and proteinuria

Surveillance for preeclampsia

Screening for gestational diabetes

Labor and delivery

Vaginal delivery is optimal; cesarean delivery for obstetric reasons

Postnatal

Intensive monitoring of immunosuppressive drug levels for at least 3 months postpartum, especially if dosages increased during pregnancy

Monitor graft function closely; graft dysfunction may require biopsy

Breastfeeding discussion

Contraception counseling

Table 4
NTPR: Selected pregnancies fathered by male transplant recipients

	Kidney	Liver
Number of recipients	623	82
Pregnancies	973	131
Outcomes[a]	992	138
Live births, %	92	86
Mean gestational age, wk	39.1 ± 2.2	39.1 ± 1.9
Mean birthweight, g	3337	3182
Newborn complications, %	17	17
Birth defects, %	3	3.9

[a] Includes multiple births.
Data from National Transplantation Pregnancy Registry. 2014 annual report. Philadelphia: Gift of Life Institute; 2015.

Male Transplant Recipients and Parenthood

Male sexuality and fertility are adversely affected by chronic organ failure.[71] Successful kidney transplantation improves reproductive function quickly after the surgery, enabling male transplant recipients to father children.[72] Increase in libido and improvement of reproductive function after transplant have also been reported in liver recipients.[73] Sirolimus has been shown to impair fertility in male transplant recipients, with a decreased proportion of motile spermatozoa and decreased rates of impregnation.[51]

Overall, the outcomes of pregnancies fathered by transplant recipients seem similar to those of the general population. Outcomes of pregnancies fathered by male kidney and liver recipients are shown in **Table 4**.[55] Pregnancies fathered by recipients taking MPA do not confer the same risks as those seen in the pregnancies of female recipients taking MPA. In a study of 205 pregnancies fathered while the recipient was taking MPA, the incidence of birth defects was 3.1%, similar to the general population, and without any specific pattern of malformation.[74]

Long-Term Follow-Up of Offspring

Overall, participants in the NTPR have reported that their children are healthy and developing well.[55] Other reports demonstrate that children of transplant recipients have comparable neurologic development to control subjects.[75,76]

Continued surveillance and long-term follow-up is warranted to discern any effects of in utero exposure to immunosuppression on the reproductive or immune systems of successive generations.

SUMMARY

Transplantation is the established therapy for end-stage organ failure and results in improved functional status, HR-QOL, and reproductive health. Addressing mental, physical, and social well-being leads to better patient satisfaction and increased compliance, which can increase overall graft and recipient survival. A close partnership among transplant hospitals, rehabilitation centers, and primary care physicians could help posttransplant recovery and successful reintegration of transplant recipients into society.

Successful transplantation improves reproductive health by restoring fertility warranting the discussion of contraception beginning pretransplant and continuing afterward to avoid unplanned pregnancies. Thousands of successful pregnancies after transplantation have been reported and the overall outcomes for parent and child are encouraging. In female transplant recipients, one class of immunosuppressive drugs, MPA products, has been shown to result in an increased incidence of miscarriage and an increased incidence and a specific pattern of birth defects. With the constant advent of new developments and modifications in immunosuppressive regimens, clinicians are responsible for providing pregnancy counseling in all pretransplant and posttransplant patients of childbearing age. Continued close collaboration between transplant personnel and primary care providers will help to identify potential pregnancy risks in transplant recipients. Therefore, centers and health professionals are encouraged to report all pregnancy exposures in transplant recipients to the NTPR.

ACKNOWLEDGMENTS

The authors thank Dawn P. Armenti, BA, Lisa A. Coscia, RN, BSN, CCTC, and Carolyn H. McGrory, MS, RN, for their assistance with the preparation of this article. The National Transplantation Pregnancy Registry acknowledges the co-operation of transplant recipients and the personnel in over 250 centers in North America who have contributed their time and information to the National Transplantation Pregnancy Registry.

REFERENCES

1. Matas AJ, Smith JM, Skeans MA, et al. OPTN/SRTR 2013 annual data report: kidney. Am J Transplant 2015;15(Suppl 2):1–34.
2. Kim WR, Lake JR, Smith JM, et al. OPTN/SRTR 2013 annual data report: liver. Am J Transplant 2015;15(Suppl 2):1–28.
3. Murray JE, Reid DE, Harrison JH, et al. Successful pregnancies after human renal transplantation. N Engl J Med 1963;269:341–3.
4. Walcott WO, Derick DE, Jolley JJ, et al. Successful pregnancy in a liver transplant patient. Am J Obstet Gynecol 1978;132(3):340–1.
5. Deshpande NA, James NT, Kucirka LM, et al. Pregnancy outcomes in kidney transplant recipients: a systematic review and meta-analysis. Am J Transplant 2011;11(11):2388–404.
6. Deshpande NA, James NT, Kucirka LM, et al. Pregnancy outcomes of liver transplant recipients: a systematic review and meta-analysis. Liver Transpl 2012;18(6):621–9.
7. Campagna F, Montagnese S, Schiff S, et al. Cognitive impairment and electroencephalographic alterations before and after liver transplantation: what is reversible? Liver Transpl 2014;20(8):977–86.
8. Griva K, Thompson D, Jayasena D, et al. Cognitive functioning pre- to post-kidney transplantation: a prospective study. Nephrol Dial Transplant 2006;21(11):3275–82.
9. Pinson CW, Feurer ID, Payne JL, et al. Health-related quality of life after different types of solid organ transplantation. Ann Surg 2000;232(4):597–607.
10. Mosconi G, Cuna V, Tonioli M, et al. Physical activity in solid organ transplant recipients: preliminary results of the Italian project. Kidney Blood Press Res 2014;39(2–3):220–7.
11. Patcai JT, Disotto-Monastero MP, Gomez M, et al. Inpatient rehabilitation outcomes in solid organ transplantation: results of a unique partnership between

the rehabilitation hospital and the multi-organ transplant unit in an acute hospital. Open J Ther Rehabil 2013;1(2):52–61.

12. Tzvetanov I, D'Amico G, Walczak D, et al. High rate of unemployment after kidney transplantation: analysis of the United Network for Organ Sharing database. Transplant Proc 2014;46(5):1290–4.

13. Saab S, Wiese C, Ibrahim AB, et al. Employment and quality of life in liver transplant recipients. Liver Transpl 2007;13(9):1330–8.

14. Weng LC, Chen HC, Huang HL, et al. Change in the type of work of postoperative liver transplant patients. Transplant Proc 2012;44(2):544–7.

15. Joseph JT, Baines LS, Morris MC, et al. Quality of life after kidney and pancreas transplantation: a review. Am J Kidney Dis 2003;42(3):431–45.

16. Matas AJ, Halbert RJ, Barr ML, et al. Life satisfaction and adverse effects in renal transplant recipients: a longitudinal analysis. Clin Transplant 2002;16(2):113–21.

17. Muehrer RJ, Becker BN. Life after transplantation: new transitions in quality of life and psychological distress. Semin Dial 2005;18(2):124–31.

18. Yang LS, Shan LL, Saxena A, et al. Liver transplantation: a systematic review of long-term quality of life. Liver Int 2014;34(9):1298–313.

19. Valderrabano F, Jofre R, Lopez-Gomez JM. Quality of life in end-stage renal disease patients. Am J Kidney Dis 2001;38(3):443–64.

20. Hathaway D, Winsett R, Prendergast M, et al. The first report from the Patient Outcomes Registry for Transplant Effects on Life (PORTEL): differences in side-effects and quality of life by organ type, time since transplant and immunosuppressive regimens. Clin Transplant 2003;17(3):183–94.

21. Kugler C, Gottlieb J, Warnecke G, et al. Health-related quality of life after solid organ transplantation: a prospective, multiorgan cohort study. Transplantation 2013;96(3):316–23.

22. Cukor D, Rosenthal DS, Jindal RM, et al. Depression is an important contributor to low medication adherence in hemodialyzed patients and transplant recipients. Kidney Int 2009;75(11):1223–9.

23. Johnson CD, Wicks MN, Milstead J, et al. Racial and gender differences in quality of life following kidney transplantation. Image J Nurs Sch 1998;30(2):125–30.

24. Yildirim A. The importance of patient satisfaction and health-related quality of life after renal transplantation. Transplant Proc 2006;38(9):2831–4.

25. Cetingok M, Hathaway D, Winsett R. Contribution of post-transplant social support to the quality of life of transplant recipients. Soc Work Health Care 2007; 45(3):39–56.

26. Dew MA, Switzer GE, Goycoolea JM, et al. Does transplantation produce quality of life benefits? A quantitative analysis of the literature. Transplantation 1997; 64(9):1261–73.

27. Overbeck I, Bartels M, Decker O, et al. Changes in quality of life after renal transplantation. Transplant Proc 2005;37(3):1618–21.

28. Czyzewski L, Sanko-Resmer J, Wyzgal J, et al. Assessment of health-related quality of life of patients after kidney transplantation in comparison with hemodialysis and peritoneal dialysis. Am J Transplant 2014;19:576–85.

29. Griva K, Davenport A, Newman SP. Health-related quality of life and long-term survival and graft failure in kidney transplantation: a 12-year follow-up study. Transplantation 2013;95(5):740–9.

30. Rogal SS, Dew MA, Fontes P, et al. Early treatment of depressive symptoms and long-term survival after liver transplantation. Am J Transplant 2013;13(4):928–35.

31. Wyld ML, Clayton PA, Jesudason S, et al. Pregnancy outcomes for kidney transplant recipients. Am J Transplant 2013;13(12):3173–82.

32. Holley JL, Schmidt RJ, Bender FH, et al. Gynecologic and reproductive issues in women on dialysis. Am J Kidney Dis 1997;29(5):685–90.
33. Cundy TF, O'Grady JG, Williams R. Recovery of menstruation and pregnancy after liver transplantation. Gut 1990;31(3):337–8.
34. French VA, Davis JS, Sayles HS, et al. Contraception and fertility awareness among women with solid organ transplants. Obstet Gynecol 2013;122(4):809–14.
35. Krajewski CM, Geetha D, Gomez-Lobo V. Contraceptive options for women with a history of solid-organ transplantation. Transplantation 2013;95(10):1183–6.
36. Constantinescu S, Gomez-Lobo V, Davison JM, et al. Pregnancy and contraception in transplantation. In: Kirk AD, Knechtle SJ, Larsen CP, et al, editors. Textbook of organ transplantation, vol. 97. London: Wiley-Blackwell; 2014. p. 1161–78.
37. McKay DB, Josephson MA, Armenti VT, et al. Reproduction and transplantation: report on the AST consensus conference on reproductive issues and transplantation. Am J Transplant 2005;5(7):1592–9.
38. Coscia LA, Constantinescu S, Moritz MJ, et al. Report from the National Transplantation Pregnancy Registry (NTPR): outcomes of pregnancy after transplantation. Clin Transplant 2009;103–22.
39. Fraser FC, Sajoo A. Teratogenic potential of corticosteroids in humans. Teratology 1995;51(1):45–6.
40. Park-Wyllie L, Mazzotta P, Pastuszak A, et al. Birth defects after maternal exposure to corticosteroids: prospective cohort study and meta-analysis of epidemiological studies. Teratology 2000;62(6):385–92.
41. Hviid A, Molgaard-Nielsen D. Corticosteroid use during pregnancy and risk of orofacial clefts. CMAJ 2011;183(7):796–804.
42. Sifontis NM, Coscia LA, Constantinescu S, et al. Pregnancy outcomes in solid organ transplant recipients with exposure to mycophenolate mofetil or sirolimus. Transplantation 2006;82(12):1698–702.
43. Constantinescu S, Axelrod P, Coscia LA, et al. Pregnancy outcomes in kidney recipients who discontinued mycophenolic acid products prior to conception. J Am Soc Nephrol 2013;24:861A [abstract].
44. Coscia LA, Armenti DP, King RW, et al. Update on the teratogenicity of mycophenolate mofetil. J Pediatr Genet 2015;4(2):42–5.
45. Cleary BJ, Kallen B. Early pregnancy azathioprine use and pregnancy outcomes. Birth Defects Res A Clin Mol Teratol 2009;85(7):647–54.
46. Armenti VT, Ahlswede KM, Ahlswede BA, et al. National Transplantation Pregnancy Registry: outcomes of 154 pregnancies in cyclosporine-treated female kidney transplant recipients. Transplantation 1994;57(4):502–6.
47. Bar Oz B, Hackman R, Einarson T, et al. Pregnancy outcome after cyclosporine therapy during pregnancy: a meta-analysis. Transplantation 2001;71(8):1051–5.
48. Kainz A, Harabacz I, Cowlrick IS, et al. Review of the course and outcome of 100 pregnancies in 84 women treated with tacrolimus. Transplantation 2000;70(12):1718–21.
49. Framarino dei Malatesta M, Corona LE, De Luca L, et al. Successful pregnancy in a living-related kidney transplant recipient who received sirolimus throughout the whole gestation. Transplantation 2011;91(9):e69–71.
50. Jankowska I, Oldakowska-Jedynak U, Jabiry-Zieniewicz Z, et al. Absence of teratogenicity of sirolimus used during early pregnancy in a liver transplant recipient. Transplant Proc 2004;36(10):3232–3.
51. Zuber J, Anglicheau D, Elie C, et al. Sirolimus may reduce fertility in male renal transplant recipients. Am J Transplant 2008;8(7):1471–9.

52. Veroux M, Corona D, Veroux P. Pregnancy under everolimus-based immunosuppression. Transpl Int 2011;24(12):e115–7.
53. Centers for Disease Control and Prevention (CDC). Update on overall prevalence of major birth defects—Atlanta, Georgia, 1978-2005. MMWR Morb Mortal Wkly Rep 2008;57(1):1–5.
54. Coscia LA, Constantinescu S, Davison JM, et al. Immunosuppressive drugs and fetal outcome. Best Pract Res Clin Obstet Gynaecol 2014;28(8):1174–87.
55. National Transplantation Pregnancy Registry (NTPR). 2014 annual report. Philadelphia: Gift of Life Institute; 2015.
56. Martin JA, Hamilton BE, Ventura SJ, et al. Births: final data for 2010. Natl Vital Stat Rep 2012;61(1):1–72.
57. Davison JM. Pregnancy in renal allograft recipients: problems, prognosis and practicalities. Baillieres Clin Obstet Gynaecol 1994;8(2):501–25.
58. Correa A, Gilboa SM, Besser LM, et al. Diabetes mellitus and birth defects. Am J Obstet Gynecol 2008;199(3):237.e1–9.
59. McKay DB, Josephson MA. Pregnancy after kidney transplantation. Clin J Am Soc Nephrol 2008;3(Suppl 2):S117–25.
60. Constantinescu S, Axelrod P, Coscia LA, et al. Pregnancy outcomes in kidney recipients after retransplantation. Am J Transplant 2012;12(Suppl 3):155 [abstract]. A430.
61. Constantinescu S, Coscia L, Armenti D, et al. Pregnancy outcomes in female kidney transplant recipients: does ethnicity have an influence? Am J Transplant 2015;15(Suppl 3) [abstract].
62. First MR, Combs CA, Weiskittel P, et al. Lack of effect of pregnancy on renal allograft survival or function. Transplantation 1995;59(4):472–6.
63. Sturgiss SN, Davison JM. Effect of pregnancy on the long-term function of renal allografts: an update. Am J Kidney Dis 1995;26(1):54–6.
64. Armenti VT, Ahlswede KM, Ahlswede BA, et al. Variables affecting birthweight and graft survival in 197 pregnancies in cyclosporine-treated female kidney transplant recipients. Transplantation 1995;59(4):476–9.
65. Blume C, Pischke S, von Versen-Hoynck F, et al. Pregnancies in liver and kidney transplant recipients: a review of the current literature and recommendation. Best Pract Res Clin Obstet Gynaecol 2014;28(8):1123–36.
66. Coscia LA, Davison JM, Moritz MJ, et al. Pregnancy after liver transplantation. In: Doria C, editor. Contemporary liver transplantation. Switzerland: Springer International; 2015. p. 1–20.
67. Nagy S, Bush MC, Berkowitz R, et al. Pregnancy outcome in liver transplant recipients. Obstet Gynecol 2003;102(1):121–8.
68. Armenti VT, Herrine SK, Radomski JS, et al. Pregnancy after liver transplantation. Liver Transpl 2000;6(6):671–85.
69. Kubo S, Uemoto S, Furukawa H, et al. Pregnancy outcomes after living donor liver transplantation: results from a Japanese survey. Liver Transpl 2014;20(5):576–83.
70. Constantinescu S, Pai A, Coscia LA, et al. Breast-feeding after transplantation. Best Pract Res Clin Obstet Gynaecol 2014;28(8):1163–73.
71. Holdsworth S, Atkins RC, de Kretser DM. The pituitary-testicular axis in men with chronic renal failure. N Engl J Med 1977;296(22):1245–9.
72. Handelsman DJ, McDowell IF, Caterson ID, et al. Testicular function after renal transplantation: comparison of cyclosporin A with azathioprine and prednisone combination regimes. Clin Nephrol 1984;22(3):144–8.
73. Madersbacher S, Ludvik G, Stulnig T, et al. The impact of liver transplantation on endocrine status in men. Clin Endocrinol (Oxf) 1996;44(4):461–6.

74. Jones A, Clary MJ, McDermott E, et al. Outcomes of pregnancies fathered by solid-organ transplant recipients exposed to mycophenolic acid products. Prog Transplant 2013;23(2):153–7.
75. Schreiber-Zamora J, Kociszewska-Najman B, Borek-Dzieciol B, et al. Neurological development of children born to liver transplant recipients. Transplant Proc 2014; 46(8):2798–801.
76. Nulman I, Sgro M, Barrera M, et al. Long-term neurodevelopment of children exposed in utero to cyclosporine after maternal renal transplant. Paediatr Drugs 2010;12(2):113–22.

Index

A

Acarbose, 541, 543
Acetaminophen toxicity, transplantation for, 453–454
Acute cellular rejection
   in kidney transplantation, 494–495
   in liver transplantation, 479–480
Acute Kidney Injury Network staging system, 489–490
Acute rejection, of kidney allograft, 496–497
Acute tubular necrosis, in kidney transplantation, 492–493
Acyclovir, prophylactic, 594–595
Age factors
   in living donor, 601, 603
   in transplant recipient, 469–470
Alanine aminotransferase, in liver allograft dysfunction, 478
Albiglutide, 542–544
Albumin level, in MELD score, 451
Albuminuria, in kidney allograft dysfunction, 489
Alcohol abuse, 460, 481, 577
Alemuzmab, 439, 512
ALERT (Lescol in Renal Transplantation) Trial, 526–527
Alkaline phosphatase, 478, 576
Allograft dysfunction
   in kidney transplantation, **487–503**
      causes of, 488–489
      diagnosis of, 488–491
      early (up to 6 months), 491–496
      later, 496–499
      symptoms of, 488
   in liver transplantation, **477–486**
      causes of, 478
      definition of, 478
      differential diagnosis of, 478–482
      monitoring of, 482
      recurrence of, 482
      treatment of, 483–484
Allopurinol, 510
Alogliptin, 542–543
Alpha-glucosidase inhibitors, 541, 543
Alport syndrome, 470
American Association for the Study of Liver Diseases guidelines, 453–454
American College of Cardiology, coronary artery disease guidelines of, 468–469

Med Clin N Am 100 (2016) 631–645
http://dx.doi.org/10.1016/S0025-7125(16)33781-6
0025-7125/16/$ – see front matter © 2016 Elsevier Inc. All rights reserved.

medical.theclinics.com

American Heart Association, coronary artery disease guidelines of, 468–469

Anemia, 510, 527

Angiography, for renal artery stenosis, 497

Angiotensin receptor blockers, 524

Angiotensin-converting enzyme inhibitors, 523–524

Animal studies, 440

Anogenital cancer, 554, 560

Anti lymphocyte globulin, history of, 441

Anti proliferative agents, 509–511, 538

Antibiotics, 513
    drug interactions of, 509
    prophylactic, after transplantation, 594–595

Antibody-mediated rejection, in kidney transplantation, 494–495, 497

Anticonvulsants, 510

Antifungal agents, 509, 513

Anti-glomerular basement membrane disease, 470

Antihypertensives, 513

Antimetabolites, 509–510

Antineutrophil cytoplasmic antibody vasculitis, 470

Antithymocyte antibodies, 512

Anxiety, 514

Art, Surgery and Transplantation, 439

Ascites, in MELD score, 451

Aspartate aminotransferase, in liver allograft dysfunction, 478

Aspergillosis, 593

Atorvastatin, 526

Autoimmune hepatitis, 454, 481

Avascular necrosis, 574, 581

Azathioprine, 509–510
    bone disease and, 575
    history of, 439, 441, 506
    in pregnancy, 618–620
    side effects of, 516

B

Banff criteria, 492–493

Basal cell carcinoma, 553–555

B-cell lymphomas, 555–556

Belatecept, 439, 511–512, 516
    diabetes mellitus due to, 539
    in pregnancy, 618

Beltzer, Folkert, 442

Beta blockers, 513, 524

Bile leaks, in liver transplantation, 479, 483

Biliary complications, after liver transplantation, 479

Biliary obstruction, after liver transplantation, 483–484

Bilirubin level, in MELD score, 451

Bilomas, after liver transplantation, 479

Biomarkers, bone, 576

Biopsy
   bone, 577
     572
   of kidney allograft, 491, 497
Bisphosphonates, 580–581
BK virus nephropathy, 493, 593
Bladder, cancer of, 558–559
Bladder dysfunction, in kidney allograft, 494
Bone densitometry, 576
Bone loss. *See* Metabolic bone disease.
Borel, Jean, 439, 506
Bortezimib, 445
Breast cancer, 560
Breastfeeding, 622
Brescia, Michael, 438

C

Calcidiol, 580
Calcineurin, action of, 507
Calcineurin inhibitors
   bone disease due to, 574
   diabetes mellitus due to, 538–539
   drug interactions with, 507, 509
   in pregnancy, 618–619
   mechanism of action of, 506–507, 509
   nephrotoxicity of, 498–499, 507, 509
Calcitonin, 579–580
Calcitriol, 580
Calcium, supplementation of, 577–578
Calcium channel blockers, 509, 513, 523–524
Calne, Roy, 439, 441
Canagliflozin, 542, 544
Cancer. *See* Malignancies.
Cannon, Jack, 439
Cardiac catheterization, 468–469
Cardiomyopathy, 468–469
Cardiovascular disease, **519–533**
   epidemiology of, 520–521
   in immunosuppressive therapy, 515, 517
   in kidney transplantation, 467–469
   risk factors for, 521–529
Cardiovascular examination, 457–458
Carotid arteries, stenosis of, 469
Carrel, Alex, 436, 505
Casts, in kidney allograft dysfunction, 490
Cerebrovascular disease, 469
Cervical cancer, 560
Child-Turcotte-Pugh score, for liver transplantation decisions, 449–451

Cholangiocarcinoma, transplantation for, 456
Cholangitis, 593
Cholestasis, bone disease in, 572
Chronic allograft nephropathy, 498–499
Chronic kidney disease, transplantation for, **465–476**
    evaluation for, 466–475
    kidney allocation system for, 465–466
    wait list for, 466
Chronic Kidney Disease Epidemiology Collaboration equation, 488–489
Cimino, James, 438
Cinacalcet, 580
Ciprofloxacin, 513
Cirrhosis, transplantation for, 454–455
Citalopram, 514
Claudication, 469
Clonidine, 524
Coagulopathy, in MELD score, 451
Cognitive function, after transplantation, 614
Cold remedies, 514
Collaborative Transplant Study, 522
Colorectal cancer, 554, 559
Computed tomography
    for bone density, 576–577
    for kidney allograft dysfunction, 490–491, 494
Congestive heart failure, 521
Constant region (Fc), of antibodies, 512
Contraception, after transplantation, 617
Contraindications, to kidney transplantation, 466
Conversion immunosuppression, 515
Coronary artery disease, 457–458, 468–469
Corticosteroids, 511
    avoidance of, 579
    bone disease due to, 573–574, 579
    diabetes mellitus due to, 538
    history of, 439
    side effects of, 516, 527–529
Costimulation blockade, 511–512
C-reactive protein, 527
Creatinine level, in kidney transplantation, 488, 496
C-terminal telopeptide of type 1 collagen, 576
Cyclosporine
    bone disease due to, 574
    diabetes mellitus due to, 538–539
    history of, 439, 506
    in pregnancy, 618–620
    mechanism of action of, 507–509
    side effects of, 495–496, 516, 527–529
Cystitis, 592
Cytomegalovirus infections, 480, 483–484, 592–594
Cytotoxic T-lymphocyte 4, 511–512

D

Dapagliflozin, 542
Decompensation, MELD score in, 454
Dehydroepiandrosterone, 579
Delayed allograft function, in kidney transplantation, 492–493
Denosumab, 580–581
Dense deposit disease, 470
Depression, 514
Desensitization, 473
Detemir, 541
Diabetes mellitus, **535–550**
    after transplantation, 523–524
    bone disease in, 571
    groups of, 537
    in living donors, 604
    new-onset after transplant (NODAT), 515, 523–524, **535–550**
        bone disease in, 575
        definition of, 537–538
        diagnosis of, 537–538
        immunosuppressive drugs and, 538–539
        risk factors for, 538
        treatment of, 539–545
Dipeptidyl peptidase-4 inhibitors, 543–544
Domino transplantation, liver, 443
Donation Service Areas, 452
Donors
    for transplantation, 442–444
    infections in, 590
    living, 442–444, **599–613**
Doppler studies, of carotid arteries, 469
Drug(s)
    bone disease due to, 571
    hepatotoxicity of, 482–483
Drug abuse, 460, 472
Dual energy x-ray absorptiometry (DEXA), 576–577
Dulaglutide, 543–544
Dyslipidemia, 514, 524–526

E

Echocardiography, 457–458, 469
Elion, Gertrude, 506
Empagliflozin, 542, 544
Employment, after transplantation, 615
Encephalopathy, in MELD score, 451
Entecavir, prophylactic, 594–595
Epstein-Barr virus, 555–556
Escitalopram, 514
Estimated glomerular filtrate rate, in kidney allograft monitoring, 488–490
Estimated Post-Transplant Survival Score, 466
Estradiol, replacement of, 579

European Renal Best Practice Advisory Board guidelines, 556
Everolimius, 510–511
    bone disease due to, 575
    in pregnancy, 618–619
    nephrotoxicity of, 499
    side effects of, 516, 527–529
Exenatide, 542–544
"Extended criteria" donors, 442–443

F

Familial amyloidotic polyneuropathy, 454
Fenofovir, prophylactic, 595
Fertility, after transplantation, 617–624
Final Rule, 438
Focal segmental glomerulosclerosis, 470, 498
Fractures. *See* Metabolic bone disease.
Functional recovery, after transplantation, 614–615

G

Genital cancer, 554, 560
Glargine, 541
Glinides, 541
Glipizide, 541, 544–545
Glomerulonephritis
    in allograft dysfunction, 497–498
    membranoproliferative, 470
    recurrent, 469
Glucagon-like peptide 1 receptor agonists, 543–544
Glucocorticoids. *See* Corticosteroids.
Glyburide, 541

H

Head and neck cancer, 554, 556
Health-related quality of life, after transplantation, 614–617
HELLP syndrome, 621
Hematologic disorders, in antimetabolite therapy, 510
Hematoma, in allograft dysfunction, 493–494
Hematuria, in kidney allograft dysfunction, 490
Hemolytic uremic syndrome
    atypical, 470
    in allograft dysfunction, 495
Hepatic artery, thrombosis of, 478–479, 483–484
Hepatic osteodystrophy, 572
Hepatic vein, thrombosis of, 479
Hepatitis, autoimmune, 454, 481
Hepatitis A, evaluation for, 459
Hepatitis B, 454
    evaluation for, 459, 472
    in liver transplantation, 481, 483–484

prevention of, 595
Hepatitis C
    evaluation for, 471–472
    in liver transplantation, 480, 483–484
Hepatitis E, 482–483
Hepatocellular carcinoma, 559
    after liver transplantation, 483–484
    recurrence of, 481
    risk factors for, 554
    screening for, 459
    transplantation for, 455–456
Hepatopulmonary syndrome, 454–455, 457–458
Herbal medications, 510, 514
Herpes simplex virus, 593
Herpesvirus-6, 593
Histocompatibility, 473
Histomorphometry, 577
Historical perspective, **435–448**
    animal studies, 440
    earliest attempts, 435–436
    government approval, 441
    legal aspects, 438–439
    milestones in, 437–439
    moratorium, 440–441
    nineteenth century, 436
    organ allocation, 442–443, 450–452
    organ supply and demand disparity, 441–442
    pioneers, 439
    tacrolimus introduction, 441
    transplant center, 444–445
    twentieth century, 436–438
Hitchings, George, 506
Hodgkin lymphoma, 555–556
Holman, Emile, 505
Homocysteine, 527
Hormone replacement therapy, 579
Human herpesvirus-6, 555
Human immunodeficiency infection
    bone disease in, 571
    evaluation for, 459, 471
Human leukocyte antigens, 473, 493
Human papillomavirus, 555, 560
Hydralazine, 524
Hydronephrosis
    in allograft dysfunction, 493–494
    in kidney transplantation, 491
Hydroureter, in allograft dysfunction, 493–494
Hyperacute rejection, of kidney allograft, 492
Hyperlipidemia, 514, 524–526
Hyperoxaluria, primary, 454
Hyperparathyroidism, 571–573, 575

Hypertension, 521–523, 604
Hypertriglyceridemia, in immunosuppressive therapy, 511
Hypogonadism, 574
Hypophosphatemia, 573

I

Ibandronate, 580
Immunoglobulin A nephropathy, 470
Immunosuppressive therapy, **505–518**. *See also individual drugs.*
    adjunct agents with, 513–514
    bone disease due to, 573–575
    cardiovascular disease and, 527–529
    complications of, 515–517
    diabetes mellitus due to, 538–539
    future of, 445
    history of, 438–439, 441, 505–506
    infections in, 590
    malignancies due to, 553
    mechanism of action of, 506–507, 509
    pharmacokinetics of, 513
    phases of, 507–509
    teratogenic risks of, 618
    within immune system, 507–512
INDIGO (Kidney Disease Improving Global Outcome) guidelines, 522, 575
Infections
    evaluation for, 459, 471
    posttransplant, 479, **587–598**
        active, 589–590
        after six months, 593–594
        between one and six months, 592–593
        diagnostic tools for, 588–589
        in first month, 591–592
        in pregnancy, 618
        latent, 589–590
        microbiology of, 588
        prevention of, 594–596
        principles of, 588–589
        risk factors for, 589–590
        symptoms of, 588
        timeline of, 590–591
        treatment of, 589
        variety of, 588
Infliximab, 512
Insulin, 536–537, 539–541, 544
International Consensus Guidelinex, for NODAT, 523–524, 537
Israel Penn International Transplant Tumor Registry, 459

J

Jaboulay, Mathieu, 505

K

Kaposi sarcoma, 555
Kidney, cancer of, 558–559
Kidney allocation system, 465–466
Kidney Disease Improving Global Outcome (INDIGO) guidelines, 522, 575
Kidney Disease Outcomes Quality Initiative, 575
Kidney Donor Profile Index, 466
Kidney transplantation
  cardiovascular risk in, **519–533**
  diabetes mellitus care after, **535–550**
  for advanced chronic kidney disease, **465–476**
  historical perspective of, **435–448**
  immunosuppressive therapy for, **505–518**
  infections after, **587–598**
  living donors for, **599–611**
  malignancies after, **551–567**
  metabolic bone disease after, **569–586**
  outcomes of, **613–629**

L

Labor and delivery, in transplant patients, 621
Lescol in Renal Transplantation (ALERT) Trial, 526–527
Lifestyle changes
  for bone disease, 577
  for diabetes mellitus, 539
Linagliptin, 543
Liraglutdide, 542–544
Liver failure, acute, transplantation for, 453–454
Liver function tests, in allograft dysfunction, 478
Liver transplantation
  allograft dysfunction in, **477–503**
  cardiovascular risk, **519–533**
  diabetes mellitus care after, **535–550**
  historical perspective of, **435–448**
  indications for, **444–467**
  infections after, **587–598**
  living donors for, **599–611**
  malignancies after, **551–567**
  metabolic bone disease after, **569–586**
  outcomes of, **613–629**
Living donors, 442–444, **599–611**
  indications and contraindications for, 601–608
  postoperative care of, 605
  preparation of, 601
  psychosocial outcomes in, 608
  risks for, 605–608
Lung cancer, 554, 556–558
Lupus nephritis, 470
Lymphocele, in allograft dysfunction, 493–494
Lymphomas, 555–556

M

Macrolides, 513
Magnetic resonance imaging, for kidney allograft dysfunction, 490–491
Male transplant recipients, parenthood in, 624
Malignancies, **551–567**
    in immunosuppressive therapy, 517
    incidence of, 552–553
    mortality in, 552–553
    posttransplant lymphoproliferative disorder, 555–556
    risk factors for, 553
    skin, 553–555
    solid organ tumors, 556–560
    surveillance for, 560–561
Mammalian target of rapamycin inhibitors
    diabetes mellitus due to, 539
    side effects of, 527–529
Mammalian target of rapamycin kinase, action of, 507, 510–511
Medawar, Peter, 438
MELD (Model for End-Stage Liver Disease), 444, **449–464**
    benefits of, 451
    exceptions for, 452
    for evaluation, 456–460
    for indications and, 452–456
    historical perspective of, 450–452
Membranoproliferative glomerulonephritis, 470
Membranous nephropathy, 470, 498
Mental health, drugs for, 514
6-Mercaptopurine, 509–510
MESSAGE (MELD Exception Study Group and Conference), 444
Metabolic bone disease, post-transplant, **569–586**
    biochemistry of, 575–576
    causes of, 570–575
    epidemiology of, 570
    monitoring of, 575–577
    pathophysiology of, 575–576
    treatment of, 577–581
Metabolic syndrome, 527
Metastasis, from hepatocellular carcinoma, 456
Metformin, 540–542, 544–545
Methylprednisolone pulse therapy, 581
Microangiopathy, thrombotic, in kidney allograft, 495
Miglitol, 541, 543
Milan Criteria, for hepatocellular carcinoma, 455–456
Minoxidil, 524
Model for End-Stage Liver Disease. See MELD (Model for End Stage Liver Disease).
Modification of Diet in Renal Disease study, 488
Monoclonal anybodies, 439, 512
Moore, Francis, 440
Murray, Joseph, 436, 439, 506, 600
Mycophenolates, 509–510

bone disease and, 575
history of, 439
in pregnancy, 618–619
side effects of, 516
Myocardial infarction, 468–469, 521

N

Natetlinide, 543
National Institutes of Health, transplantation approval by, 441
Nephritis, lupus, 470
Nephropathy
BK virus, 493
membranous, 470
Nephrotoxicity, of drugs, 507, 509, 515
NODAT. *See* Diabetes mellitus, new-onset after transplant.
Nucleotide synthesis, in calcineurin action, 507
Nutrition, evaluation of, 459–460
Nystatin, prophylactic, 594–595

O

Obesity, 472, 527
in living donors, 604
screening for, 460
Opportunistic infections, 592–594
OPTN final rule, 444
Organ allocation policy, historical perspective of, 450–452
Organ Procurement and Transplantation Network, 438, 601
Organ Procurement Organization, 452
Osteoblasts, corticosteroid effects on, 573–574
Osteoclasts, corticosteroid effects on, 574
Osteocytes, corticosteroid effects on, 574
Osteodystrophy
hepatic, 572
renal, 571–572
Osteonecrosis, 574, 581
Osteoporosis. *See* Metabolic bone disease.
Outcomes, of solid organ transplantation, **613–629**
functional recovery, 614–615
health-related quality of life, 614–617
pregnancy, 617–624
Oxalosis, 470

P

Pancreas, transplantation of, with kidney transplantation, 473–475, 573
Parathyroid dysfunction, 571–573, 575
Patient education
for diabetes mellitus, 537
for kidney transplantation, 467

PELD (Pediatric End-Stage Liver Disease) system, 444
Penile cancer, 560
Peripheral vascular disease, 469
Physical function, after transplantation, 614–615
Pioglitazone, 543
Pneumocystis jiroveci, 594
Pneumonia
    after liver transplantation, 479
    in immunosuppressive therapy, 511
Polyclonal anybodies, 512
Polycystic kidney disease, 469
Polyneuropathy, familial amyloidotic, 454
Portopulmonary hypertension, 454–455, 457–458
Posttransplant lymphoproliferative disorder, 554–556
Pravastatin, 514, 526
Prednisone
    history of, 441
    in pregnancy, 618–619
Pregnancy, after transplantation, 617–624
Preventive health care, 514
Primary biliary cirrhosis, bone disease in, 572
Proglitazone, 541
Pro-oncogenic viruses, 553
Prostate cancer, 558–559
Proteinuria, in kidney allograft monitoring, 488–490
Pulmonary examination, 457–458
Pulmonary function tests, 472
Pulmonary hypertension, 469
The Puzzle People, 439–440

R

Radionuclide imaging, for kidney allograft dysfunction, 490–491
Redundancy, of immune system, 506–507
Rejection
    antibody-mediated, 497
    in pregnancy, 621
    of kidney allograft, 492
    of liver allograft, 479–480, 483
Renal artery
    stenosis of, 497
    thrombosis of, 491–492
Renal cell carcinoma, 558–559
Renal osteodystrophy, 571–572
Renal transplantation. *See* Kidney transplantation.
Renal vein, thrombosis of, 492
Repaglinide, 541, 543
Repeat transplantation, kidney, 473
Reproductive function, after transplantation, 617–624
Return to work, after transplantation, 615
Rituximab, 512

Rosiglitazone, 541, 543
Rosuvastatin, 514, 526

S

Saxagliptin, 542–543
Scientific Registry for Transplant Recipients, 442–444
Scribner, Belding, 438
Sensitized persons, 473
Sepsis, after liver transplantation, 479, 483
Sexuality, after transplantation, 617–624
Share 35 policy, 444, 452
Simvastatin, 526
Sirolimus, 510–511
    bone disease and, 575
    diabetes mellitus due to, 539
    in pregnancy, 618–619
    nephrotoxicity of, 499
    side effects of, 516, 527–529
Sitagliptin, 541, 543
Skin cancer, 553–555
Slush technique, 442
Smoking, 472, 526–527, 577
Sodium-glucose cotransporter 3 inhibitors, 544
Solid organ transplantation. *See also* Kidney transplantation; Liver transplantation.
    cardiovascular risk in, **519–533**
    diabetes mellitus care after, **535–550**
    historical perspective of, **435–448**
    immunosuppressive therapy for, **505–518**
    infections after, **587–598**
    living donors for, **599–611**
    malignancies after, **551–567**
    outcomes of, **613–629**
Southard, James, 442
Squamous cell carcinoma, 553–555
Starzl, Thomas, 439–441, 450
Statins, 514, 525–526
Stenosis, of renal artery, 497
Stents, urinary, for allograft dysfunction, 493
Stress testing, 468–469
Sulaglutide, 542
Sulfomethoxazole-trimethoprim, drug interactions of, 496
Sulfonylureas, 541–543
Surveillance, for malignancies, 560–561
Syphilis, evaluation for, 459, 471
Systemic lupus erythematosus, bone disease in, 571

T

Tacrolimus
    bone disease due to, 574

Tacrolimus (*continued*)
    diabetes mellitus due to, 538–539
    history of, 439, 441–442
    in pregnancy, 618–620
    mechanism of action of, 507–509
    side effects of, 495–496, 516, 527–529
T-cell lymphomas, 555–556
Teriparatide, 580
Testosterone therapy, 579
Tetracyclin double-labeled transiliac crest bone biopsy, 577
Thiazide diuretics, 513, 524
Thiazolidinediones, 541, 543
Thrombocytopenia, in immunosuppressive therapy, 511
Thrombophilia, 473
Thrombosis
    of hepatic artery, 478–479, 483–484
    of hepatic vein, 479
    of portal vein, 479
    of renal artery, 491–492
    of renal vein, 492
Thrombotic microangiopathy, in kidney allograft, 495
Thyroid cancer, 556
Tissue culture, replacement organs from, 445
Tobacco use, 472, 526–527, 577
Transient ischemic attacks, 469
Transplant centers, 444–445
Transplant renal artery stenosis, 497
Transplantation. *See* Kidney transplantation; Liver transplantation.
    offspring produced after, 624
    pancreas, with kidney transplantation, 474–475, 573
Transplantation Act of 1987, 450
Transthyretin gene mutations, 454
Trimethoprim-sulfamethoxazole, prophylactic, 594–595
Tuberculosis, evaluation for, 459, 471
Tumors. *See* Malignancies.

U

Ullman, Emerich, 436, 505
Ultrasonography
    for cancer, 558
    for kidney allograft dysfunction, 490–491, 494
    for renal artery stenosis, 497
Unagliptin, 542
Uniform Anatomic Gift Act of 1968, 438
United Network for Organ sharing, 438, 450–455, 519
United States Renal Data System, 520–521, 523–524
Ureter, stenosis of, in allograft dysfunction, 493–494
Ureterostomy, for allograft dysfunction, 493
Urinalysis, for kidney allograft dysfunction, 489–490
Urinary leaks, for kidney allograft dysfunction, 493

Urinary obstruction, for kidney allograft dysfunction, 493
Urinary tests, for kidney allograft dysfunction, 489–490
Urinary tract infections, 592
Urinoma, in allograft dysfunction, 493–494
Urolithiasis, in kidney allograft, 494

V

Vaccinations, 514, 595–596
   before kidney transplantation, 471
   before liver transplantation, 459
Vaginal cancer, 560
Valacyclovir, prophylactic, 594–595
Valgancyclovir, prophylactic, 594–595
Variable region (Fab), of antibodies, 512
Varicella zoster virus, 593
Vascular complications, after liver transplantation, 479
Vasculitis, antineutrophil cytoplasmic antibody, 470
Venography, for renal vein thrombosis, 492
Venous outflow obstruction, after liver transplantation, 483–484
Ventricular hypertrophy, left, 521–523
Viruses, pro-oncogenic, 553
Vitamin D, supplementation of, 577–580
Vulvar cancer, 560

W

Wait lists
   for chronic kidney disease, 466
   for liver transplantation, 449–450
Welch, C. Stuart, 439

Y

Yuronoy, Yu Yu, 436

Moving?

Make sure your subscription moves with you!

To notify us of your new address, find your **Clinics Account Number** (located on your mailing label above your name), and contact customer service at:

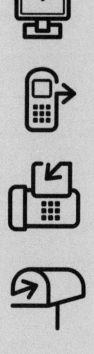

Email: journalscustomerservice-usa@elsevier.com

800-654-2452 (subscribers in the U.S. & Canada)
314-447-8871 (subscribers outside of the U.S. & Canada)

Fax number: 314-447-8029

Elsevier Health Sciences Division
Subscription Customer Service
3251 Riverport Lane
Maryland Heights, MO 63043

*To ensure uninterrupted delivery of your subscription, please notify us at least 4 weeks in advance of move.

Printed and bound by CPI Group (UK) Ltd, Croydon, CR0 4YY

03/10/2024

01040398-0004